Understanding
BREASTFEEDING
and How to Succeed

Elisabet Helsing and Anna-Pia Häggkvist

Understanding Breastfeeding and How to Succeed

Elisabet Helsing

Anna-Pia Häggkvist

Hale Publishing, L.P.
1712 N. Forest St.
Amarillo, TX 79106-7017
806-376-9900
800-378-1317
www.iBreastfeeding.com

Library of Congress Control Number: 2011945817

ISBN-13: 978-0-9847746-0-9

Printing and Binding: Malloy, Inc.

TABLE OF CONTENTS

PART 3.
GLIMPSES INTO THE HISTORY OF BREASTFEEDING: WHAT HAPPENED AND WHY?

APPENDICES

PREFACE

Once in a while a remarkable person comes out with a remarkable book devoted to a profoundly important issue, an issue that affects the survival of millions of infants and brings joy and happiness and also good health to infants and mothers. The senior author, Dr. Elisabet Helsing, has devoted decades of her life bringing to bear her skill in nutrition knowledge and working from her dedicated positions in the United Nations and many other big and small organizations.

This book is a wonderfully readable, yet comprehensive guide to and review of the womanly art of breastfeeding. Dr. Elisabet Helsing is extraordinarily well qualified to do this. We believe that she is the single person most responsible for making Norway the most baby and mother friendly country on earth. This was not always the case. But this one person's dedication, knowledge, hard work, and humanity achieved this. She led a European country away from the disastrous course taken by almost all other industrialized countries. That course, particularly in countries whose governments were increasingly wedded to industry, allowed a bottle-feeding culture to become dominant. Today, Norway is an inspiring model of what can be achieved. Dr. Helsing's achievements in this and related fields was recognized by the King of Norway in 2003, when he awarded her the "King's Gold Medal for Services to the People." Now, in this new book written in close collaboration with Anna-Pia Häggkvist, an experienced nurse and International Board Certified Lactation Consultant (IBCLC), the authors provide very broad, yet deep information and guidance on all aspects of infant and young child feeding. All of this is based on their scientific knowledge and years of practical experience in assisting mothers to breastfeed successfully. The text is full of detail, but all this is presented in a very understandable and inviting manner. Without it being dogmatic, one can sense throughout this book the authors' very strong belief that breastfeeding is a baby's right and a mother's duty.

Dr. Helsing, like both of us, has been a loyal member and supporter of the World Alliance for Breastfeeding Action (WABA) since it was founded. She is currently Co-Chair of WABA's International Advisory Council and continues to inspire us with her passion, dedication, and competence.

We commend this book, knowing the contribution it will make global-wide towards the protection, support, and promotion of breastfeeding and the support it will give the work of WABA and its core partners—the World Health Organization (WHO), UNICEF, and breastfeeding groups everywhere.

Professor Dr. Michael C. Latham †
Co-chairperson, International Advisory Council
World Alliance for Breastfeeding Action (WABA)
c/o Division of Nutritional Sciences
Cornell University
Ithaca, USA

Professor Anwar Fazal
Chairperson Emeritus
World Alliance for Breastfeeding Action
c/o Right Livelihood College
Universiti Sains Malaysia
Penang, MALAYSIA

FOREWORD

Breastfeeding is a major element in a baby's first encounter with its mother and in a mother's first encounter with her baby.

All mammals produce milk for their young–hence their name, from the Latin *mamma*, meaning the breast. The human race has, however, contrived to complicate the matter for itself, and breastfeeding has, in consequence, been under threat for several decades and from various directions. Those of us who work to provide information and guidance on breastfeeding find ourselves, at times, criticized for our eagerness, for supposedly ignoring real problems, and for our belief that breastfeeding is so simple and so natural. In the press and other media, it is asserted that today's women are being unreasonably pressured to breastfeed. At the same time, breastmilk substitutes are aggressively promoted in much of the world, even to the point where in some situations, the feeding bottle dominates the scene, and feeding at the breast becomes the exception. That has not been the case in Norway, where a very high proportion of mothers today breastfeed. This is due to the fact that in the 1970's so many valiant souls came forward to help mothers to believe in their talent as natural breastfeeders at a time when the practice of breastfeeding had fallen to its lowest ebb in many western countries.

This book starts with the ambitious aim of showing how breastfeeding has always been universal among the world's mammals, and a natural and necessary part of human existence. We go on to provide, in practical language, sound advice on the path to successful breastfeeding, as well as guidance to those who experience problems on the way, and some encouragement to those who may need it.

If we succeed in this, it will in no small measure be thanks to the valiant support from loyal friends, advisers, and helpers. They include many who are both mothers and experts in this or related fields: Kristin Engh Førde (social anthropologist and journalist), Kristine G. Hardeberg (breastfeeding consultant and photographer), Eli Heiberg (social anthropologist), Dr. Elisabeth Kylberg (nutrition physiologist, Sweden), Kari Paalgaard Pape (physiotherapist), and Ingrid Eide (sociologist). Kaia Engesveen has advised us on the text in her capacity as a nutrition physiologist. For certain chapters, we were able to benefit from expert advice provided by Professor Lars Å. Hanson (pediatrician) and Dr. Bergljot Børresen (veterinarian). At Norway's National Breastfeeding Centre, Anne B. Baerug (nutrition physiologist and Director) and Elisabet Tufte provided material and guidance. Anne Hagen Grøvslien, head of the milk bank at Oslo's National Hospital, has at all times provided help and information relating to milk banks. Liv Tønjum, at the Norwegian publisher, Fagbokforlaget, enthusiastically supported the publication of the corresponding Norwegian volume. We are immensely grateful to Fagbokforlaget itself for graciously agreeing to our use in the present book of much of the material that originally appeared in the Norwegian version. The illustrations were provided free of charge by Ingerid Helsing Almaas (architect and technical journalist), Ellen Wilhelmsen (artist and journalist), and Pollyanna von Knorring (technical drawings).

Various breastfeeding consultants from a range of countries have commented on particular sections of the text. In particular, we would like to thank Ruth Wester (Wellstart, Vermont, USA) and Denise Fisher (Director, Health e-Learning, Australia), who commented on the entire text, as well as Dr. Julie Smith and Dr. Virginia Thorley (Australia). Many other friends around the globe have encouraged us on our way; they came from Swaziland, Guatemala, India, Saudi Arabia, and last, but not least, Malaysia, where the World Alliance for Breastfeeding Action (WABA) is based.

Our thanks are due, too, to those Norwegian mothers who came forward and allowed us to cite their own experiences: Anne Marit Thorsrud, Anne Lise Robak, Eva Grønstrand, Nina Grundell, and Kristin Engh Førde.

Finally, we must thank all those whom we have encountered along our way and who have shared their knowledge with us, as well as provided us with invaluable insight into all the facets and challenges of breastfeeding.

Elisabet Helsing

Anna-Pia Häggkvist

Oslo, November 2011

Part 1.

Preparing for Breastfeeding: Useful, But Not Strictly Necessary Things to Know

Chapter 1.
WHAT BREASTFEEDING IS

To fully understand breastfeeding, you may need to know a little about the process itself. Not every detail is important, but it is good to have a clear picture of what goes on when a baby is put to the breast. Breastfeeding and breastmilk are not mysteries, and one can actually enjoy knowing a little more about them. We also learn a lot from looking at the same process where our closest relatives in nature–the other mammals–are concerned.

THE IDEA OF BREASTFEEDING

Breastfeeding is, of course, a means of providing food, but it is a great deal more than that. To put it briefly, breastfeeding is the natural means by which young humans are provided with:

- The food they need to survive and develop.

- The ability to deal with microorganisms ("bacteria" – whether good or bad), both within the body and in its surroundings.

- The human contact and care that every baby needs.

When we look a little more closely, we can see that breastfeeding comprises a whole chain of events, flowing seamlessly from one to another. First, the mother produces the milk, and then with the help of her reflexes, most of which are localized in her breasts and her brain, she puts it within easy reach of her baby. At this point the baby's reflexes, mostly acting around the mouth, come into play. Like any newly born mammal, the baby begins to search for a source of milk and soon finds the breast. As it does so, it stimulates the mother to release the milk. After which, the baby's reflexes help it accept the milk and send it into its system. And all the time, it is the baby that inspires and regulates the continuing flow of milk from the breast.

Perhaps as an extra precaution, this entire process is almost completely automatic, rather than being under the control of the will. A reflex is defined as "an automatic response to the stimulation of nerves."[1] The fact that these events are not controlled by the will has its advantages, but also some drawbacks. With the help of all the various reflexes, the baby finds its way to the food it needs, searching as long as necessary until it finds what it is looking for, as surely as if it had a built-in autopilot. And having arrived at the breast, it is the baby that unlocks the production of milk.

Can All Mothers Produce Milk?

Almost every woman will find that *once her baby has been born, she will have milk in her breasts.* Looked at physiologically, lactation is a fairly straightforward bodily function and very little can go wrong with it. Remarkably, even a woman who has never been pregnant can produce milk, though not always a great deal. The only conditions being that she wants to breastfeed, that a baby is put to her breast, and that the baby is willing to patiently suckle the breast, even though it gets little milk at first.

However, even though it is true that almost all healthy women can produce milk, one must add that some women still struggle to *continue* breastfeeding successfully. While many succeed in getting milk from the first day onwards without experiencing serious problems, others unfairly find themselves wrestling with all sorts of difficulties. It is sometimes completely unclear why one woman has more problems than another; it may happen that a highly motivated woman who is well prepared encounters difficulties, while her happy-go-lucky neighbor with no special desire to breastfeed sails through the entire process without a hitch.

There are, in other words, situations in which exclusive and full breastfeeding does not succeed, despite the mother's desire, good will, and expertise, and with support and encouragement from all around her. A very few women cannot fully lactate for anatomic or physiological reasons. A small number of others find it difficult, especially in the first few days. Unfortunately, however, too many women *mistakenly believe that breastfeeding is impossible for them*, and give up without ever looking for good advice and practical help.

---

1   The Concise Oxford Dictionary of Current English, Ninth Edition, Clarendon Press, Oxford 1995.

We hope this book will provide you with the information you need to be confident that you can produce – and go on producing – the milk that is quite certainly coming in.

PHYSIOLOGICAL OR ANATOMICAL BARRIERS TO BREASTFEEDING ARE RARE EVENTS

No one knows precisely how many women have anatomic or physiological barriers that make it impossible for them to breastfeed successfully; the data quoted proves to be based on guesswork or limited experience. This important question has never been properly studied. But it is true that some mother-child couples are faced with an uphill battle to breastfeed, and sometimes they do not really succeed. With such exceptional cases in mind, we are fortunate that we do have alternatives to breastfeeding and that we have the knowledge to help the child concerned by adapting milk from another species, such as that produced by our long-term friend, the Dairy Cow, who has been with us for 6000 years.

A LOOK AT THE BREAST: THE TIME BEFORE PREGNANCY

In the case of a woman who has never been pregnant, the breast (or the "mammary gland" as scientists like to call it) consists largely of connective tissue, fat deposits, some milk passages, and undeveloped "milk cell tissue." The size and shape of the breasts and nipples at this time give no clue as to how successful they will be at producing milk and delivering it to a baby. The important elements for breastfeeding are the milk producing cells needed to *make* the milk and the milk containers or "alveoli" where it will be briefly *stored* until it is wanted (Geddes, 2007). Both of these are scattered in the ten to 15 separate "segments" in which the breast is divided (see Figure 1.1). Each of these segments, with its own alveoli, milk ducts, and passages leading to the nipple, is an *independent* unit, capable on its own of producing and storing milk, and delivering it through the nipple. Not all the segments need to be active at the same time (Ramsay, Kent, Hartmann, & Hartmann, 2005). A great many women are able to provide more milk than a single baby is likely to need at any given moment; therefore, some of the segments are likely to be in a resting phase, only becoming active when there is a need for them. Having such a reserve capacity can be useful, for example, if the pregnancy produces twins and there is an extra mouth to feed. With such an arrangement, we can see why even a woman who has had a part of an over-large breast removed by plastic surgery can still hope to feed her baby if the surgeon has left untouched a number of the breast segments, each with its own nerves and blood supply. Naturally, one cannot guarantee success, but it will soon become clear how well the remaining segments of the breast can perform on their own.

Changes in the Breast During Pregnancy

When a woman becomes pregnant, a series of important changes begin to take place in her breasts. She will usually notice that they become larger. The nipples become more prominent, and as a rule, they become darker in color, as does the surrounding area–the areola. These are all signs the body is getting ready to feed the baby who is now on the way.

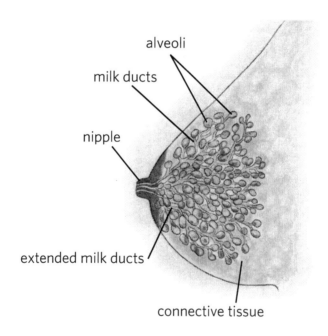

Figure 1.1. *Simplified view of anatomy of the breast early in pregnancy based on research by Dr. Peter Hartmann and colleagues in Australia.*

Source: Drawing by Pollyanna von Knorring. Used with permission.

During the first three months of pregnancy (the "first trimester"), the connective tissue and milk ducts become more prominent and extensive. Next, the milk-producing tissue develops. Towards the end of pregnancy, you may be able to express colostrum – the "golden milk." Colostrum has a series of important functions:

- It provides the newborn baby with its first nutritious food.

- It equips the baby with its first defenses against the intricate world of infectious microorganisms into which it has arrived.

The network of blood vessels in the breast similarly becomes more extensive during pregnancy. All the elements that are needed to feed and protect a baby are carried by way of the blood, from stores in the mother's body to the milk-producing cells. Here they will be processed and mixed to form the complex liquid tissue we know as milk.

By the time pregnancy is complete, some of the fat that was originally present in the breast will be gone to make way for more connective tissue, milk ducts, and alveoli. And around each of the alveoli, comprising a cluster of milk-producing cells, one now finds a fine network of smooth muscle fibers, ready to contract under the influence of the hormone oxytocin and expel the milk towards the nipple (see Figure 1.2). Finally, one finds that the network of nerves throughout the breast has similarly developed as the pregnancy has run its course.

Contrary to what some people believe, there is no point in avoiding breastfeeding for fear of its spoiling the shape or elegance of the breasts. The most important changes in the breast have already happened during the course of pregnancy; they are almost all inside and hidden from view, and breastfeeding will produce no further visible alterations. Also, breastfeeding will not make the breast less sensitive to the pleasures of erotic stimulation - something many mothers would not want to forgo.

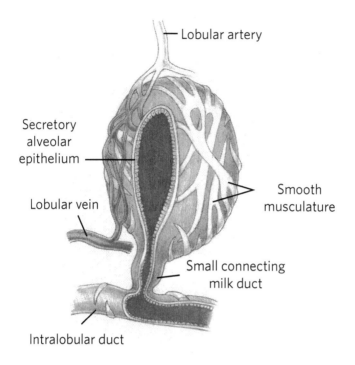

Lobular artery

Secretory
alveolar
epithelium

Lobular vein

Smooth
musculature

Small connecting
milk duct

Intralobular duct

Figure 1.2. *Anatomy of the breast following birth. The illustration shows an alveolus with milk-producing cells, capillary blood vessels, nerve fibers, and smooth muscle.*

Source: Drawing by Pollyanna von Knorring. Used with permission.

The Ingenious Feeding Process

It is striking how perfectly the baby and the breast are attuned to one another. One can also imagine that this very close physical and psychosocial bond created between baby and mother, with the skin of the baby against the warm and welcoming breast of the mother, is an ideal means of easing the baby's transition from the security of the womb to the vast and unexpected world outside. Of course, there can be physical closeness in the absence of breastfeeding, but with breastfeeding the contact is inevitable, frequent, and guaranteed. Even a mother who has scarcely realized how much need her baby has of skin-to-skin contact and intimacy will find herself providing it because it is a built-in element in the feeding process.

PRODUCTION OF MILK

Like all the other processes associated with pregnancy and birth, the production of milk is regulated by the body's chemical messengers known as hormones. One of the most important hormones in this particular connection is *prolactin* - the name literally means "for milk." Prolactin is first released within the mother's body as early as the second half of pregnancy. Its role at this time is to stimulate the growth and development of the milk glands. At this early stage, it does not cause milk to be produced, since at the same time the placenta releases other hormones (progesterone and estrogen) that block the milk-producing effect of prolactin. The levels of these two hormones in the mother's system are higher at this time than at others. However, once the baby is delivered, the placenta is promptly expelled, and with it goes the main source of progesterone and estrogen, leaving the prolactin free to act fully on the milk glands and induce the secretion of milk.

Where and How Is Milk Made?

The production of milk takes place in the cells that make up the walls of the small "milk containers" or "milk chambers," known as the alveoli, which lie in clusters throughout the breast.

The network of fine hair-like blood vessels that surround these alveoli bring the hormone oxytocin into close contact with the "smooth musculature" – small muscles that are not under the control of the will. This same network also supplies the milk-producing cells with the components needed to make milk: fat, sugars, and the building blocks for protein (amino acids), as well as vitamins and minerals, all arriving by way of the blood. Once they enter the milk-producing cells of the alveoli, all these substances are built into complex molecules. They may be very large as molecules go, but they are still far too small to be seen with the naked eye. These molecules have their own special tasks, in particular to protect the baby's stomach and intestines. Other similarly large molecules arrive ready-made from the mother's body and find their way through the narrow spaces between the milk-producing cells and pass directly into the milk. This is the way immune globulins from the mother's blood form part of the immune defense system.

We still do not know what role every component of mother's milk plays, despite all the thorough scientific studies that have been carried out in recent years. Over the last half century, more than 10,000 articles on this subject have appeared in the scientific literature. You can access these articles by doing a search in the medical database PUBMED, using the term "Milk, human."

How Is the Milk Stored?

As the milk is produced, it is stored until it is needed; most remaining in the alveoli, and some accumulating in the milk passages that empty into the nipple. As the breast progressively fills with milk, pressure builds, and the walls of the milk cells and alveoli are stretched. The idea has been raised that the milk-producing cells have receptors of their own which detect the increasing pressure and stop the production of milk. At any rate, because of the back-pressure less blood is able to enter the breast, and this, in turn, causes the production of milk to decrease–fortunately, one might say.

All this explains why there is no point in trying to "save up" milk by skipping a breastfeed in the hope that this will make it possible to give the baby more milk later on. That is not the way things work. The only effective approach is to *give your baby as much milk as you can at all times.* Studies show that as a rule you have more milk in your breasts than you think. The baby very rarely empties the breast completely – commonly 10-20% is left in the breast (Dewey, Heinig, Nommsen, & Lønnerdahl, 1991). Immediately after the baby has taken milk from the breast, the pressure in the alveoli is at its lowest (think of an almost completely deflated balloon), more blood flows in bringing more oxytocin, and the milk cells start producing milk much more actively than they did when the breast was full.

At this point, we need to consider some ***Golden Rules of Breastfeeding.***

Golden Rule Number 1

The more milk the baby takes, the more milk you will make.

Breastfeeding is a generous process, and humans belong, as we will see presently, to the group of "continuous feeders." The fact that milk is continuously removed from the breast provides a signal to the body to produce more.

At the same time, reflecting the fine physiological balance between supply and demand, mother and baby, another Golden Rule comes into play:

Golden Rule Number 2

The more often you put the baby to the breast to remove milk and stimulate your hormone production, the more milk you will make.

What is meant by "more often" naturally depends on how frequently you are already giving the breast.

The number of breastfeeds given in a day will vary from one mother to another and for any given mother over time. Many women feed ten or 15 times a day – sometimes more often, so one cannot lay down any "ideal" frequency.

Babies that *do not put on weight* and *do not seem satisfied,* even though they are given the breast very often and despite good positioning, need a check-up. Contact your local health center, and if they find the baby's weight is satisfactory, there is no reason for concern. If they are not satisfied with what they find, both you and the baby may need further guidance on positioning and ensuring the baby is properly attached. Do this before even considering the use of artificial feeding.

These golden rules relate to *complementary processes that work together* to adjust the mother's production of milk to the child's needs:

- The first process is mechanical: the baby takes milk from the mother's breast, reducing the pressure in and around the milk-producing cells.

- The second process is hormonal: every time the baby is put to the breast, it leads to a new hormonal stimulus in the mother's body to produce milk.

- In other words: the more milk is taken from the breast, the greater the stimulation to produce even more.

These processes *work in harmony with one another,* eventually making sure the mother's milk production corresponds to her baby's needs.

How Does Your Baby Obtain Your Milk?

One very basic thing that has to be understood about breastfeeding is that a baby–for that matter any young mammal – *does not suck the milk out of the breast,* though the word "sucking" is often used and reflects the traditional belief that it does (Cowie, 1972). The form and structure of the milk glands is different from one species of mammal to another, but the basic process of getting milk from the breast is the same in all of them. *All mammals are dependent on the milk let-down reflex (the "oxytocin reflex") which actively delivers the milk into the offspring's mouth.* The milk is not waiting near the surface, ready to be sucked up; it is relatively deep in the breast, in the milk containers (the alveoli), and when these are filled to capacity, it accumulates in the milk ducts as well.

DOMESTIC ANIMALS: TRUE MILKING PROFESSIONALS

The cow and the goat possess an ingenious "milk chamber" just where the teat joins the udder, which makes the milking process very simple for the calf or kid (to say nothing of the milkmaid). In the case of the mouse, all the various milk passages within a breast segment feed into a single duct. In the human breast, on the other hand, one finds only a modest widening of the milk passages just before they feed into the nipple. None of these various arrangements allow the offspring to *suck* the milk actively from the breast, as one sucks lemonade through a drinking straw – that would simply not be possible according to the laws of physics and physiology. Sucking alone, even if it were possible, would not be sufficient to extract milk from the breast. The milk produced there and stored in the alveoli, milk passages, and milk sacs has to be actively expelled by the mother when the baby is ready and waiting for it. All the baby mammal needs to do is to set the process in motion, rather like turning on a tap.

The Mother's Let-Down Reflex in Action

Many mothers experience from time to time that, in spite of knowing she has plenty of milk, her baby does not seem able to get to it. The baby lies there, endlessly pushing and pulling at the nipple, and now and again screaming impatiently because nothing seems to come out. What has gone wrong? Fairly obviously, *the milk let-down reflex* has failed to perform.

One cannot always expect a process like this to start immediately. After the mother has put her baby to the breast, a little while may elapse before she can hear her baby taking in the milk and swallowing it with audible gulps. The mother may at the same time feel a mild sensation of pricking in her breast, and it may become harder to the touch. What is going on?

Put simply, it is like this: when a mother puts her baby to the breast and the baby begins to suckle the nipple, a signal goes up through the nervous system to her brain. There is a small gland called the posterior pituitary that begins to secrete the hormone oxytocin. One property of this hormone is that it causes *smooth muscle* to contract. This sort of muscle is not subject to the will, but it plays an important role in various parts of the body, including the uterus. It plays a vital role in birth itself, and experienced mothers know that oxytocin is responsible for the after-pains they may feel in the uterus during breastfeeding. There is also a network of smooth muscle fibers around each of the breast's alveoli and along the milk passages. When the oxytocin released from the brain arrives in the breast, it causes the small muscles around the alveoli to contract, and those along the largest ducts to relax (Uvnäs-Moberg & Eriksson, 1996). All this sets the milk release in motion, first into the small milk passages, and then into the wider passages which feed into the nipple. In the final stage of the let-down reflex, the walls of these passages relax under the influence of oxytocin. The effect may often be so strong that the milk literally sprays out of the breast. Newer research using ultrasound has shown multiple let-down reflexes during one feed, but mothers usually just sense the first one (Ramsay, Kent, Owens, & Hartmann, 2004).

With this reflex in motion, the baby hardly has to make an effort; all it needs to do is accept the milk and divide it into small portions, each just enough to be passed on and swallowed.

This ingenious milk production system may take a few days to get fully into motion after birth, and the baby is therefore equipped with a reserve store of energy and nutrients to help it through the first few days. Even before the whole breastfeeding process is operative, however, the baby will certainly succeed in taking a few teaspoonfuls of colostrum, just enough to prepare the right environment for "friendly bacteria" in the baby's digestive system; encouraging them to settle there, where they can stimulate the development of the child's own immune defense system. The baby's stomach is too small at this time to hold very much milk.

Influencing the Let-Down Reflex - For Better or for Worse

Although the let-down reflex has been recognized for many years in milk-producing farm animals, it was only recognized as existing in human mothers in 1948. It was in that year the married couple, Niles and Michael Newton (1948), a psychologist and a physician, carried out some novel experiments to define the nature of the let-down reflex. Niles Newton was the experimental subject, backed up by the couple's seven month-old breastfed baby. At the moment when she began the breastfeeding session, her husband would expose her to various unexpected and unpleasant stimuli and note the result. At one moment she might, for example, have ice-cold water poured over her feet–a stimulus sufficient to cause the flow of milk to stop acutely, as a result the baby would release the nipple and start screaming. A similar effect could be elicited by posing unpleasant questions, calculated to irritate the mother and make her angry; this too was sufficient to arrest the active flow of milk.

The explanation for these effects on the let-down reflex is clear: the hormone adrenaline, which is involved in a whole series of bodily processes, controls the function of various organs by causing the smallest blood vessels to contract, reducing the local blood circulation. If the mother is frightened or angry, her body will at once mobilize all its resources to resist or to flee from danger; at such a moment, it will be the muscles in her arms and legs that call for more blood. Conversely, the small vessels in those parts of the body (such as the breast) that play no role in fighting or fleeing will contract, and the local blood supply will be reduced. This means the oxytocin coming from the brain will not reach the vessels supplying the smooth muscle tissue around the milk sacs, and the milk will not be expelled through the nipple. Essentially, there will be no let-down reflex, no milk supply, a desperate baby, and an equally desperate mother. Not a kind experiment, but clear proof of the central part played by the let-down reflex in successful breastfeeding.

A True "Conditioned Reflex"

The let-down reflex, as we explained earlier in this chapter, is a "conditioned" reflex (some readers may have heard the term "Pavlovian reflex" for this type of reaction, named after the Russian scientist who discovered it). It may be triggered by any of the stimuli capable of setting it in motion. It may even be triggered by the mother thinking or talking about her baby. Many a breastfeeding adviser will recall how many mothers attending a breastfeeding get-together, where the conversation is about breasts and babies, ultimately display decorative milk stains on their dresses.

THE BABY'S MIRACULOUS ABILITIES

Every baby is born with an innate ability to find and take food. The same can be said of every newborn mammal on earth; it has a programmed ability to find nourishment and thereby survive. This ability relies on a chain of inborn reflexes, which equip the newborn baby to react automatically to certain signals without the need to think about them and interpret them first. This chain of processes is what we call the "milking reflexes," and they swing into action as soon as the baby is born. Below, we will take a look at the various links in the chain – the complex, yet readily understood process that ensures the transfer of milk from mother to baby. Many people throughout the years have overlooked this fascinating process, simply assuming – quite mistakenly – that a baby takes its milk by sucking it from the breast, as it would suck it from a feeding bottle.

The Searching and Crawling Reflex

When we look at the way breastfeeding begins in various mammals other than ourselves, it is striking that as a rule the young infant animal begins to hunt actively for the mother's nipple as soon as it is born. When a litter is being delivered, the first of the young may already be on the nipple, while the later arrivals are still being born. At one time it was believed that human babies did not display any such "searching and crawling" reflex – we humans, it was thought, had advanced beyond such processes, picking up our babies and putting them to the breast ourselves. Then came the revolutionary discovery in the 1980's that human babies also have this same ready-programmed ability to search for the breast as soon as they come into the world. It was a research team of Swedish midwives who alighted upon the truth in 1987 (Widström, Ransjö-Arvidson, Christensson, Matthiesen, Winberg, & Uvnäs-Moberg, 1987). They found that if a newborn baby was placed on the mother's naked skin immediately after delivery and preferably on the upper abdomen, it would start to creep, crawl, and struggle upwards towards the nipple, however far away it might be. The "searching and crawling reflex" guides the baby's movements in the direction of the breast, perhaps influenced by the slight odor produced in "Montgomery's glands" which surround the areola, the sight of the dark areola itself, or the prominent nipple, obvious as a lighthouse, guiding the baby on its way.

The Seeking and Rooting Reflex

The rooting and seeking reflex is elicited as soon as the baby senses a slight movement or touch in the area close to its mouth. Promptly, the baby turns its head towards the stimulus and searches for it, its mouth open. Already the young human has come much of the way. Now, as if it senses something delicious is nearly within reach, it begins to salivate, just as any other human might do when thinking of a good meal. It waves its arms and grabs seemingly at random with its hands, bringing them up towards the mouth. In the process, the baby will touch the nipple. The touch of the baby's hands causes the nipple to become erect and to tighten, so it becomes more prominent and easy to grasp. The baby's head begins to move, at first hesitantly from side to side, until at a given moment it is very close to the nipple. As the nipple touches the chin, the last phase of the reflex swings into action—the baby roots with its mouth open until it is able to take the nipple and a part of the breast into its mouth.

The Extrusion or "Welcoming" Reflex

During the first few months of life, any baby put to the breast will exhibit a little "greeting" to the nipple, using its tongue. As its lips touch the nipple, the mouth opens wide and the tongue thrusts forward, folding into a trough. From that moment, the upper lip and the tongue grasp the nipple firmly on all sides, and the nipple is pulled into the mouth. All these movements are part of the "welcoming reflex." As soon as the tip of the breast is sufficiently close for the baby's mouth and tongue to take a firm grip on it, the mother's let-down reflex is set in motion, the first milk is ejected into the baby's mouth, and breastfeeding is initiated. This "extrusion reflex," as it is also called, persists throughout the first four to six months of life, after which it fades away.

Once the nipple is so far into the baby's mouth that it touches the junction between the hard and soft palate, a new set of reflexes comes into motion—and the baby truly begins to milk the breast.

The Milking Reflex

The next step is a complex chain of well-coordinated movements of the baby's tongue, somewhat similar to the wave-like motion by which the gut moves food along during digestion. If you think back to our description of the breast's anatomy, you will recall that just below the areola (the dark area around the nipple) one finds the terminal section of the milk passages. It is precisely this part of the breast that the baby works on to get access to the milk.

Golden Rule Number 3

The baby is not sucking; it is primarily the mother who is ejecting the milk.

The Swallowing Reflex

As a portion of milk reaches the back of the baby's mouth, it sets off the "swallowing reflex" – often very audibly – and it is this reflex that delivers the milk to its destination, downwards through the esophagus into the stomach. On the way, it briefly passes the palate, and although the palate seals off the nasal passages, where the milk has no business to be, the contact is just enough for the baby to briefly experience whatever odor or taste the milk may carry with it. Dr. Julie Mennella (2009), who has taught us a great deal about the newborn baby's sense of smell and taste, has suggested that some of the scents of the food the mother has eaten may in this way become familiar to the newborn infant. The idea that the baby is learning to appreciate garlic or custard may seem a little strange, but it's never too early to learn.

What About the Sucking Reflex?

The ancient idea of "sucking" may have been exaggerated, but there *is* a sucking reflex. The role of this reflex is primarily to *hold the breast* firmly in the baby's mouth. If the baby feels it is losing its grip on the breast (which may, for example, happen if the mother is not holding her child sufficiently close), it will react by sucking actively to avoid losing its grip. The baby is quite able to maintain a firm and airtight hold on the breast. The suction can be remarkably strong, sometimes sufficient to produce reddish or purple marks (petechiae) on the unfortunate portion of the breast that is exposed to it, making life very uncomfortable for the nipple that is well equipped with sensory nerves. For that reason, it is truly important that the mother hold her baby sufficiently close to her to make sucking action almost unnecessary. The less the baby is obliged to create a negative pressure in order to maintain its grip on the breast, the less chance of hurting the skin on and around the nipple.

Sucking: Nice, Nice, But Oh, So Dangerous....

To say that the baby "sucks" at the mother's breast is therefore a little misleading- "suckle" would be a better term to use. It is a fact that young babies love to suck on something. They suck their fingers with great enthusiasm, sometimes even before they are born—it probably feels good in the mouth and satisfies some deep desire that we retain throughout life. It is a very simple process involving only a few muscles of the mouth. Compared with the chain of reflex acrobatics that are necessary to ensure that milk flows, is ingested, and swallowed, sucking is—if one may use the term—child's play. That is probably why bottle-feeding using a rubber teat is so popular with the babies exposed to it—they need only to suck to get the milk. But, as we have seen, sucking is not always harmless, and you need to take care that it does not become painful.

So what role does sucking really play during breastfeeding? Quite simply, sucking creates suction or negative pressure that should mainly serve to hold the nipple and breast within the baby's grip.

The Art of Coordination

The task of coordinating all these reflexes can hardly be a simple one for an individual who has just arrived in the world, but the breastfeeding baby is resourceful and learns unbelievably quickly. Naturally, babies differ to some degree; one baby will manage to master the art of breastfeeding a little more rapidly than another does. A baby born prematurely may need many days (and sometimes weeks) of effort before all these reflexes get established through the nervous system, while a baby born at term may confidently take control from the start.

MILKING THE BREAST - NOT SUCH A SIMPLE BUSINESS! (A SUMMARY)

When the baby feeds at the breast, its mouth handles the gland expertly, stimulating the sensitive nipple so the hormone oxytocin is released from a gland in the mother's brain.

The hormone is transported to the breast through the bloodstream. As soon as it reaches the network of smooth muscle fibers in the alveoli, the latter contract and fire off the mother's *milk let-down reflex.*

Pressure then builds up in the alveoli and milk ducts, causing the milk to be ejected from the breast.

Some mothers consciously experience this reflex, others may not. But in either case, it is effective, as evidenced by a change in the swallowing rhythm of the baby as the milk begins to flow.

Having first *stimulated* the breast, the baby's mouth now proceeds to *milk* it actively, i.e., to breastfeed in the true sense of the word. The pressure within the mother's breast, built up under the influence of the let-down reflex, ejects the milk from the nipple with force.

While the baby's lips and gums hold the breast firmly in place, assisted by the necessary suction, the *milking reflex* is set in motion – the baby's tongue rhythmically presses the nipple and breast up against the palate.

The baby lies and receives the milk, while movements of the tongue divide it into convenient portions for swallowing. The tongue holds back any excessive flow of milk until it is ready for it, and the next wave of milking begins.

Before it is swallowed the milk passes the nasal passage, where the baby has the chance to sense the taste and odor of the milk it is about to swallow. Newborn babies are, as we now know, much more capable of distinguishing smell and taste than was once believed (Mennella, 2009).

Cream for Dessert?

It seems to be the case that, particularly if the baby is only put to the breast relatively infrequently, once every three or four hours or so, the milk in the breast will separate into portions of different nutrient composition: watery milk, delivered first, and fattier energy-rich milk that will be provided towards the end of a feeding session. Many mothers have noticed that the first milk released by the breast is almost transparent and somewhat bluish—resembling skimmed cow's milk, while if you express a little of the residual milk after the baby has finished feeding, it is positively creamy (Czank, Mitoulas, & Hartmann, 2007). No doubt it is delicious, and some researchers have suggested that this variation in the composition of the milk during feeding may actually be of importance in learning to regulate appetite in later life (Hall, 1975). However, it is equally possible that when a baby is fed more frequently, the difference in milk composition during feeding is less noticeable, and it may actually nearly disappear. This is important: if your baby is gaining weight and is happy with life, you can forget about the content of fat – or other nutrients – in your milk.

THE MOTHER - AFTER BIRTHING

We can quite clearly see the whole chain of processes or reflexes that we have just described if a baby is placed on the mother's exposed body directly after birth. There, the baby will experience the mother's skin, her body warmth, and maybe the heartbeat with which it has long been familiar. In research work, mothers may often be asked to remain more or less passive towards their babies, so it is easier to compare events in different families. The natural situation, however, would be for a mother who has just experienced a normal birth to immediately take her baby in her arms and lay it close to the breast, while she gently dries it off (important so the baby can remain warm), caresses and becomes familiar with it – counting its fingers and admiring its hair, and talks to it. Other mammals lick their newly born young, but that is perhaps a trifle farfetched for most human mothers. Whatever she chooses to do, it seems very likely that by fondling and encouraging her baby, she will provide it with a stimulus to reach the breast more rapidly than if it were left to fend for itself. Most mothers are curious to experience their babies and soon discover to their joy that they have been blessed with the world's most perfect baby. It may still be a greasy and bloody little thing, but there is hardly a mother who will not want to fondle and care for it.

If Things Don't Progress Quite as They Should

This whole process—where the baby finds its way to the breast and begins to feed as soon as it is born—runs most smoothly if mother and child are in constant physical contact after delivery. The inborn reflexes have the necessary time and opportunity to swing into action, one by one and in the right order, just as they are supposed to do. Even picking the baby up to be weighed and measured, or to be dressed, may disturb the process. The baby's reflexes may also be weakened if during the delivery, the mother has been treated with pain-relieving or tranquilizing medicines (Nissen et al., 1997). There are clear differences in the occurrence of feeding problems if we compare babies who have had uninterrupted skin-to-skin contact with the mother and those who have been taken for washing and dressing, or some other routine, without first having the chance to do what they have been programmed to do, in other words to seek a new form of contact with their mother as soon as the umbilical cord has been cut.

... There Is Always a Later Train...!

Some babies are born professional milkers. They seem to know precisely how a breast should be approached once it is presented. Others simply cannot figure out what it is they are supposed to do, even given the best of opportunities.

The occasional baby may be ill, or it may simply be a slow reactor, needing to take its own time. For any of these reasons, things may not start off as one had hoped and intended. Never despair! If it is not possible to allow the baby all the time it seems to want to find the breast in its own sweet way, or if the baby seems to be puzzled or hesitant about this whole business about mouths and nipples, that does not mean breastfeeding will be impossible.

One thing worth trying is simply to enact the start all over again. Give the baby a second chance. Lay the baby in direct skin-to-skin contact with you, where it can easily find its way to the breast. You will need to take your time, be patient, and use all available familial support while things sort themselves out. If given this new chance, many babies will be able to start afresh, comprehend what is intended, find the breast, and take to it as if there had never been any problem at all. (See chapter 5 for more detail.)

BREASTFEEDING – A CONFIDENCE TRICK

Breastfeeding can be successful and enjoyable if some conditions are met:

- First, a mother must *want* to breastfeed (or at least not be uncomfortable with the idea).

- Second, she must have ready access to good information and wise help, if and when she has need of it.

- Third, she needs to have persons around her who have a clear and positive view of things, who really know what they are talking about and radiate confidence.

- Fourth, but not in the last place, almost every new mother needs a little genuine admiration, praise, and support. This will build her self-confidence and her conviction that breastfeeding is something which others have managed and mastered, and which she is also going to be able to do.

This is not simply something we believe. Danish nursing researchers, Kronborg and Vath (2004) have published a study that confirms earlier findings. They were able to show that the greater a mother's confidence, her accumulated knowledge, and her earlier experience of breastfeeding, the greater is the likelihood that she would succeed.

What Is Good Breastfeeding Practice and Unrestricted Breastfeeding?

Today, it may seem obvious that mother and baby should continue to be together in the days after birthing, just as they have been inseparable for the previous nine months. The artificial separation of mothers from their children, which was once a routine practice in many countries (and in some countries is still practiced) all too often means that the mother lies for hours with congested breasts, longing for her baby that has been taken to be cared for in a separate ward. This is contrary to the idea of "good breastfeeding practice" and makes free and unrestricted breastfeeding impossible. *"Free breastfeeding"* (also called *"unrestricted breastfeeding,"* *"breastfeeding on baby's demand,"* or *"baby-led breastfeeding"*) is a sound modern principle with many names, which is in keeping with the baby's physiological needs. When a young infant needs food, it gives some very clear signals to that effect.

"Baby-led breastfeeding" simply means that these signals are respected; the baby is given the chance to breastfeed whenever it needs, and for as long as it needs. To achieve this, mother and baby must obviously be close to one another at all times.

Not everyone understands that the human mother, like other primate mothers, is by nature a free breastfeeder, giving her milk *whenever* it is needed. It *should* be no problem to put this into practice, and you have a right to do so. But when you feel you really need a rest, never hesitate to occasionally ask for and accept help in taking care of the baby. For the parents of a newborn baby, sleep is sometimes the most precious of gifts!

Chapter 2.
WHY FEED AT THE BREAST?

Breastfeeding is a feeding strategy that many of nature's species have developed in order to survive and multiply throughout the world. The instinct to ensure the species will continue by producing offspring and by protecting and feeding those offspring until they can care for themselves is probably one of the most fundamental elements in life. Many forms of reproduction have been developed over millions of years; some have failed, while others have succeeded brilliantly. To begin with, let us concentrate on those feeding strategies which have turned out to be quite successful – the production of eggs and the making of milk – and consider how, in our own time, they still make it possible to protect and nourish one generation after another.

EGGS

To lay and hatch eggs – as birds and reptiles do – may be said to be an ambitious approach to feeding, but one that involves considerable risks. All the nutrients needed to produce a new member of the race are packed, alongside the germinal tissue, inside a protective shell, and then the egg is put to mature and hatch under the more or less watchful eye of a parent. That is all fine so long as it remains undisturbed, but an egg is a tempting package of food for other species. Should it be taken, and the rate of loss is high, everything the mother has consigned to the egg from her own body will be lost. Laying and hatching eggs, in other words, can and often will turn out to be uneconomic – and very much subject to variations of fortune.

MAKING MILK

Making and providing milk is the approach adopted by mammals. The offspring is born at a very early phase of its existence, well before it is able to care for itself. During its early life, the mother provides it with all its food, essentially corresponding to what one finds in the yolk and white of an egg of other species, but here taking the form of specially constituted mother's milk. The "milk strategy" may be more risky for the still immature young, but it demands less of the mother's energy than the constant laying of eggs. Should anything go wrong, for example if the offspring is taken or killed, the mother will soon cease to produce milk, thereby sparing herself unnecessary loss of resources. Milk production and transfer, however, also has a series of other functions, as we saw briefly in Chapter 1 (the anatomy of the breast; Figures 1.1 and 1.2).

THE FUNCTIONS OF BREASTMILK AND BREASTFEEDING: CARE, PROTECTION, FOOD

The role that breastfeeding plays in *care*, and how one can ensure that such care continues when breastfeeding proves difficult or even seems impossible, is a theme we will return to time and again in this book.

The *protective* role of breastfeeding and of milk centers on the part milk plays in building a baby's immune defenses. We will take a broad look at this process in this Chapter and compare ourselves with the mammals of the animal kingdom. Later, in Chapter 3, you will learn a little more about mother's milk and its impressive immunological properties. In that same Chapter, we will also consider more closely the role played by breastmilk as *food* and as a *special diet*, both in man and animals.

Care, Closeness, Contact, Consolation - and Love

Man is a family animal; and whether a mother is consciously aware of it or not, breastfeeding provides the baby with an assurance of care and of belonging, of security and of love – so important for every child. That assurance is provided in a series of clear signals (skin-to-skin contact, attention, closeness), which obviously can also be provided without breastfeeding. Any mother – or father – can provide them in other ways as well. But if the baby is not fed at the breast, the parents will have to make a conscious effort to ensure that this indeed happens. With breastfeeding, the closeness of contact and the assurances of care are provided automatically. A mother who is breastfeeding will automatically pass along to her offspring the message: "Here you are safe." This is a bonus that breastfeeding delivers, and one that can actually be traced back to the hormones that stimulate the milk flow. Animal studies involving rats have taught us that oxytocin has a direct effect on the mother's *will* to devote herself to her offspring, though not necessarily on her *ability* to do so. Obviously, there is quite a gap between rats and humans, although oxytocin is active in lactation in both species – indeed in all mammals. Perhaps one can best express this by saying that because it is intrinsic in the feeding situation, a mother who succeeds in breastfeeding will find that the process provides her with a free opportunity to give her baby care, contact, and when needed, consolation.

An Invitation to Some Friendly Germs

Any newborn is faced with both visible and invisible challenges. The bacteria, viruses, and other microorganisms that surround us are a natural and essential part of our ecological environment, everywhere on earth. They are of many different types – dangerous, harmless, useful, and in some instances, even essential. Present in vast numbers and numerous varieties on and in every animal and its surroundings, these microorganisms are ready, waiting, and anxious to colonize the newly born and still sterile mammalian offspring. The body is ready to invite many of them in: moist skin and membranes (for example, the lining of the nose and mouth) provide a welcome environment for them, with plenty of warmth and foodstuffs within reach. From here many bacteria will pass more deeply into the body, ready to play a useful role there, for example, digestion. The more fully the body is colonized with these useful bacteria, the less room there is for those that are less welcome, such as the germs that cause disease. At the same time, the young body begins to build up its own immune defenses to keep unwelcome micro-visitors at bay.

Protecting and Feeding the Offspring

Not enjoying the protection afforded by a hard eggshell, the mammalian species is obliged to develop very early in life other tools to protect itself from harmful influences from the outside, especially disease-causing bacteria, while remaining capable of attracting helpful microorganisms. The first stage of protection is provided by the mother directly. During her life she has built up immunological protection, and through the milk, she is able to share her protective tools – substances capable of immobilizing or killing dangerous bacteria, virus, and fungi – with her baby. Most of these "antibodies" passed through the milk, along with defensive cells and enzymes, are made up of nutrients: proteins, fats, and a series of sugars. Once they have served their protective purpose, they can be digested as foods. The milk of all mammals has this double function – feeding and providing protection – even though the composition of the milk varies a great deal from one species to another.

The milk produced by each individual species of mammal is thus specially constituted for its purpose, complex, active in defense, and appropriate in terms of the food that the offspring needs. It is constructed to meet each species' requirements for growth and protection in the environment in which the mother and child find themselves. The raw materials needed to put the milk together are found throughout the mother's body – which constitutes a large store on which the milk glands can draw upon to provide precisely the food the offspring will need to grow and develop. Through her own diet, the mother will need to replace all the nutrients her body has provided to make the milk. All the same, the production of milk costs her remarkably little energy!

And the mother has built up her own immune protection against the microorganisms in her surroundings and passed it on to her baby, who, living in the same environment, is in need of precisely the same protection.

CHANGING PERSPECTIVE: LET'S IMAGINE SOME RATHER UNUSUAL SCENARIOS...

- **Felicia,** the mother cat, returns home from her nightly hunt, bringing with her twelve milk-producing mouse mothers, whom she has caught alive. Proudly, she declares that she proposes to feed her sick kitten mouse milk, for that is what the veterinary surgeon has suggested. Mouse milk for kittens – well, why not?

- The mother of **Jumbo,** the young elephant, has taken into her head that since she is accustomed to eat only plants and hay that are low in protein, her milk cannot possibly be sufficient to ensure that little Jumbo will grow into a big, strong, and healthy elephant. She considers that tiger milk would be better for him, for tigers eat a great deal of protein-rich meat. Even if it is problematic to obtain tiger milk for him, parents will do everything possible for their baby.

- **Buttercup,** the dairy cow, one day hits on the notion that if animal rights mean anything at all, her little calf should be provided with human milk. Why not? Her own sisters are milked daily to provide milk for human babies, so isn't it fair to turn things around for a change?

And so we lay these three stories before a nutrition physiologist. What does she say about them?

> Dear friends, she says, dear Felicia, Jumbo-mama, and Buttercup – Haven't you all stopped to think that your babies may not tolerate milk from mice, humans, or tigers? Their milk, you have to remember, is made for their own species, and you can't expect it to provide the sort of protection against the microorganisms to which hunters like your kitten, grass eaters like Buttercup's family, or jungle-dwellers like Jumbo are exposed. Every animal species makes its own special milk – because that is what is needed.

And presently, we will consider why that is so…

Species-Specific Milk: What It Is and Why …

Scientific work on human milk and its properties has taught us a great deal about ourselves. The family of mammals has been on the earth for something like 200 million years (Attenborough, 1992). Humans – and our friends the apes – have been around for several million of those years, and they have taken that time to perfect the art of breastfeeding.

After it became clear in the 1970's that women's breasts were still going to produce milk for as long into the future as we could see, and with research pointing ever more clearly to the fact that human milk was ideally adapted to the needs of human children, human milk acquired new admirers. It has nearly reached the point where one might wonder whether the songs of praise raised for human breastmilk are not perhaps a little overdone. Zoological history is full of examples of the diverse and incredible initiatives devised by mammals to ensure their defenseless offspring's survival through the perilous time of childhood (see examples later in this chapter). Let us consider for a moment how other mammals have survived–and thrived. That may give us perspective and perhaps rather more confidence in the wisdom of parents (and more especially mothers) in raising their own offspring.

Why the Cow?

Let us be clear from the start that the "breastmilk substitutes" you find on the supermarket shelves have nothing whatsoever to do with human milk, despite the name. The great majority are made from cow's milk, with some adaptation; a very few are made from soybeans.

The reason why our friend the cow was honored with the job of providing a replacement for human milk has nothing to do with her milk's supposed suitability for meeting the needs of little children. If these needs were to be the starting point, and one had really tried to find some form of animal milk that was close to human breastmilk, one would never have chosen the cow. Milk from the chimpanzee, donkey, or horse (in that order) would have been more appropriate nutrient-wise. Still, cow's milk has been used preferentially for baby feeding since around the year 1900, primarily *because it was available.* The cow had been a domestic animal for thousands of years. What is more, the cow had obviously developed nerves of steel. Most mammals (including humans) become nervous and unhappy if anyone but the baby handles their nipples or mammary glands, and as a reaction, they have problems with their *milk let-down reflex* – in other words, *the milk refuses to flow.* The cow, on the other hand, is perfectly content to be milked by strangers. What is more, with selective breeding, the cow has become unbelievably productive. After the birth of a single calf, a cow will produce sufficient milk to feed several calves at a time.

The milking machine, which was invented in 1895, made it profitable for farmers to produce and deliver vast amounts of what had originally by Nature been intended as food for calves. Dairy farming and meat production developed into large industries. These were and are the reasons why children are still offered cow's milk in their bottles and cups. It is quite simply the cow's tolerant mood and prolific productivity that has made her the leading producer for the massive world market that constitute today's infant feeding culture.

Breastmilk – Simply and Naturally

For the sort of reasons we have just considered, it is rather surprising that, even today, it may still be necessary to argue with people in order to persuade them that *the best way of raising healthy human children is to feed them species specific milk, i.e., human milk.* There are even countries where politicians have found it necessary to lay down in the law a mother's right to breastfeed in particular situations and places. It happens that it is regarded as perfectly acceptable to bottle-feed a baby with cows' milk in public, while breastfeeding is sometimes regarded as indecent and unacceptable. In the scientific literature, comparisons of cow's milk and human milk are routinely made. Obviously, this is of interest to the manufacturers of substitute products, as their sources of raw materials are essentially limited to various suppliers of dairy milk and soybeans, which the milk firms modify in some modest way, so that human babies will tolerate them better. Beyond that, comparisons between human milk and substitutes are hardly helpful to anyone; the relevant differences between human babies' food and calves' food remain gross and basic. Let us just imagine that someone set out in earnest to compare the milk of elephants with that of the shrew, and then sought support from an animal rights' movement to modify elephant milk on a global scale and sell it in powdered form to alleviate the task of the poor little shrew in raising its offspring. The absurdity is obvious, and the shrew has not asked for assistance. But it is not more absurd than the situation we now have with a massive activity to feed human infants with milk from the cow.

Mammals, Milk, and Breastfeeding: Similarities and Differences

We are called mammals because we breastfeed: "Mamma" is simply the Latin term for the breast. Feeding at the mother's breast is a central part of the reproductive strategy of the group of species to which we belong, and it has at least three basic functions:

1. Breastfeeding stimulates the pituitary gland in the mother's brain to produce the milk-producing hormone prolactin and the milk-expelling multi-function hormone oxytocin (also known as the love hormone).

2. This contact with the breast stimulates the offspring to attach to the breast and to swallow the milk produced, which, in turn, provides a further stimulus to the mother's milk production and the offspring's own existence. In some species, this entire process is speeded up to meet the demands of a hectic existence – a rabbit mother has very little opportunity to sit still and relax for more than a few minutes, but because breast contact with the offspring fires off the let-down reflex in the mother's system things can happen very quickly indeed.

3. Breastfeeding can delay a further pregnancy and thus the arrival of a new competitor at the mother's breast (see Chapter 7).

Mammals are to be found on land and in the water, and the milk glands can work under a variety of different conditions, as we will see from the examples below.

BREASTFEEDING STORIES

Breastfeeding under water...

The whale - that massive water mammal – constantly remains in the presence of its young. It feeds under water, but close to the surface, three or four times an hour. The blue whale is enormous–the largest animal to ever have existed on the planet. Its body weight of 120,000 kg equals that of 40 breastfeeding elephants, 2000 breastfeeding human mothers, or 48 million similarly occupied shrews. It has been estimated that the young may ingest as much as 600 liters of whales' milk daily. Breastfeeding can continue for between six and 12 months, depending on the sub-species of whale involved.

To set the milk let-down reflex in motion, the young nudges its mother's milk gland with its snout. Since the gland lies close to the anal opening, the young receives a useful dose of harmless intestinal bacteria as it feeds. There is no nipple to which the young can be latched on, but the initial stimulus by the snout of the young sets the mother's oxytocin production in motion, and the let-down reflex follows with such force that the milk is sprayed through the water and directly into the young whale's mouth–a striking demonstration of how important this reflex is under very variable conditions (Oftedal, 1997).

OUR CLOSEST RELATIVES

Gorillas and Other Apes

The mother ape is highly protective of her offspring, carries it with her at all times, and keeps curious neighbors at a distance, at least during its first five months of life. In some subspecies, such as the silk monkey, it is the father that carries the young, but he hands it over to its mother at the first sign the baby needs to feed. Among other apes, it is most often the young that takes the initiative to feed – it begins to feel its way towards the nipple and the mother reacts by taking it in her arms and making sure it is well positioned. Mother apes are expert in handling their young, never, for example, turning them around to face the big world head-on. They are always carried with their vulnerable chest and stomach up against her body – "soft side in."

HERD ANIMALS

Herd Animals as a Group...

Most animals accustomed to living in herds have strong social instincts regarding their offspring, infant care, and the survival of the species. In some, there is even a form of social breastfeeding, with a young animal happily taking the occasional meal from an animal other than its own mother. All the same, mother and young recognize one another, even at some distance, by sight, sound of voice, and smell, acquiring these mutual signals immediately at the time of birth. In animals such as *sheep*, which have two mammary glands and two teats, problems can arise if there is a triplet birth, which is not uncommon. In that case, the farmer must do his best to find a foster mother, hoping that both she and the young animal will be willing to accept one another. Something similar can happen in the pig with its eighteen nipples, should it deliver more than eighteen live young piglets, each convinced that it has a right to a particular nipple. The film "Babe" is the story of the extra piglet in a litter, pushed aside by his stronger siblings, but happily saved by the farmer's son and a diet of milk, no doubt, from the cow. The pig, like the human, is omnivorous.

EGG-LAYING MAMMALS

A Curious Discovery or a Missing Link?

Australia is the home to two remarkable members of the breastfeeding sisterhood. Both may have been roaming the earth since the days of the dinosaur; they are the echidna and the platypus. Both represent a transitional form between the egg-layers on the one hand and the mammals on the other, suggesting a long-term experiment in the art of reproduction. Both of them lay eggs having relatively soft shells, which hatch within a few weeks. The young are far from ready to take care of themselves, but in both species, the mother has simple milk glands on the abdomen from which high-fat milk flows when the let-down reflex comes into play in response to the licking, hunting, and searching motions of the young animal. In the case of the platypus, the milk is directly made ready for the waiting young, while with the echidna, the milk flows first into a small storage chamber on the mother's abdomen. In both species, the young lap up the milk – the echidna from the storage chamber and the platypus from among the mother's hair and fur, while it clings firmly to her.

The moral of all this is that there really is no moral to be drawn from it. We simply cannot generalize when it comes to breastfeeding patterns among mammals and related species. One thing is, however, clear: the same physiological mechanisms are at work in all of them, with prolactin and oxytocin at the heart of it all. In all these various species, the milk comes replete with immunoglobulins, anti-bacterial agents, and modulators of various types, all there to provide protection.

Whatever the difference in behavior and surroundings, we usually see the mammalian mother succeed in breastfeeding, at least provided she has enough nipples for all the young she has delivered. Only where these animals have been reared in an artificial environment, such as a circus or a zoo, can things become more difficult. That may be because the mother in this environment lacks role models – elder sisters, a mother, or wise women – to show her the way. In such an environment, any mammal – and any woman – may become unsure what she is supposed to do with this little bundle of life that has been entrusted to her. But so long as a mother, and in some cases a father, manage to react suitably to the infant's signals and a breast is at hand, feeding will go very much as it is supposed to go.

Variation in the Composition of Milks

What about the differences in the composition of the milk that we touched on above? Why is it that some mammals produce creamy protein-rich milk, while others deliver watery milk, looking as if it has been skimmed? There has been a deal of speculation on the matter and several theories have been put forward.

Different Rates of Growth

Some writers have suggested that there may be a link between the amounts of fat and protein in the milk and the rate at which the young are likely to grow. Comparisons have been made, for example, between the composition of the milk and the time it takes the young individual to double its birth weight (Lozoff, Brittenham, Trause, Kennell, & Klaus, 1977), without, in fact, demonstrating any clear relationship.

Differences in Immune Defenses

One might set out to explain differences in the protein content of the milk produced by the various species as follows: The body's immune defenses are largely built of substances with a high protein content. Enzymes, hormones, and immunoglobulins are large packages of amino acids, the building blocks of all proteins. Differences in the protein content of milk could well reflect differences in the types and number of microbes in the various environments in which different species of animals live, and consequently differences in the type and degree of protection that is needed if unwelcome microbes are to be prevented from entering and injuring the infant's body. No one has studied this, so it simply remains an interesting theory (Hall & Oxberry, 1977).

Differences in Water Requirements

It has also been pointed out that as man is believed to have descended from equatorial species, we need to be prepared for a level of water intake demanded in hot climates around the equator. Therefore, it is argued, human milk is watery and suitable for quenching a tropical thirst (B. Børresen, personal communication, May 4, 2006).

Differences in Feeding Patterns

Thomas Ljungberg (1991), a Swedish developmental psychologist, has raised an interesting theory on links between the composition of the milk and the frequency of breastfeeding. In his opinion, the composition of the milk is determined both by the infant's need of food and the number of opportunities it has to breastfeed in the course of a day. It is not difficult to determine how frequently different species do breastfeed, and the differences are quite striking. At one extreme, we have animals like hares and rabbits, with nervous and busy mothers that only get to their young now and again – perhaps once a day or even only on alternate days – for a few minutes of feeding – and the rest of the time hardly dare to visit them for fear of putting hungry predators on their scent. Ljungberg calls these mothers "intermittent breastfeeders" – we would prefer the more descriptive "sporadic breastfeeders." It is striking that animals whose milk is rich in fat and protein (such as the reindeer and the walrus) allow their young access to the nipple only a few times a day, e.g., on four or five occasions, which is perhaps rational in the severe cold in which they are brought up. The young of the "sporadic feeders" need to take their meal rapidly, before the mother hurries out again, and the milk needs to be rich in energy. It is striking that, although the rabbit breastfeeds only about once a day, the calorie level of the milk is nearly four times as high as that of human milk. Mammals producing less energy-rich and more watery milk, containing relatively little protein and fat, as is the case with humans and apes, must put their young to the breast very frequently – sometimes almost continually – which is what the offspring needs if it is to acquire sufficient energy (Neville & Neifert, 1983). Such frequent small feeds are also better suited to the smallness of the newborn's stomach – only large enough to take a thimbleful of milk at a time. Humans and apes are adapted to an intensive program of infant care with frequent breastfeeds – often several times an hour, each lasting 10-15 minutes. Such offspring must therefore have almost unlimited access to the breast, involving continual breastfeeding contact with the mother throughout early life. Bears in hibernation provide another example of this – the young are delivered in the lair and the breasts are always within reach of the young. The higher primates – the apes and humans – are also "continuous feeders." The young are born at a very early stage of physical development, and in order to keep up with the flock, they have to be carried continuously by an adult, generally the mother. The infant seeks the breast not only in order to obtain food, but also for social reasons: it needs comfort, security, and learning. All this is of fundamental importance, particularly for primates kept in confinement. If they have not experienced maternal contact and have not observed it among others of the same species, they are likely to become confused when later faced with the need to care for their own young, not knowing, for example, how to put the baby to the breast (Hess, 1996).

Studies from the last century of breastfeeding among hunter-gatherers, who had perhaps perpetuated the breastfeeding pattern of man's early ancestors and ensured the survival of the race through the millennia, point to frequent and unrestricted breastfeeding contact (Konner & Worthman, 1980). Even today, one will encounter this pattern in some countries and cultures; the mother carries her child on her body, and offers the baby the breast whenever it is desired.

Ljungberg, we feel, has provided us with the most credible explanation for the differences in the composition of the milk between species.

And so...when irritated voices around you ask whether you intend to breastfeed this baby all day long, you can, if you wish, with our relatives in nature's kingdom in mind, answer: "That is precisely what I intend to do."

THE WORLD CHAMPION OF BREASTFEEDING

Let us get this straight from the start: Proud of ourselves though we may be, the undisputed breastfeeding champion of the world is the female kangaroo and her near relative the wallaby. Both deliver their performance in Australia, a continent with severe challenges where nutrition is concerned and extremely variable conditions to battle with.

Delivery in the case of the kangaroo is remarkably easy – the miniature "joey," as it is known, is hardly larger than a bumble-bee and is born after a gestation of a mere 26 days. On its own, it must find its way through its mother's fur to her pouch, but once having arrived there, it finds in the very bottom of the pouch a choice of four nipples of varying size. It attaches itself to one of these, holding on by firm suction sufficient for it to resist any alien attempt to dislodge it. The joey will remain in the pouch for nearly 200 days (Figure 2.1). At first, it receives a continuous flow of clear, nutritious kangaroo milk from the milk gland, but as time goes by, the nipple enlarges and the milk changes to become much more similar to cow's milk (see Table 3.1). After the long stay in the pouch, Joey I is ready to take an occasional trip outside to explore the world. By this time, however, a second young joey (Joey II), conceived a month before, is ready to make its perilous way toward the pouch and to a free nipple, duly attaching to it to take the clear starting milk. Joey I, in the meantime, continues on its "milk for big kangaroo babies" from the nipple that it originally selected, and will have grown appreciably in the meantime. And by then, the mother will have copulated yet again, but she keeps the fertilized egg waiting in her uterus until the first Joey has successfully left the pouch and the conditions food-wise are favorable. A kangaroo mother takes no chances!

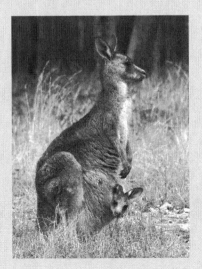

Figure 2.1. *Kangaroo mom & baby. Source:* ©*Fotolia.com*

So we see how this remarkable mother is capable not only of producing two different types of milk, but also of delivering it separately to two of her young through two different let-down reflexes:

- A low-level reflex – operating continuously to ensure that Joey II has as much as he needs of the clear early milk, and

- A stronger let-down reflex, fired off several times daily when Joey I needs richer milk from his own particular nipple.

And all this time, the industrious kangaroo mother is moving around, taking three meter high obstacles in one leap after another, and reaching speeds of 60km an hour – fully capable of escaping from most of the threats she may encounter, yet never losing the Joeys from her pouch. Now and again, she will pause for a vegetarian meal of grasses and leaves– and perhaps an occasional snack from the farmer's fields.

Truly, a world champion of breastfeeding – even if the Australian farmer may not entirely share our enthusiasm for her…

The Birthing Process Is Only Complete When Your Baby Is Weaned from the Breast

It is time to draw some conclusions before we go further.

The human baby spends a relatively short time of its expected lifetime in its mother's body. As one sees across the mammalian family, it is born early, but with the prospect of breastfeeding to follow as a second phase of dependence on and support from its mother. In the mother's body, it has, like a chicken still in its shell, lived an existence protected from microorganisms and with unlimited access to all the nutrients it needs to become a small human being. Once it is born, the direct blood link to its mother's body provided by the placenta and umbilical cord is broken. At that moment, however, the child has not yet received everything it needs to begin an independent existence without its mother's support. It is far from ready to consume the same food as that taken by adults. A child at this stage has been described as an exterogestate fetus, or *"fetus outside the uterus"* (Jelliffe & Jelliffe, 1978). It is at this point that the milk gland, or the breast, provides the infant with what we call milk, a product that offers both protection and all that it needs in the way of nutrition. As is sometimes said, an infant is born in an unripe state, and it remains in a "pre-physiological" stage until it has been weaned from its mother's breast. Only at that moment has the new life, with the help of its mother, completed the process of physical and mental formation that began in the uterus. From that tiny beginning, the mother has devoted her body and her soul to the creation of a living and viable new member of the human race.

Chapter 3.

MILK

During the first 50 years of the 20th century, there was strikingly little interest among researchers for either human milk or the physiology of breastfeeding. Feeding babies from the breast, it was considered, had had its day; it was now finally and firmly on the way out. And then, around the mid-70s, it became apparent that a great many mothers in a great many countries had not the slightest intention of abandoning breastfeeding. The practice, it now appeared, was very far from being confined to the history books and the museums. Once that was realized, the idea of studying human milk suddenly became interesting. By that time, new methods of investigation had arrived, making it possible to study the individual processes concerned and the various components of milk in much greater detail and with more accuracy than ever before (Lai, Hale, Simmer, & Hartmann, 2010). Suddenly it was all new and fascinating.

MILK AND BREASTFEEDING AMONG MAMMALS: SIMILARITIES AND DIFFERENCES

It costs the human mother much less in terms of energy to produce milk for her offspring than is the case with most other mammals. She needs only about 25% more calories in her daily diet than she did before her pregnancy, while an animal mother with a large litter, such as the sow and the rat, may need up to 300% more energy than before (Prentice, Goldberg, & Prentice, 1994).

ONCE MORE: THE ELEPHANT AND THE SHREW

Mother Elephant, who may weigh several tons, gives birth to a small Jumbo, weighing some 70 kg. But within a matter of eight months, the little one is capable of putting on about 500 kg of extra weight, simply and solely thanks to the mother's milk. Exclusive breastfeeding indeed – and on the basis of what sort of a diet? A varied and well-balanced food intake? In fact, it will mainly consist of a mixture of available twigs, straw, leaves, grasses, and various sorts of foliage. The mother elephant's milk glands are fully capable of transforming this mixture into high quality elephant milk. As to her energy needs – at this time, they are a third greater than before her pregnancy.

Mother Shrew is, given her size, an even more remarkable performer. She weighs only about 11 grams, but she delivers eight tiny shrews, each of which weighs half a gram. They will, in the course of three weeks, grow seven grams each in weight. What this means is that the mother shrew must provide enough milk to build shrew bodies equivalent to five times her own body weight (Brambell & Jones, 1977). During this period, her energy needs rise by 500%. Perhaps there is among the shrews a market for milk substitutes based on elephant milk after all?

The milk produced by each species of mammal is distinct from that of any other species because it is specially constituted to meet the needs of its own young. Babies of shrews and whales, tigers and sows, humans and wolves – each of these is provided with milk adapted to its own bodily needs and its environment – that holds true not only as far as nutrition is concerned, but also as regards to the ability to welcome friendly microflora from their environment and repel the less friendly, whether they be bacterial, viral, or parasitic.

Not that the milk necessarily differs very much in appearance from one species to another; all these milks behave similarly – forming curds or cheese or cream – and all will, by and large, contain the same major nutrients, though in very different amounts and proportions.

The Let-Down Reflex and Oxytocin

Every mammalian mother relies on the let-down reflex to release the milk to her young. And the hormone oxytocin, as we have discussed in chapter 1, is central to this process in every species.

Oxytocin: The Love Hormone?

Oxytocin can, in fact, achieve more than just expelling milk from the breast. Researchers have studied various aspects of maternal behavior, both in humans and other mammals, and found that there is a remarkably close link between the oxytocin levels in the blood and the extent to which a parent is interested in and concerned with the young (Pedersen & Prange, 1985). That is the case with fathers as well as mothers – when a father handles his child, there will be more oxytocin than otherwise in his bloodstream. It seems likely that this hormone plays an important role in the development of emotional links between child and parent (Uvnäs-Moberg, 2003).

MOTHER SOW AND THE JOY OF BREASTFEEDING

If, at this point, anyone is still in any doubt as to the role of the milk let-down reflex in the various species, it is worth glancing at the sow's striking story. She may have delivered up to 18 piglets, for she has 18 nipples awaiting them. To ensure that each finds a place for itself, she has to lie on her side. As soon as she is ready to receive them, she emits a very special "food-is-ready" grunt that they soon recognize, and with that, they promptly come running. Should she have delivered more than eighteen this time, a battle will ensue, for the law of the strongest prevails, and no one of them is willing to share its rightful place. At first, each piglet nudges and licks at the nipple it has secured, sparking the let-down reflex to the accompaniment of ever more grunting from Mother Sow, while the young milk and swallow for dear life. And so it continues until the reflex begins to fade, Mother's grunting calms down, and the young content themselves by suckling the unyielding teats.

But ... now and again it will happen that Mother Sow, whatever the book of unwritten rules may say, is not particularly inclined to provide a feed, but perfectly inclined to have some family fun. When that is the case, she sets up an inviting grunt of a different kind. The piglets come running up, but she does not set off the let-down reflex – and the young are simply left to satisfy themselves at the teats for a while. Whether Mother Sow does this for her own pleasure or for that of her young, we are left wondering – for no one has ever asked her. What does seem clear is that piglets, like human babies, simply like being at the breast, and they too seem to enjoy the closeness to their mother...

One might add that such behavior has been noted in various species of animals, which is why one can conclude that for all of them breastfeeding has in some way social and psychological dimensions – it is more than just a physical process.

> But if, in that respect, there is a difference between sows and human mothers, it is that for the former this is completely unproblematic - and there is no one around to criticize her for being indulgent to the little ones, spoiling them in the process... (Shillito Walser, 1977).

THE COMPOSITION OF MILK

How Do We Study Milk?

Milk has more than 200 different components, many of which are specific to the species for which the milk is composed. Some of these are active components, such as enzymes (that cause other substances to change) and hormones, others have mainly a nutritive function, and yet others just happen to be around, for example, as residue from the milk-making process (such as fragments of ruptured cell membranes), but the great majority of them are there with good reason. All this means is that in its natural state milk is complex to an almost confusing degree, certainly when one compares it with the homogenized and standardized mixtures that are sold as "breastmilk substitutes" (see Figure 3.1).

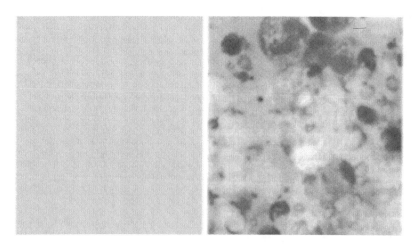

Figure 3.1. *A comparison of formula (left) and human milk (right). Human milk is a dynamic colloidal solution of perfect nutrient and growth factors for infants. Formula is a totally homogenized solution of nutrient chemicals.*

Source: *Lawrence & Lawrence, 2005. Used with permission from Ruth Lawrence and Nancy Wight.*

In the breastfeeding literature, one finds many descriptions of the composition of milk made by various species, but the figures vary a lot, probably depending on how accurately the analysis has been carried out. The milk of 150 different species has so far been examined in the laboratory, but the milk of 4000 other species of mammals has yet to be studied. The samples examined so far are, as one might expect, those from humans and from species providing milk that has market value, notably the cow. Other work has been carried out on milk from experimental animals (such as the rat and the mouse), as well as from species important in animal husbandry, notably the water buffalo, goat, sheep, horse, and camel.

There are obvious practical difficulties to be faced in obtaining representative samples of milk from whales, bears, and more generally, those species that are not so amicably disposed to man. Even milking a mouse can be tricky – but it has been done!

The tables of results, however impressive, do not as a rule indicate how the samples were obtained–a question that should arise in your own mind when you look at a table such as the one presented below (Table 3.1). For a truly typical picture of the components of any milk, one should ideally take all the milk produced by a single breast, udder, or gland; the milk should be collected over a period, e.g. 24 hours, it must be mixed well, and particular care must be taken to collect the full content of fat that all too readily gets deposited on glass or similar surfaces. Only after that should the samples be analyzed. Obviously, all this demands much meticulous laboratory work. The results in a table such as the one below therefore need to be looked at with some caution. Note the variation in the figures quoted.

Table 3.1. Average Content of Nutrients in Milk of Various Species and Strains of Mammals

(Classified in order of carbohydrate content in grams per 100 ml)

Species or Strain Studied	Carbohydrates (esp. lactose)	Fats	Protein	Energy (kilocalories per 100 ml)
Seal (Pinnipedia)	0.1 - 0.8	43.9 - 49.4	10.2 - 11.2	465
Whale (Cetacea)	0.9 - 1.6	29.6 - 42.3	10.9 - 13.2	328
Rabbit (Lagomorpha)	1.4 - 1.8	12.2 - 17.4	10.4 - 23.7	266
Mouse (Muridae)	1.8 - 3.0	13.1 - 14.7	9.0 - 12.0	206
Cat (Felidae)	3.4 - 4.1	10.5 - 10.9	7.6 - 11.1	169
Elephant (Proboscidae)	4.2 - 5.3	8.0 - 10.5	3.7 - 4.9	141
Beef cattle (Bovidae)	4.6 - 4.7	3.7 - 5.2	3.4 - 3.6	99
Kangaroo and other Marsupials (Marsupalia)	Trace - 3.9	2.1 - 4.8	6.2	94
Camel (Camelidae)	5.1 - 5.4	4.1 - 4.9	4.9	87
Ape and man (Primates)	5.9 - 6.9	4.1 - 4.5	1.0 - 1.6	79
Horse (Equidae)	6.1 - 6.8	1.6 - 1.7	2.5 - 2.7	54

*Not indicated in the original paper
Sources: Jones, 1977, p. 87.

THE ROLE OF MILK AND BREASTFEEDING IN PROTECTION AGAINST ILLNESS

The Immune System: Protecting the Individual and Preventing Disease

The world is full of dangers, both visible and invisible. Here we are particularly concerned with the very smallest forms of life: microbes, bacteria, viruses, and other parasites. Invisible to the eye though they may be, we are in contact with them every day in the food we eat, the water we drink, and the air we breathe. What is more, we carry them with us throughout life: the whole surface of the body is saturated with them, including the internal surfaces hidden from view (if you think of the body as having the shape of a doughnut, the hole in the middle represents the digestive canal from the mouth down to the anus, all of it lined with moist surface material). In the intestinal tract alone, a human adult harbors more than 100 billion microorganisms weighing a total of a kilogram and representing more than 500 species of organisms. By and large, we can be content with them. We provide them with a home, and they bestow on us many useful services, staying, as a rule, at their appointed sites and not obstructing our life at all. So long as everything remains in balance, as it generally does, these friendly microorganisms are a blessing, filling up the sites that might otherwise be colonized by harmful (pathogenic) organisms capable of causing disease. In the struggle for survival, these pathogenic microorganisms are quite simply our adversaries, forever waiting to pounce on whatever site in the body is unoccupied, feasting and pillaging dangerously on whatever they find there.

For such reasons, any living being that has a hope of maintaining its place on this planet, because of the challenge posed by this vast army of pathogens, must build up an effective set of defenses against them. It is obvious that pathogens not encountering such resistance will penetrate the organism and have no inhibitions whatsoever about injuring or destroying it. It is, however, a fact that invading organisms do, in practice, encounter a complex defense system, which we term the immune system. These built-in defenses against invasion need to be specifically attuned to the type of invader they are likely to meet, and however complex this process is, it is vital to survival.

SOME DEFINITIONS:

Immune defense, immune system, immune competence: Each of these terms refers to the ability of the organism to challenge and overcome invasion by unwanted elements, in particular microorganisms.

Immunoglobulins, antibodies: Proteins supplied initially in the breastmilk, which attack and immobilize or destroy unwanted invaders, including bacteria, viruses, and fungi.

Cells: Structural elements of which the body is composed. Many cells are capable of producing immunoglobulins, and some are even capable of ingesting foreign microorganisms and destroying them.

Enzymes: Special proteins which work in tandem with other components in the process of immune defense. More generally, an enzyme is a protein that promotes biological reactions or causes other substances to break down or become altered.

Lactoferrin: A protein acting locally and attacking the cell walls of certain common bacteria, viruses, and fungi.

Colonization of the Newborn (Summary)

So long as a mammal remains in its mother's uterus, it is sterile. The moment it comes into a world teeming with bacteria, however, it must learn, as we have all learned in our early lives, to find a way of living in harmony with the bacteria around it. That process begins the moment the young life leaves the uterus, for in a flash, the bacteria will have arrived and will seek to "colonize" it–in other words, to make it their home. What this means is that all sorts of bacteria, both benevolent and ill-intentioned, will begin to live here and hope to thrive, especially at first, on and around those surfaces where the infant's body is in direct contact with the surroundings–especially in the lungs, gut, and on the surface of the skin. At that moment, it is vital that the young organism be capable of maintaining an internal environment that tolerates or welcomes benevolent bacteria, but repels and attacks those that are less well intentioned and capable of causing disease. The very first bacteria to present themselves at the moment of birth are, or should be, those from the mother's anus–vital right at the start.

Immune Defense - The Walls of the Fortress

By the time we come to adulthood, we already have spent many years waging this battle against the world of microorganisms, and in the process, our bodies have created a formidable defense force of antibodies (immunoglobulins) designed to counter microorganisms arriving from the outside. When a woman becomes pregnant, many of the antibodies that her body has already acquired can be shared with her developing baby through the bloodstream. That is sufficient to provide the baby at birth with a starting kit of immunoglobulins with which to enter the world. They are not ideal for the purpose, since they can cause some inflammation when they are brought into action, but their role is, fortunately, only a temporary one.

The Second Starting Kit

Very soon, these antibodies are replaced with other antibodies from the mother, which have been provided in the milk. That is just as well, for it will still be a while before the young individual is capable of building up a fully immunocompetent system of its own.

So it is the mother's milk, particularly the colostrum, that is there before the mature milk itself appears, that provides the baby with its second supply of antibodies against all the various microorganisms to which its mother has been exposed, and against which she has been obliged to build her own defenses (Hanson, 2004). This time, rather than providing the baby with second-hand antibodies, the mother's body prepares them on the spot. Some of the special immunocompetent cells, which the mother has built in her system at various points (for example, in the airways and intestine), migrate to the milk glands in her breast. In the breast, they become attached and continue to manufacture fresh antibodies against bacteria and viruses. The antibodies can be fed continually into the milk as it is secreted and passed on to her baby, making them immediately available to provide protection both in the digestive canal and wherever else they may be needed. This unbelievably complex mechanism is still the subject of much research, and further findings continue to appear. We are far from knowing how all these immunocompetent cells act, but it would seem that they attach themselves to the moist mucous membranes in the child's intestine and elsewhere, forming a lining so that enemy bacteria are unable to become affixed to the intestinal wall–the first step towards penetrating more deeply into the body.

Milk produced by women living under poor sanitary conditions, with many and diverse microorganisms all around, will naturally contain antibodies against a wider range of bacteria than milk produced by women spending their time in clean and hygienic homes. Any baby is, however, likely to find itself very much in the same environment as that to which its mother has been accustomed, and will therefore need more or less the same range of defensive antibodies to keep hostile bacteria and viruses at bay.

FOR THOSE WHO LIKE TO DIG A LITTLE DEEPER - SOME EXAMPLES

The Lactoferrin Strategy

The protein known as lactoferrin is one of the cavaliers of the immune defense regiment, working in tandem with the enzyme lysozyme; both are present in breastmilk. Together they assault the cell walls of bacteria, viruses, and fungi, especially the mold *Candida Albicans* that causes yeast infections (thrush). Directly after birth, there is a high level of lactoferrin in the colostrum (some 5 -7 grams per liter); it falls to 1-3 grams over the first two weeks as the milk matures, but by that time, the baby is taking more milk, so the supply of lactoferrin provided to the baby remains roughly the same.

While proteins are, as a rule, broken down by digestive processes when they reach the gut, this does not happen with lactoferrin. This particular protein seems to act locally, preventing bacteria from getting a grip on the gut wall. Lactoferrin acts smoothly and kindly–while some substances induce inflammation when they attack a microorganism, lactoferrin seems to be capable of preventing this from happening. What is more: when the lactoferrin molecule is finally worn out and disintegrates, the fragments that remain may still play a useful role. Such fragments are found in the urine of breastfed children, and this *could* explain why breastfed babies are less prone than others to develop urinary infections. A beautiful theory is, however, one thing, and proof is another – that is one of the eternal dilemmas of science.

Enzymes

Many of the proteins present in breastmilk have enzymatic properties. Under the microscope, enzymes look like large clumps of protein that are continuously breaking open and reuniting, just as is the case with the cells and other structures that compose our body. Some of these enzymes render the milk more readily digestible for a young child, i.e., starting the digestive process. Other enzymes protect one another and the immunoglobulins from being digested before they have performed the task for which they were intended. Yet others have an inhibitory effect on the growth of bacteria – a particularly good example of this being lysozyme. Lysozyme is also found in tears, and as we have just seen, it works with lactoferrin to attack the cell wall of many bacteria. There are far higher quantities of lysozyme in breastmilk than in fresh cow's milk – to say nothing of pasteurized milk (see Figure 3.1 at the beginning of this chapter).

Taking all these things together, one can truly conclude that the innocent bluish-whitish fluid that we call breastmilk is a hive of activity. It is a product that deserves respect.

HIV and Other Viruses in the Milk

Milk can also harbor some less desirable components that have found their way into it, such as unwanted viruses, bacteria, and fungi. Since it also provides defenses – antibodies – against these very same invaders, a baby will, as a rule, suffer no severe ill consequences from ingesting such milk. Or, should some degree of infection occur, the defenses conferred by the milk will be on hand to suppress it, in effect acting like a vaccine or an antiserum.

To every such generalization, there are unfortunately exceptions, and one of the infections that can be transferred in breastmilk is so fearful that one will want to run no risk at all of encountering it – the Human Immunodeficiency Virus – HIV – the agent that can lead to AIDS.

A HIV-infected mother is faced with the painful dilemma of having to choose between breastfeeding her baby, with the risk of transmitting the infection to it, and the likewise considerable risk to the child of depriving it of the protection provided by its mother's milk. The latter risk is particularly marked in low-income countries where conditions such as malnutrition and diarrhea pose a constant threat to child health.

"HIV and breastfeeding" is an area where there is considerable research on new medical therapies. It is important to be aware of new recommendations. The World Health Organization provides updated advice on this matter. At the time of writing (May 2011), the recommendation for infant feeding is that it is possible to lower the risk of HIV transmission by breastfeeding with appropriate drug treatment, reducing the risk of HIV transmission from 9.5 to 5.6%, based on a study of an international consortium of researchers (Kesho Bora Study Group, 2011).

According to WHO, the choice for each mother seems to be either to:

Breastfeed and receive antiretroviral therapy, or

Avoid all breastfeeding, as the strategy that will most likely give infants the greatest chance of HIV-free survival (WHO, UNAIDS, UNFPA, & UNICEF, 2010, p.2).

To "avoid all breastfeeding" is not really an alternative to breastfeed and receive antiviral therapy. Breastfeeding also has a social function – a mother who avoids all breastfeeding also signals that she has reason to do so, that she is HIV-infected.

WHO also recommends the following:

"Even when ARVs are not available, mothers should be counseled to exclusively breastfeed in the first six months of life and continue breastfeeding thereafter unless environmental and social circumstances are safe for, and supportive of, replacement feeding" (WHO et al., 2010, p.3).

If the mother chooses breastfeeding, the best evidence today is that her baby should be *exclusively* breastfed during the first six months (i.e., the baby is given no other form of food at this time).

Limits of Our Knowledge

When Elisabet published the first edition of her Norwegian *The Book about Breastfeeding* in 1970, it included a very tiny section cautiously entitled: *"Does breastmilk protect the baby against illness?"* At that time relatively little was known on the matter and the answer had to be a subdued: "It indeed looks like it – but we don't know how." Now there is a great deal of information on the mechanisms possessed by the body to recognize and battle against undesirable organisms trying to gain entry. Many characteristics of the battle that ensues when these assailants and defenders meet on the battlefield have been described. Immunologists also know more than ever before about the curiously harmonious relationship that exists between the body and its allies in the microscopic world. One could tell a great deal more about these things, but let us instead refer the interested reader to one of the finest books of all on the matter: *Immunobiology of Human Milk: How Breastfeeding Protects Babies* by Lars Åke Hanson (2004; see literature list at the back of this book).

Undoubtedly, we will in the near future come to know even more about the constituents of breastmilk and the many and various protective mechanisms that it provides against numerous and assorted dangers. This protective process, involving the transfer of *passive immunity* from mother to baby, is of the greatest importance during the first six months of a child's life, before its own immune system has become fully mature. The baby's new immune system is thus accorded a breathing space as it comes progressively into contact with this perilous world. It can take its time to develop as the child grows and matures, ready to tackle the new challenges that still lie beyond its horizon.

What Influences the Bacterial Flora?

The whole story of the "bacterial flora," as it is so charmingly termed, is very clear and well established. The bacterial flora of a baby reared only on breastmilk will be quite different, both internally and externally, from that of a baby that has received mixed feeding. This difference is readily apparent from the baby's stools. Adding even a little food other than breastmilk to the diet will be sufficient to replace the slightly acid scent prevalent during breastfeeding with a quite different odor.

Also contributing to the growth of the flora is the fact that the child uses the sensitive area of its mouth to explore the world around it. Once it has gained sufficient control over its movements and has mastered that tricky "hand-must-grasp-it and then straight-to-the- mouth" maneuver, there will be no limits to what a baby is capable of finding and putting into its mouth. With those objects come loads of (local) bacteria, and they can play an important role in building up the corresponding bacterial flora of the intestine.

THE ROLE OF MILK AS FOOD

Whatever else it may be, breastmilk is also a food – and of all the numerous foods we encounter during our lives, this is the only one that has truly been designed with humans – and only humans – in mind. It provides a child with all the energy (calories) it needs to grow and develop. As we noted earlier, no one disputes the fact that, of all foods, human milk is the one best capable of providing a child with "the highest attainable level of health." It is the perfect *designer food* – an all-in-one menu. It is quite simply ideal. For human children!

The Fat in Milk

Fat consists mostly of fatty acids, which are molecules of varying size and length. Fat takes part in the process of building up tissue, but is, at the same time, a valuable source of energy to keep the whole body going through a series of processes of "internal combustion" – rather like burning, but without the fire and flames! Milk also contains a fair quantity of cholesterol, one form of fat. In recent years, we have been told a lot about cholesterol, with emphasis on the view that it isn't a particularly desirable substance, especially when there is too much of it floating around in the blood. For adults, that is more or less true, for our bodies are no longer growing, and we are simply maintaining a body that is already complete. As a result, we have a limited need for cholesterol. For an infant, it is entirely different – there is a great deal of tissue to be built up, and for that purpose, cholesterol is an ideal building-block and completely harmless.

Fat, particularly in the form of long chain fatty acids with formidable names (just think of "docosahexanoic acid, fortunately abbreviated to DHA), is another brick in the structure, being indispensable when it comes to building the child's brain and nervous system. The types of fat you eat as a breastfeeding mother will be reflected in the fats that find their way into your milk. If you, for example, eat a lot of fish or cod liver oil, some of the long chain fatty acids they contain will end up in the milk – and benefit your baby (Rønneberg & Skåra, 1992). A lot of attention has been paid to the fat in breastmilk, since the manufacturers of substitutes have been eager to copy it – or even to try and improve upon it. Adding some single fatty acids to a product is fairly simple, but pointless because, as Ruth Lawrence and Robert M. Lawrence (2005) emphasize, the fatty components of breastmilk work together. There is no evidence that these individual fatty acids are individually effective, as when they are added to breastmilk substitutes, or that "more is better."

Fully mature breastmilk contains, on average, about the same amount of fat as cow's milk, although many mothers have difficulty believing it. Viewing the first few drops that appear from the nipple, they may get the impression that the milk is pathetically watery compared with the milk they know from the kitchen. That is literally true, but only because the milk with the highest levels of fat – the cream – does not arrive until later in a feeding session, particularly if there are not many breastfeeds in a day. Most of the energy in breastmilk – around 50% of all the calories the milk provides – is from fat. The composition of the milk varies somewhat from one mother to another, from the beginning of a feed to the end, from hour to hour, and also over time during the whole period of nursing (Mitoulas et al., 2002). The fat content will go up and down from day to day and month to month, and there may be more or less fat in the milk a mother produces for one of her children and that which she makes for another. To get anything like a reliable picture of the fat content of milk at a given time, you would need to pump or hand express all the milk produced by a breast in the course of 24 hours and mix it before sending it for analysis.

Golden Rule Number 4

The baby controls your production and its own intake very precisely according to need, by demanding to feed either more or less frequently.

The moral of all this, to put it simply, is that you should not go along with anyone who tries to persuade you to have a sample of your milk analyzed for its nutritional value; the information obtained from a single sample will be of no use at all. Many, many studies have been carried out to set the variability of mother's milk alongside the baby's need for energy and nutrients. All of them conclude quite simply that the baby adjusts the volume of milk to meet its own needs. If the milk contains less fat or lower amounts of other components than it needs, it will simply take more of it, and that is that (Dewey, Heinig, Nommsen, & Lönnerdal, 1991).

Golden Rule Number 5

There is no reason to have your milk analyzed to determine its nutritional content.

Protein

Many of the "active" components of breastmilk, such as cells and enzymes, are to a large extent made of protein. Protein is also present in the hormones and immunoglobulins that are at work in the baby's gut and elsewhere in its body. Proteins are made of long chains of amino acids, and most proteins are complex molecular bundles, which have entirely specialized functions. Once such a protein is heated, as is the case during pasteurization (heating to 60°C) or sterilization (boiling at 100°C), it is *denatured*, i.e., the chains lose contact with one another and the bundle falls apart. The protein is then no longer able to fulfill its role, for example, as an active enzyme, globulin, or carrier for other materials. Much the same, but to an even greater extent, happens when a protein is exposed to digestive fluids in the gut. In the case of proteins serving as foods, that is very necessary. Before proteins can be absorbed through the intestinal wall and enter the child's system, they have to be broken down into small and more readily handled single amino acids, or at least into small amino acid chains known as peptides.

The proteins in breastmilk have a double function. In their original form as large compound molecular bundles or as constituents of living cells, they play an active role, not only in the baby's stomach and gut (which has long been known), but also elsewhere in the young body, where foreign microorganisms either present a threat or are welcome and can be invited to take their place in the system. Once the various hormones and enzymes have played out this active role as immunological *defenders,* they are accepted as components of the *food* and gratefully digested.

The Amount of Protein in the Milk Varies Between Species

The concentration of protein in the milk may be ten times higher in one species than in another. We can only offer guesses as to *why* this should be so. Might it be that the various animal species come into the world with different needs as regards to their immune protection? When we look at the way different proteins are made, i.e., the types of amino acids they contain, we find much closer similarities between humans and great apes than between humans and cows. The amino acid pattern of the cow's milk protein is much closer to that found in sheep's and goat's milk. However, the last word on that subject is yet to be written – much more research is still needed (Davis et al., 1994).

Interestingly enough, scientists working on these matters have found no differences in the amino acid structure in the milk of mothers from different races around the world. The fact that the amino-acid make-up of their diets differs greatly seems to have no influence on the milk. On the other hand, we know that the milk of Pakistani women contains a wide range of antibodies, all ready to face far more bacterial challenges than, for example, the milk of Swedish mothers (Hanson, 2007). We may also note that there is no difference in this respect between milk produced in the right and the left breasts (Jenness, 1979).

Lactose

Lactose, also known as milk sugar, is a member of the same family of substances as ordinary white sugar (sucrose). Milk sugar is composed of two linked molecules, glucose and galactose, the latter of which is only found in milk. Most of the sugar in breastmilk is lactose, and the amount increases during the first ten days after birth. It is likely that the high lactose content of mother's milk accounts for much of its taste; anyone who has tasted breastmilk will recall its sweetish taste, even somewhat sickly sweet when compared with cow's milk. Lactose also plays an important part in ensuring that the water content of the milk is sufficiently high. This is one reason why breastfed infants, even on hot days or in tropical climates, do not need any additional intake of water. Human milk contains more lactose than the milk of any other mammal. The galactose component of lactose is also important in the build-up of the brain and nervous system (Peaker, 1977).

As already noted, anyone who has cared for both breastfed children and children receiving infant formula will have noticed that the stools are quite different. In breastfed infants, they have a slightly acid odor (mothers sometimes describe it as "fresh," but they are of course biased), as a result of the digestion of lactose and the presence of the *bifidus factor*, which creates a particular bacterial environment in the breastfed baby's digestive system.

Vitamins

To some extent, the level of vitamins in the milk reflects the vitamin situation in the mother's own body. If the mother begins to take vitamin tablets while she is breastfeeding, this will have little direct effect on the amounts of the various vitamins getting into her breastmilk.

Mothers who, as a rule, follow a normal diet can be sure that their milk will contain all the vitamins their baby needs (see also Chapter 4). The only vitamin that there may be some point in giving to a baby directly, to supplement what is present in the milk, is Vitamin D. Ideally, a child will be able to synthesize this vitamin in the skin when exposed to sunlight. In very northerly and southerly climates, however, a child is not likely to have enough exposure to the sun, especially during the colder part of the year, which is why the official nutritional advice is often to give a breastfed baby some Vitamin D in the form of drops or cod liver oil. If your baby (and you) likes fish liver oil, you can both happily take it; it will provide not only Vitamin D, but also some of those useful long-chain fatty acids. It will also contain Vitamin A, which you do not need to supplement, but it is naturally present in fish liver oil because the fish liver has put it there. Alternatively, you can buy plain Vitamin D in the form of drops for your baby to take. *But be careful here!* In large doses, vitamin D is rather poisonous and can cause calcium deposits in the child's tissues (Helsing, 2000). In the right dose, it is fine and perfectly safe, but never think that more might be better for the baby–the reverse may be true!

Minerals

The concentration of minerals in breastmilk varies over time and is higher in some mothers than in others, probably because women differ in the amount they take in the diet and the quantity stored in the body. The infant readily absorbs whatever minerals it receives in the milk. The more minerals a mother gives away in her breastmilk, the more minerals she is likely to absorb from her diet, particularly if her own bodily reserves are on the low side. Quite apart from the absolute levels of minerals, the relative proportions in which they are present can be important.

Breastmilk contains variable amounts of iron, but the baby absorbs it very efficiently, and with exclusive breastfeeding, the quantity provided will usually be sufficient (Saarinen & Siimes, 1979). It is unusual for a breastfed child under the age of six months to suffer from iron deficiency. A little later in childhood, the supply from milk alone may tend to run short of what some children need, though in most cases, the iron in the milk will be sufficient up to the ninth month. As a rule, it is now considered sensible to provide some iron, in the form of solid food, from around the sixth month (Siimes, Salmenperä, & Perheentupa, 1984). It is a fact, however, that from the time solid food is introduced, the absorption of iron from the gut becomes less efficient. Don't become unnecessarily worried about the iron levels if your baby's blood, when examined at the health center, shows what seem to be relatively low levels of iron-containing hemoglobin. Remember that children normally do have somewhat lower hemoglobin levels than adults, something that is too readily forgotten. Not until around the time of puberty does hemoglobin rise to adult levels.

In some countries, health workers are more concerned about iron levels than in others. The fact that we have differing ideas from place to place as to what is important for small children, particularly at the moment when mixed feeding is introduced, simply reflects the fact that we don't know everything, and that all of us, health workers included, tend to err on the side of caution, stressing the things with which we have been confronted and in which we have put our faith.

Trace Elements

Alongside the major components of any diet, we also recognize the *trace elements* – substances that are always needed, though only in miniscule quantities. They must not be entirely overlooked, but whether lack of them causes problems in practice varies quite markedly from one place to another. To take the case of iodine: there may be a severe shortage of it in the diet in some inland mountainous areas, though governments have often ensured that it is added to kitchen salt or other "vehicles," even industrial salts, to prevent deficiencies. The problem does not arise in countries with a long coastline and a high consumption of fish, since seawater (and hence seawater fish) contain high levels of iodine. Normally, adequate amounts of iodine will be present in breastmilk. As with other minerals, the levels of trace minerals in breastmilk are quite variable over time and from one mother to another. As with so many other things, the breastfed child of a mother taking a normal healthy diet is very unlikely to suffer from any deficiency of trace elements.

The Role of Breastmilk as a Special Dietary Food

The mother's system is capable, within limits, of adapting the composition of breastmilk to meet the special needs of her baby:

- Colostrum is one example. It is stored in the breasts at body temperature for a period of months without being infected – indeed it provides a degree of protection against infection. As the newborn baby has an immediate need to bolster its immune system, the colostrum provides a rich store of all that is needed.

- Another example of the ability to adapt: The mother of twins will often feed each twin from its "own" breast. When this happens, one is likely to find that there are differences between both the quantity and composition of the milk produced on the two sides (Akre, 1999).

- Mothers who deliver a preterm baby produce during the first few weeks after birth an enriched form of milk containing enhanced quantities of all those substances that we know a preterm infant is particularly likely to need, especially components that provide support to the immune system. Among other things, it has a higher content of protein, especially in the form of immunoglobulins, and fat. This is highly significant in practice since these very small children need particularly strong protection against infection (which the immunoglobulins will supply) and extra amounts of energy, provided in the form of fat (Riordan, 2010). It has also been shown scientifically that these very small preterm babies are most ready and able to digest their mother's breastmilk and that this milk is particularly valuable in promoting the further development of the neurological and motor systems (Hurst & Meier, 2010). Preterm babies have fewer digestive upsets and grow faster when fed on human milk than when fed infant formula. If the baby is still insufficiently mature to breastfeed directly, health personnel should help the mothers of these babies to express their milk, so it can be fed to their babies. (See also Chapters 8 and 10.)

- Finally, during the normal period of breastfeeding, the composition of the milk will be found to change progressively, beginning with colostrum as an introduction to this world and culminating with the most mature form of milk, suitable for a child that has learned to live among us.

MILK BANKING IN SCANDINAVIA

In Scandinavia, even very small preterm babies are fed human milk from the first hours of life onwards. They get either their mother's own expressed milk or milk from other mothers, provided through a milk bank. Mothers providing milk for this purpose must be prepared to answer very direct and penetrating questions as to their lifestyle, similar to those used by blood banks, and their milk will be examined for possible bacterial content and tested for viruses, such as HIV and CMV. The milk is frozen, but is not routinely heat-treated before use provided the bacterial tests are satisfactory (Norwegian Board of Health, 2002).

Heat treatment in Scandinavia is avoided wherever possible since it will destroy some of the immunoprotective properties that the milk possesses. This necessitates a milk banking system in which every sample of milk can be traced back to the original donor.

Colostrum: Golden Drops

Right from the baby's first attempt to feed at the breast, it will obtain milk, taking a little of the golden colostrum. It may seem that it takes very little, but the newborn baby has very little space in its tiny stomach. In the early days, the baby's stomach is no larger than half the size of your thumb. Soon it will become larger, the size of an entire thumb. One can readily appreciate that the newborn infant's digestive system during these early days and weeks is best suited to almost continuous feeding of small quantities, rather than to periodic intake of large feeds. And however small the amount of colostrum it receives, it will be sufficient to meet its needs. These few golden drops are vital, for colostrum is a veritable magic potion, as the fairy tales put it. The ingredients and the quantities in which they are present are very different from those of the milk which is to follow. It is adapted both to the conditions under which it has been made and stored (spending several months in a lukewarm breast) and to the newborn baby's immediate needs for food. The golden-yellow fluid contains, for example, the provitamin beta-carotene (a precursor of Vitamin A, which also endows the colostrum with its characteristic color) in ten times the concentration that will be present in the mature milk. Colostrum is also capable of setting the baby's digestive process in motion. Even more important is its ability to encourage benevolent bacteria to settle in the baby's stomach and intestines, fully occupying a place that would otherwise be promptly colonized by the pathogenic microorganisms that are always lying in wait close by.

The colostrum also provides active defenders, ready to tackle and destroy intruders. As we pointed out earlier, the newborn baby borrows some of its mother's immune defenses until it is ready to build up protective mechanisms of its own. One is, therefore, not surprised to discover that colostrum is richly provided with cells which can both do battle directly with unwanted microorganisms and which can produce antibodies aimed against those hostile bacteria that the mother has encountered in the recent past – bacteria that are all too likely to be lying in ambush, ready to challenge the new individual.

It is remarkable that, down through the ages and all over the world, people have tended to view this first form of milk with deep suspicion, often discarding it, probably because of its brilliant yellow color (Edmond et al., 2006). In its place, the unfortunate newborn has often been fed all manner of dubious concoctions, sometimes as part of a ritual to welcome it into the world.

Maternal Infectious Disease and the Milk

A mother who has contracted an infectious illness will, during the course of her recovery, produce bacteria-inhibiting substances and antibodies to counter her infection. These, like other protective materials, will naturally be passed into her milk, providing her child with the necessary defense against her illness. As a rule, this natural mechanism works seamlessly, which is not to say that one can afford to completely overlook the need to keep the infant healthy. It will be as necessary as ever to avoid coughing and sneezing in the baby's face as if it were impervious to any form of infection!

One Mammal's Milk - And Another's....

In many countries around the world, people are thoroughly accustomed to a regular milk supply. But do we realize sufficiently what milk – and in particular processed milk – really is? The question is particularly important when we consider the feeding of young children. Man is the only mammal that systematically uses the milk of another species as a replacement for its own. In the course of the ages, substitute milk has been provided from any convenient species of animal that has been at hand. Apart from the cow, milk has been obtained from the goat, buffalo, camel, mare, and donkey. Milk from the latter two, we might note, is closer in composition to human milk than is that of the cow.

The experience of staff responsible for animal nutrition in zoos shows that it is possible to use the milk of one species to feed the young of another. To have a reasonable hope of success, however, the milk should be interchanged preferably between species which produce milk of reasonably similar composition, and to avoid digestive upsets, the milk should be administered at intervals similar to those normal for breastfeeding in the recipient species. Cow's milk modified using modern techniques can also be used in other species, not only in human infants. One must, however, know what one is doing, and such artificial feeding must be guided by proper knowledge of what the donor species' milk can offer and what the recipient needs to receive.

MANUFACTURING BREASTMILK SUBSTITUTES - CURRENT AND FUTURE PROBLEMS

The baby food industry constantly strives to improve its products. Some of the improvements introduced are genuine; others are of little more than promotional value. It has been said that baby feeding is an experiment in progress. As far as the nutrient composition and nutritional value of the products are concerned, there has been progress over the last decades. The large-scale production of milk powder or liquid milk will, however, always involve a number of problems, whether these products are prepared from cow's milk or (to provide for children who are allergic to bovine milk protein) from soya beans. But particular vigilance is certainly called for as this product may well be an infant's only food for some months of its life. The mass production of milks for babies may involve difficulties concerning bacterial contamination or the addition of exact amounts of various nutrients (especially minerals and vitamins). There have been instances both of contamination and faulty dosage of ingredients added to milk substitutes, the most notorious being the large-scale contamination with melamine of Chinese dairy products, including formula, in 2008 (Liu et. al, 2010). When such faults are detected, the batches in question will be withdrawn from the market, but not always in time to avoid the tragic consequences of the contamination. The case of melamine in infant formula resulted in thousands of casualties and an unknown number of long-term complications.

During the period 2000-2005, the consumer-based International Baby Food Action Network (IBFAN) registered through its International Code Documentation Centre 20 instances of batch contamination involving milk substitute powders, each leading to withdrawal of the product concerned. This is, however, in all probability only the tip of an iceberg. It is likely that some contaminated batches are sold and used without production faults being detected, unless many children become severely ill with an easily diagnosable disease as a consequence. This latter situation arose in 2001 and 2002 when milk substitute powder contaminated with the microbe *Enterobacter sakazakii* reached the market, leading both in Belgium and the USA to the deaths of children who had been fed the infected product (Weir, 2002; Van Acker et al., 2001).

Will It Ever Be Possible to Manufacture True "Artificial Breastmilk"?

From time to time, the claim is published that genetic manipulation of domesticated animals can now produce strains capable of secreting human breastmilk. Such claims are usually based on success in producing one or more components of human milk in this way, components that could then in theory be added to powdered milk substitute. So far as one knows, no product based on this principle has ever been marketed, probably because it would be extremely expensive to produce a breastmilk substitute of this type and because no health benefit has been demonstrated. Again, the necessary technology exists to synthesize the enzyme lysozyme. Applying this technology on an industrial scale would, however, be expensive, in addition to which it would introduce new risks. Lysozyme, for example, is prepared from the egg white of the domestic hen, and it is difficult to guarantee that the product is free of residues of this substance, a potent allergen to which some children might react violently.

What renders it impossible to produce industrially or through genetic manipulation a product that is identical to human milk, or closely similar to it, is the fact that genuine breastmilk possesses a host of active, *living* properties as described in this chapter (see Figure 3.1). Carbon copies of breastmilk, or substances closely similar to it, will never emerge, even from the most sophisticated and up-to-date factory in the world.

One venture seeking to produce "humanized" milk in China is noted in the box below.

CAN COWS BE ADAPTED TO PRODUCE "HUMANIZED" MILK?

According to a newspaper report published in April 2011 (Gray, 2011), a group of scientists at the China Agricultural University have genetically modified 300 cows to cause them to produce "human-like milk." The resultant milk contains lysozyme, lactoferrin, and alpha-lactalbumin, which are all found in human milk. In other work, the fat content has been raised by 20%, and there have been changes in the levels of milk solids. It is claimed that the modified milk will promote a baby's immune protection and have improved nutritional value. Research will continue and the "humanized" product is, in due course, to be commercialized, perhaps within a decade.

Are approaches like this safe, sensible, necessary, and affordable? In much of the world, the safety of genetically modified foods for human use – even in adults – is still strongly challenged; campaigners also point to the environmental risks, since genes from modified species will escape into the world at large, upsetting normal biology. Modifying cow's milk in this way will tackle only a few of the many differences that exist between human milk and that of animals. Babies are unlikely to experience real benefit–and what about the unfortunate calves? Even the Chinese researchers declare that human milk is the ideal food for human babies. And will the altered milk, the product of costly research, marketing, and high-tech industrial production, result in a product that can compete cost-wise?

It may be possible to provide breastmilk substitutes with one or two of the components hitherto unique to human breastmilk, but such an advance would scarcely render these substitutes in any real sense comparable to genuine breastmilk, with its hundreds of active components, all specifically adapted to the human condition. There is a point at which insignificant scientific advances become the subject of extravagant commercial fairy tales. The contribution to human health of a "human" lactoferrin prepared laboriously from the milk of Buttercup the Dairy Cow is minuscule, if it exists at all; it is scarcely a miracle of man's invention. It is conceivable that this entire scientific stage show has been enacted in order to provide the ultimate purchaser with the impression that we now have before us a product closely resembling human breastmilk. And even a flimsy suggestion of progress can serve the ends of commercial promotion.

Such claims have been advanced before (70 years ago a manufacturer was offering "humanized truefood") and they will no doubt be made again. When one bears in mind that breastmilk contains literally hundreds of substances and active agents specifically designed to set a new human life on the road to maturity and health, the arrival of a single copy of an enzyme is hardly revolutionary and its practical value negligible. The producers of breastmilk substitutes must in any case keep their costs in check, always asking themselves whether the expenses of any innovation will not outweigh even its supposed benefits to health. Breasts are perhaps old-fashioned, but they are unbelievably efficient, and they provide their milk totally without an eye to profit.

Chapter 4.

WHAT SHOULD A BREASTFEEDING MOTHER EAT?

THE MESSAGE DOES NOT CHANGE

The basic principle that applies to your baby's diet holds equally true for your diet: there are no miracle foods, no quick fixes, no smart diets. After all the breakthroughs that have been announced over the years and the wonder diets (often not very scientifically based) that have come and gone again, one becomes pretty sober when it comes to the way we should be feeding ourselves. Not that the promises will cease to flow; somewhere in the background there are usually some people rubbing their hands and counting the money.

But if you think that you have a reasonably healthy diet, have read a little about food and nutrition, and have kept away from magic diets, there is really no need for you to read this chapter. Its central message will be that as a breastfeeding mother with a history of eating good, varied food, you need not change your current pattern of eating at all. *Moderation in all things* is a sound principle; Hippocrates recognized it over 2000 years ago and up to now no one has disproved it.

BUILDING YOUR BABY'S BODY - WITH THE HELP OF YOUR OWN

In the first six months after birth, your baby is going to double its weight, and it is you, with your own bodily resources, who will make it happen. Your milk contains everything that is needed to bring it about.

Just as was the case during pregnancy, it is the baby's needs that have priority during breastfeeding, unless, of course, you are not properly nourished, in which case, it is equally important for your own sake to put that right. What the baby needs will be taken automatically from you, with your body serving as a storehouse for the purpose. The gross composition of your milk is, in the short run, unlikely to be affected by anything you do or don't do with your own diet.

NO SPECIAL FOODS

Now and again, it will be claimed that breastfeeding is expensive, since you have to eat specially selected food – and plenty of it – for as long as you have your baby at the breast. Don't believe a word of it. Firstly, many women put on some weight in the form of extra fat while they are pregnant, and that provides a useful reserve that can be used during breastfeeding. It has been shown that breastfeeding mothers tend to lose more weight, certainly if feeding continues for more than three or four months, than do women who are not feeding their babies at the breast (Baker et al., 2008). But you need no special foods for this purpose; your body is able to make milk from potatoes and bread, from carrots and salad, from hamburgers and cola – and more. In other words, Mother Human is quite as adaptable as Mother Elephant who happily makes her milk from twigs and leaves.

The old saying that during pregnancy and breastfeeding you are "eating for two" is strictly speaking correct, but it certainly doesn't mean that you should eat twice as much as before. The other person on whose behalf you are eating is not an adult, but a very tiny little being who doesn't need so very many calories, even if it is growing like a healthy cabbage.

All the same, you may find yourself eating just a little more than you are used to. If we estimate the energy needs of an average woman at around 2000 calories daily, then taking 500 or so additional calories every day will be quite enough at this time. Precisely how much you need will vary, depending on how much milk you are providing, how active you are, and what reserves you have built up while you were pregnant. The important thing is not to worry about it or start making calculations. Your own appetite will usually be the best guide, adjusting itself so that you end up eating just the right amount for the two of you (Food and Nutrition Board [U.S.], 2010).

THE BODY'S NEEDS - IF YOU WANT TO KNOW THE DETAILS

The body needs fuel, in other words, some source of energy, so that it can function. It needs to keep itself warm and to move around, and all its organs need to perform their functions. Your fuel is provided by the food you eat.

Food is composed of hundreds of different substances, but the main nutrients are usually divided into six groups: carbohydrates (sometimes called starches and sugars), fat, proteins, vitamins, minerals, and trace elements; in addition to which, we must also mention water.

Fats and carbohydrates are essentially used as fuel to keep the body running; properly fueled it will keep itself warm, move around, and carry out all the functions it should. If you provide more fuel than the body needs to do its work, the excess will be laid down in the form of fat – you will put on weight.

Proteins build up the body during the years of growth, and after that, they maintain and renew it throughout the whole of life. Proteins, as we have seen, are clumps of amino acids, and often the clump as a whole has some special task or tasks to carry out, quite apart from building and replacing tissue. During pregnancy, some of the protein a mother eats will be used to build up the baby and meet its needs. But protein will also, as we saw in Chapter 3, play an important role in forming the immune system. Not much protein is normally stored as a reserve in the body; if you eat more than you need, it will be used as fuel.

Vitamins are molecules of various kinds, which play a part in processes that are going on within the body. The name *vitamin* is, in fact, rather misleading, as it was the result of a historical misunderstanding in the 1920's. The scientist Kasimir Funk (1912), when he recognized the part played by these substances in the diet, was so delighted by this discovery that he felt they deserved a name reflecting their importance to life itself ("vita" in Latin), so no one would fail to recognize how significant they were. In that endeavor, he was successful, perhaps a little too much so, because vitamins soon developed an undeserved reputation as miracle substances. The only property that all the various vitamins have in common is that they cannot be made in the body and have to be brought in from the outside. Vitamin D is really something of exception to this rule; it is indeed important in the food supply, but it can also be built up in the deeper layers of the skin when the body is exposed to the sun with its ultra-violet light.

Most of the vitamins have more than one function in the body; Vitamin A, for example, is involved in chemical processes in the eye that enable us to see, in the multiplication of cells (which are constantly dividing to produce more), and in the immune defense system.

Minerals, such as iron, serve both as building blocks and as facilitators. They are components in many structures, but are also active in ongoing processes in the body, for example, the transport of oxygen. Iron forms an important part of hemoglobin, the red-colored substance in the blood that carries oxygen from the lungs to all parts of the system, and thus completes the process of respiration.

Calories, like the meter and the kilogram, are units of measurement, and are used to indicate the amounts of energy or heat that are released when a given amount of fuel is consumed in the body. Carbohydrates and fats (and to some extent proteins) provide this fuel. In some countries, "calories" have in recent years increasingly been replaced as energy units by "Joules" (or kilojoules, equivalent to 1000 joules). In these countries, joules rather than calories are found on food labels.

What Is a Healthy Diet?

You will sometimes run into the statement that you must "ensure you have a complete and well-balanced diet." Most people, hearing phrases like this, get the feeling that this is something rather complicated they ought to learn more about if only they had the time. But drastic measures are seldom called for. During pregnancy and breastfeeding, you may find moments when you can think a little about what your body needs and what you should eat to provide for your baby's healthy development– but don't regard it as the sort of thing you need to *study*. Terms like *complete* and *balanced* are really rather misleading when it comes to your diet. Qualified nutritionists are more likely to talk about "satisfying" or "sensible" food habits – without forgetting that essential word "tasty."

Eating sensibly simply means that the food you eat covers your physiological needs, not necessarily every day, but as an average. In any country with a normal food supply and enough food in the shops or markets, that is not difficult, at least for people with a regular income. Rather than worrying about getting too little of any particular item, many people would probably do better to take care not to eat too *much* of certain tempting things (like foods containing lots of butter, oil, and other fats, with sugar) while ensuring a good intake of foods with many nutrients, such as wholemeal grain products and vegetables. Once again the good old rule - everything in moderation - still holds true. No revolutionary miracles or magic bullets.

Some Well-Intentioned Dietary Tips

Most of us, when we sit down at the dinner table, are likely to be more interested in eating than in doing calculations. It is a human right to be able to eat in peace without being forced to do higher mathematics. The tips that follow are therefore meant as reminders – not as rigid rules.

Your Body Knows How Much It Needs

Most people have a natural saturation level – in other words, we only manage to ingest a certain number of calories each day. The important thing is the way we handle those calories. True, some people complain that it is all too easy to put on weight, but it is a fact that the majority of people regulate their food intake very well indeed, purely by physiological "instinct." Beware, however – that balance is a delicate one. If you eat just a *little* more than you need each and every day, for example, 180 kcal extra (about the amount in a small dessert spoonful of olive oil), you will find yourself gaining six or seven kilos (approximately 12 – 14 pounds) in a year!

Losing Contact with Your Body

Many women, who have so far remained slim over the years, discover after delivery that, here and there, they have acquired unwelcome pads of fat. That is because so many mothers seem to lose contact during pregnancy with the body with which they have been so familiar. Given a good appetite, this can lead them to put on weight. "Never mind," you may say to yourself when you see what has happened, "once the baby is born I will slim easily." The trouble is that while people tend to add on the ounces or grams with a smile, getting rid of the pounds or kilos can be a disagreeable process. So again, one has to trot out another of the old rules that really speaks for itself: be a little careful about accumulating the kilos or pounds. *What easily gets piled on may be rather difficult to shed.*

Generally speaking, it is the fatty and very sweet foods that cause problems, as they are full of "empty calories" that just add weight. They are tempting to eat, but they satisfy hunger without giving the body the variety of nutrients it needs, and they make it difficult to adjust your intake properly.

Breakfast: Much Overrated!

There is no firm rule about breakfasts; that is one matter in which people differ greatly. There are those who like to begin the day by shoveling large amounts of food into their systems on which they feel they can survive for hours, and they simply get unhappy if they are deprived of the opportunity. Others feel very little temptation to eat much in the morning. There is no reliable scientific evidence to show that either habit is better than the other.

What Are Eggs and Milk, Actually?

Strictly speaking, the task of the egg is to build a little bird or a reptile, and that of cow's milk is to build a calf, while that of human milk is to build a small human. Egg and milk are made specifically for animal body-building. But animal milks and eggs are also good and readily digestible items of food for humans, renowned for their high protein content. Today, the general recommendation, however, is to avoid an exaggerated intake of eggs and dairy milk – one normally gets more than enough protein in the daily diet, even without touching an egg.

Some 50% of calories found in dairy milk or human milk are derived from fat. For adults, low fat or skimmed milk is preferable; the taste is hardly different from that of full-cream milk, and the calcium level is the same. For that matter, you can ensure an adequate calcium intake during breastfeeding by drinking a couple of glasses of milk daily (around half a liter or a pint) and eating about three slices of bread well covered with cheese.

If you don't particularly like milk, take comfort in the knowledge that calcium is also found in vegetables, whole grain bread and cereals, and sardines or other small fish, which are usually eaten with bones and all. When you have a need for extra calcium, as is the case during breastfeeding, the body is fortunately better able than at other times to absorb dietary calcium.

UNDERSTANDING FOOD COMPOSITION TABLES

If your interest in foods and nutrition extends to the point where you find yourself devouring food composition tables, the most important thing is to read them correctly. The figures in such a table usually show the content of a particular nutrient present in a standard amount, for example, in 100 grams of the edible part of the food. It may, for example, seem quite impressive that there are 3.6 grams of iron in 100 grams of parsley, but if you try weighing out 100 grams of parsley leaf, discarding the stalks, you will see that you need a surprising amount to reach that weight – and few of us have such a voracious appetite for parsley that we are tempted to eat 100 grams in a day. That is why those solid, heavy, everyday foods, like rice, maize, potatoes, and bread in various forms, are so important to us – because we eat a lot of them. Whole grain rye bread, with 4.2 grams of iron in 100 grams, is therefore much more significant for our iron supply than are the few twigs of parsley we are likely to take in a meal, however much they add taste and color to what we eat. Similarly, if we look at eating patterns across the world, we will notice that rice meets half of the global population's protein needs, despite the fact that its protein content is very low. Again the point is that it is eaten widely and in very large amounts – and it is this that matters. Another point to look for when you have a food composition table in front of you is whether the figures relating to a particular food describe it in its raw state or after it has been processed. Dry white rice, for example, contains 7.3 grams of protein per 100 grams, but once it has been boiled, absorbing water, the relative protein content will be only 2.6 grams per 100 grams.

To make sense of the figures in these tables, in other words, you need to know roughly how much of a particular food you may eat in a day and in what form, what proportion of your daily diet it accounts for, and how much you are likely to eat over a longer period. But that is nutrition science – and not a very convenient means of deciding how to eat healthily every day!

DOES YOUR DIET INFLUENCE YOUR MILK?

There are plenty of venerable old wives' tales about diet and breastfeeding, but there is not one piece of credible, scientifically based advice about how to increase the quantity of milk that you produce. It may well be that some advice may persuade a mother that she can do better, and this may give her the confidence to actually do so. In reality, however, the only effective stimulus to milk production is to have a hungry baby repeatedly taking milk from the breasts, thereby encouraging the milk glands to produce more.

Can you adjust your diet to make *better* milk? Again the answer is probably not. What may play a role is how well stocked your body was beforehand (i.e., before you became pregnant) with the various substances that together make up milk.

The *fats* in breastmilk come partly from the food you eat, and partly from your own body's fat stores, while a little is made on the spot by the milk-producing cells in the breast. How much comes from each of these sources actually varies with the amount and type of fat in your diet. It is believed that the milk of an undernourished mother reflects the fat in her body stores, and the milk produced by a well-nourished woman reflects the fats of her diet. There is, in any case, a considerable amount of variation between mothers in the fat levels of their milk - two to six grams per deciliter daily is quite normal (Kent, Mitoulas, Cregan, Ramsay, & Doherty, 2006).

Protein levels in milk are not readily influenced by dietary protein intake, though some smaller proteins from your food may well turn up in your milk.

The *mineral content* of the milk is not likely to be influenced by adding mineral supplements to your food – the mineral level in your milk seems to be determined largely by the quantities stored in your system before you became pregnant.

The milk content of several of the water-soluble *vitamins* can, on the other hand, be influenced by your vitamin intake, though only to a small extent, and only within the limits of normal dietary intake. By and large, there is no point in trying to enrich your diet with large doses of vitamin and mineral supplements, whether in the form of tablets or so-called "fortified foods." They simply pass through your system, and the only improvement that results is in the quality of your urine….

The most important thing is simply to eat well and healthily for the sake of your own well-being.

Feeding the Mother of Twins or Even More Babies - No Problem at All!

The mother who is feeding twins, triplets, or even more babies generally finds that she has a voracious appetite, and quite a considerable need for energy. For once, there is no harm in her eating to her heart's content. Since her demands for energy are relatively great, her body will actively absorb all the nutrients she needs from whatever she eats, just as one sees with active sportspeople. Her thirst will normally ensure that she drinks as much as she needs.

The Renowned Mediterranean Diet

It is known that people living on the borders of the Mediterranean Sea traditionally lived particularly healthy lives, based on a wonderful diet. When it was first thoroughly studied in the 1960s, it was found that, in the absence of any deliberate policy aimed to promote healthy dietary habits, the Greeks were at that time quite simply the longest-lived nation in the world.

So what was there about the Mediterranean diet? We do not have all the answers, but it certainly had several striking characteristics:

- People ate large amounts of vegetables and fruit every day; it was an ingrained national habit. The Greeks ate many of their vegetables raw, or only lightly boiled, mixed in with the rest of the diet.

- Mediterranean people as a whole ate considerable amounts of cereals, not only in the form of bread, but also in the form of pasta and other cereal-based commodities.

- Few could afford to eat meat every day. At the time Greece joined the European Union in 1981, meat-based foods were still regarded as food only for Sundays and festivities. A great deal of fish was eaten, and small fish were eaten whole.

- The fat most widely used in Mediterranean countries was the region's own renowned olive oil. For many years, investigators displayed little interest in it. They were more occupied with the ways in which saturated and unsaturated fats influenced the cholesterol level in the blood, and since olive oil had very little effect on cholesterol, it was regarded as having no great significance for health. Today researchers realize that it is precisely the absence of any effect on cholesterol that can be the great advantage of olive oil. We also know that there are many different types of serum cholesterol, and that the various fatty acids have different effects on the levels of these sub-types. Whatever the details of the matter, the fatty acids present in olive oil seem to ensure that the blood cholesterol pattern is compatible with good health, at least in people for whom olive oil is the main dietary source of fat. But olive oil is also fat – and if you take much of it, you will ingest correspondingly more calories.

- In most Mediterranean countries, of course, people have traditionally drunk wine, particularly at meals, but in very modest amounts – this is typically the case in Greece. Women, however, commonly either abstained from wine completely or drank it mixed with water.

- Last but not least: the meals were often associated with good company and with relaxation in the form of a siesta after lunch. The fact that Mediterranean people enjoyed a necessary pause from work in the middle of the day, while the sun was at its hottest and they waited for the shadows of late afternoon, meant among other things that they had the *time* to eat those raw vegetables – it takes more than five minutes to eat a Greek salad!

Sadly, perhaps, the Mediterranean diet has today undergone change: the "good" Mediterranean diet described above was the diet common in the 1960s. As the countries around the Mediterranean Sea changed their agriculture policy as a result of their membership in the European Union, they also changed their eating pattern. Affluence, for example, brought with it increased meat consumption. Globalization led to the importation of new fats and oils that displaced the venerable olive oil that had been so central to Mediterranean food through the centuries.

The result was inevitable: chronic diseases, such as heart diseases and cancer, also increased. *Sic transit gloria mundi! (Thus passes the glory of the world.)*

All the Little Things As Well....

Vitamins and Minerals as Pills[2]?

As we pointed out above, some of the minor components of food have earned a rosier reputation than they deserve, in part because some of them were misleadingly declared to be "vitamins," somehow suggesting they were life-giving substances. Pregnant women and nursing mothers are often advised to fortify their diet to make doubly sure they are getting everything they need by taking supplements in the form of vitamin or mineral tablets or pills. From what we have said above, it is probably clear that Elisabet, who has lived a long life as a nutrition physiologist, does not consider all this necessary in countries where people have a sound diet, with the exception of taking supplementary Vitamin D in parts of the world where people – often especially women – for geographic, religious, or cultural reasons do not get a great deal of sun.

If you have been diagnosed as suffering from a lack of iron, iron supplements may be useful, but don't start using them unless you know you need them.

We do not, in fact, know very much about the consequences of taking individual substances as tablets or "pills," since in the body most such substances act both singly and in unison with others. Here and there, however, we have become cautious about unnecessary supplementation with single substances. It has been shown, for example, that taking iron tablets can reduce the levels of zinc in the blood.

One reason for an exaggerated belief in the virtues of iron during pregnancy was the long-known fact that the levels of the iron-based protein hemoglobin in the blood are at that time often lower than usual. However, this is, as a rule, merely due to the fact that during pregnancy the blood volume is greater than at other times, since it is somewhat diluted, and within limits, this is a perfectly normal manifestation of pregnancy. All the

---

2   "Pills" is, in fact, the wrong word, though it is often used. Pills were medicines formerly rolled by hand in the local pharmacy, and they had the form of small balls, often coated with sugar. All the products in use today are tablets, stamped in a machine, though some are then given a smooth coating reminiscent of the old apothecary's "pill"!

same, when a blood sample shows a reduced hemoglobin concentration, there is a natural temptation to believe that one is anemic and needs iron.

If you do have a need for some added iron, there is still no need for tablets. You can raise your intake simply by cooking your meals a few times a week in an iron pot, rather than in steel or aluminium. A little of the iron in the pot combines readily with components of the food, providing you with a selection of iron compounds that your body can use. If you are eating normal amounts of foods containing Vitamin C (ascorbic acid), this will help to promote the absorption of iron into your system. And finally, there is, as a rule, a lot of iron in the red part of meat (not in the fatty layers), and this is a type iron your body can readily use.

Fiber and Constipation

It is generally recognized nowadays that man needs more than readily digested food. In fact, it is good to have a considerable amount of indigestible material in food, so the intestine has something solid to work on and move along as digestion proceeds. Foods of plant origin are rich in fiber and other more or less indigestible substances. It may be that it is the vegetables and fruits in the Mediterranean diet that have traditionally protected the peoples of that region from one of the chronic problems besetting people further north, namely constipation.

When You Are Hungry

Most pregnant and breastfeeding women find that they have a good appetite, and the path from the living room to the kitchen cupboard (or the nearest candy shop) is short. When you feel like eating a little something, first try eating a few scraped carrots or a banana, or drinking a glass of skimmed milk. Or take a bold step in the direction of the refrigerator and make yourself a slice of bread with a little plain cheese. Don't make yourself believe that you are not eating when, in fact, you are constantly nibbling things on the side, be they chocolate biscuits or spoonfuls of jam. They add up! (That was the moral for the day.)

What About Slimming?

Even undernourished women make perfectly normal and good breastmilk. It is only if one is virtually starving over a long period of time that the amount of milk falls and perhaps contains a little less fat (Prentice, Goldberg, & Prentice, 1994).

Nature, as we have seen, has wisely ensured that women's bodies have a reserve store of energy that can be brought into use when needed, particularly during pregnancy and breastfeeding; that store is in the form of fat around the hips and thighs (Rebuffe-Scrive et al., 1985). These fat stores are so typical of a woman's figure that they have been called the "gynecoid" (feminine) depots. They are not affected by most efforts to reduce weight in the non-pregnant state, but when you are pregnant or breastfeeding, their fat may be mobilized.

There is nothing wrong in trying to slim in moderation while you are breastfeeding, but you should not lose more than four pounds (two kilos) a month. Even losing one or two pounds (0.5 to 1 kilo) a month will probably get you back to your pre-pregnancy weight if you keep it up right through the period that you are breastfeeding. If, however, you notice that you feel weak or faint when you try to diet, or if you find yourself constantly thinking about food, these are signs that your body really needs more than it is getting and that it is time to forget slimming for the moment. On the other hand, if you notice that you are thriving on a more modest diet and perhaps even that you are in a thoroughly good humor as you see the fat melt away, then carry on. As we have said, modest dieting will not affect the quality of your milk. Just realize that there is a limit; if you eat less than 1800 calories a day, your body will simply not be getting enough of all the nutrients it needs.

Slimming and Pesticides

In Germany, a country with large and heavily contaminated industrial areas, mothers were at one time advised against slimming while they were breastfeeding. The health authorities reasoned that mothers would over time have accumulated pesticides and other contaminants in their bodies, and that during slimming, these contaminants would be released into the system and pass through the breastmilk to the baby. There was no proof that this represented a real health risk to children – the reason for taking such a precaution was purely theoretical and perhaps represented excessive concern. Today, as a result of measures in many countries to clean up the environment, the measurable levels of these toxins in human body fat have been falling rapidly (IPCS, 1992). On the other hand, we are now becoming aware of new contaminants, which had escaped the attention of governments in the past – such as the flame retardants that have been incorporated in clothes and toys (see Contamination of Human Milk below).

From Slimming to a New Lifestyle

The fact that you are eating less should not proceed to the point where you are living on a bottle of cola and a bun a day. If you need to slim and positively want to do so, these are good reasons to read a little about the sort and amount of food your system needs. "Good slimming practice" as we might call it, means learning to do all those little things that are worth keeping up for the rest of your life. Examples include: learning to spread a little less butter on your bread, choosing skimmed or low-fat milk, dropping the biscuits with your morning coffee, and slicing off the fat when you have a meat cutlet on your plate. We will not mention physical activity - many mothers of small children find they get more than enough of that. When you find yourself getting hot and sweaty as you battle to get a recalcitrant little being into its rain clothing, just console yourself with the thought that the calories are streaming away by the minute!

Too Thin?

There are women who lose a fair amount of body fat during and after pregnancy. If you get the feeling that this is not only happening, but getting out of hand, so that you can't prevent your weight falling more than you want, it's time to talk to the doctor. Some women on the other hand are more than happy to see their feminine ("gynecoid") fat melting away. It is not a bad thing to weigh yourself now and again to see how you are doing – there is no better way of detecting weight gain or loss. Use the same scales each time, weigh yourself at the same time of day, and (if you don't have a head for figures) make a note of what you find.

ORAL HYGIENE DURING PREGNANCY

The solemn proverb from the old days that a woman "loses one tooth for every child" dates from an era of poor dental care and oral hygiene. Today, loss of teeth is more likely to be a problem with women who are in the habit of eating sweet things between meals. It is a fact, however, that pregnant women are more prone than others to experience problems with the gums and, therefore, need to devote extra care to their dental hygiene.

And while we are concerned with the teeth, dentists tell us that what matters here is not the quantities of sugary snacks that are eaten, but how long they stay in the mouth, and how firmly they cling to the teeth until the toothbrush removes them. In other words: eating twenty candies at a time will do less harm to the teeth than chewing the same number in the course of a day. Raisins and other dried, sweet fruits – natural foods though they may be – stick to the teeth and are not so good for them. Fizzy lemonade, cola, and other soft drinks mostly contain a lot of sugar, and they can account for a considerable sugar intake, so the "diet" and "light" varieties are preferred, although again in moderation. They contain artificial sweeteners, and there is no proof that these are harmful in pregnancy or during breastfeeding, at least in reasonable amounts.

HOW MUCH FLUID SHOULD YOU DRINK?

How much you need to drink depends on how much fluid you lose in the course of a day. You will, for example, lose a lot if the weather is particularly hot or if you strain and sweat during physical training. As a rule, your thirst is the best guide. There are some mothers who tend not to notice their thirst, and if you are one of these, you may notice if you are passing more concentrated and strongly yellowish urine. In that case, you will do well to drink a few liters of water daily. Remember that soups and fruit are also good sources of fluid. Studies have not shown any clear link between a mother's intake of fluid and the volume of milk she produces, though occasionally mothers do claim that in their experience the more they drink the more milk they deliver – and they may, for this reason, choose to drink as much as three liters more than usual every day. We have no physiological explanation as to why this should affect the milk flow. It might well be a *placebo effect* – the term used to describe something that you experience because you expect it – meaning in this case that drinking more gives more self-confidence and for that reason more milk.

Coffee, Tea, and Cocoa

It is perhaps encouraging to know that, up to the present, scientists have found no reason to criticize breastfeeding mothers for drinking coffee in moderation – in other words a few cups daily. Ideally, this should be filter coffee, espresso, or powdered coffee – not the variety made by boiling it or pressing it through a sieve. Coffee that has been standing for a while with the hot grounds in it – which is the case where coffee has been boiled

– actually raises the cholesterol in the blood, and that is not what you need, whether or not you are breastfeeding.

Tea, coffee, and cocoa contain polyphenols, which have the inconvenient habit of binding with iron and carrying it out with them into the stools. That is a good reason for taking all these beverages in moderation. Herbal tea is, in this respect, not a problem.

Alcohol

In large parts of the world, the question of drinking alcohol or avoiding it does not arise since it is not an ingrained part of social behavior, or it is outright prohibited. This section is intended for those living where alcohol is accepted in beverages that may also be consumed by the breastfeeding mother.

It is not easy to give acceptable advice on breastfeeding and alcohol. For one thing, this popular old intoxicant is set about with strong feelings and prejudices, and for another, one's own feelings on the matter tend to be colored by personal experiences, just as is the case with breastfeeding itself. For another we still lack knowledge – we know some of the relevant facts, but not all.

The Health Sector's Conclusion

To begin with the conclusion: Milk from a mother who has been drinking alcohol will contain about the same concentration as that currently circulating in her blood, and that concentration is quite low. However, we know that even small amounts of alcohol are sufficient to give a signal to the nursing baby's system. What we do not know is whether that signal is positive or negative. For that reason, we are quite simply unable to give any clear guidance to a mother as to whether one glass, or two, or three may be acceptable. So what do you do?

What you can do is to read what follows, which is a summary of *what we actually know* on the subject, so you can decide for yourself whether you reach for that drink or not (Hale, 2010; Fisher, 2010).

How Much? How Often? What? When?

To make sure that we are talking about the same thing, here are a few definitions:

First – *quantities*. For various purposes, European countries regard a "unit of alcohol" as comprising 12-15 grams of pure alcohol. This is equivalent to the quantity we find in:

- A small bottle of beer containing 330 units (ca. 4.5% alcohol).

- A glass of wine containing 120-150 units, since wine contains roughly 10-13% of alcohol by volume.

- A small glass (40 units) of any strong drink, such as vodka or whisky, which contains about 40% alcohol by volume.

We also need to consider *how often* a person indulges, and for this purpose we often classify drinkers into four groups:

- Those who drink a little at a time and only occasionally.

- Those who drink in moderation, but fairly often.

- Those who frequently drink a lot, and (usually) have an alcohol problem.

- Those who drink a lot, but not frequently, and who do not necessarily have an alcohol problem.

Strictly speaking, one needs to distinguish between exclusive and partial breastfeeding as well, when considering the possible effects on the baby, but that distinction is not usually made in the studies concerned. It is, however, relevant to consider how old the child is (more or less than six weeks).

Another thing that plays a role is the mother's body weight. A large lady of ninety kilos (200 pounds) and her thin sister weighing fifty kilos (100 pounds) have very different body volumes into which the alcohol they consume is distributed.

Effects on the Baby's Health

When we consider the question as to whether alcohol can harm a baby, we have to consider pregnancy and breastfeeding separately. During pregnancy, the baby will have precisely the same level of alcohol in its blood as does its mother. During breastfeeding, on the other hand, it is *the milk reaching the baby's stomach* that has the same alcohol level as the mother's blood, and that makes a considerable difference. We have many convincing reports about the harm done to the unborn child by drinking in *pregnancy*. Most mothers are able and willing to abstain from alcohol for those vital nine months.

There are also studies of the effects detected in the child if its mother consumes alcohol while breastfeeding. Several reports point to damage to the child's health where the mother belongs to the third or fourth category, i.e., she is one of those who drink either a lot or often, or both (Binkiewicz, Robinson, & Senior, 1978; Wyckerheld Bisdom, 1937).

Most people are, however, more interested in the first two situations, i.e., where the mother drinks more moderately, and particularly where she is only a light and occasional drinker, i.e., belonging to the first group. So what do we know about that?[3]

There are very few studies of the extent to which the mother's alcohol consumption is reflected in her milk, how long after drinking it reaches the milk, what levels it reaches, and what individual variations occur. We have the results of only two such investigations (Kesäniemi, 1974; Lawton, 1985). Both are old and limited in scope, so they do not help us in formulating good advice. However, we have learned a little more about the effects of this alcohol. One much-quoted study (Little, Anderson, Ervin, Worthington-Roberts, & Clarren, 1989) shows that the child's motor development at one year of age is less satisfactory if the mother has consumed alcohol frequently and in large amounts. Four drinks a day, as studied in that paper, must be regarded as a fairly heavy intake, meaning the child will receive a quarter of a gram of alcohol daily through the milk. Although the investigators stress that the findings need to be confirmed by further work, they suggest that the adverse motor effects could mean either that the brain of the newborn is unusually sensitive to the effects of alcohol or that alcohol for some reason accumulates in the child's system. The mothers involved in the study were picked from the records of a life insurance company, and that could naturally have influenced the objectivity of the selection.

---

3   The attentive reader will have noted that most of the references here are quite dated. This may be because the ethical committees that today have to approve studies in humans have become even more strict as breastfeeding has become more common.

Effects Mediated Through the Mother

Other work has examined the physiological effects of modest amounts of alcohol on the breastfeeding mother herself. It would seem that the baby is able to detect the odor of alcohol in the milk (Mennella & Beauchamp, 1991; Mennella, 1997). The child feeds more enthusiastically at the breast when the mother has taken alcohol than when she is entirely sober – yet the baby gets less milk (Wagner & Fuchs, 1968; Cobo, 1973). The latter could be due to the fact that alcohol weakens the let-down reflex. With doses of 1-2 gm pure alcohol per kg maternal body weight, the reflex is increasingly inhibited, and at an intake of 2 gm per kg body weight, it appears to be entirely blocked. The higher level would correspond to a total dose of 120 gm pure alcohol drunk by a 60 kg (120 pound) woman, which is the equivalent of about 10 drinks a day, so one indeed needs to drink a great deal to block the let-down reflex completely. Nomograms have been worked out to help mothers estimate how much time must elapse after consuming a given number of drinks before one can be sure of offering one's baby alcohol-free breastmilk (Ho, Collantes, Bhushan, Moretta, & Koren, 2001).

We repeat: there is much we still do not know, and for that reason alone, you need to make your own decision.

CONTAMINATION OF HUMAN MILK

One repeatedly reads in the press that samples of mothers' milk have been found to be contaminated with substances having sinister names, such as polychlorinated biphenyl's, hexachlorocyclohexane, or bromated flame retardants. When you encounter such a report, you should realize that such items are always regarded as spicy material for the news columns, with their elements of environmental poisons and innocent little children. The reason for carrying out these studies was not that there was any evidence that harm had been done to children's health. The fact that we are periodically faced with such data reflects, as a rule, efforts made by public health authorities to determine the extent to which contamination of the environment represents a burden on the population. For that purpose, one needs to know what substances are entering the body and getting stored in the body fat. Most of the substances we have just mentioned are fat-soluble, which is why they tend to end up in the fat deposits. It is, however, laborious and not particularly pleasant to go around collecting samples of body fat from hundreds of individuals – it involves inserting a wide canula through the skin and into the fat, and withdrawing samples. Examining breastmilk offers a much simpler alternative. Since it is known that a certain proportion of the fat in the milk is derived from the mother's fat deposits, it provides direct evidence of her exposure to environmental toxins and their retention in the fat. The attention devoted to all this in the press is disproportionate to any health problem that may exist. And there is very little a mother can do other than be very concerned when she hears that these substances are present both in her body and in her milk. Fortunately, some consolation is available.

Various reports from the early 1990s showed that during the preceding years the level of environmental toxins had fallen considerably, probably as a result of greater restrictions on the use of pesticides in agriculture. Such reports appeared from various countries, including Sweden (Vaz, Slorach, & Hofvander, 1993), Germany (Somoyogi & Beck, 1993), and Canada (Mes, Davies, Doucet, Weber, & McMullen, 1993).

One reason why *no ill effects on infant health* have been observed could be the fact that young infants lay down considerable deposits of fat during the first year of life. This could well mean that fat-soluble substances are simply transferred from the mother's fat stores to those of the baby, and remain there.

Where authoritative sources list the maximum concentrations of foreign substances in breastmilk which can be regarded as acceptable, they tend to set very low levels, since it would be unethical to suggest concentrations that could conceivably create risk for the child.

The World Health Organization, which is carefully evaluating current knowledge and levels of environmental toxins and their possible risks to the breastfeeding child, continues to conclude that the benefits offered by breastfeeding considerably outweigh any potential risk to the infant, and WHO continues to recommend breastmilk rather than any alternative (LaKind, Berlin, & Mattison, 2008).

Flame retardants have been found to be present in human milk, but in such small amounts that they cannot be regarded as presenting any risk to health (Hönerbach, 2005).

No Problem?

There is naturally no reason to play down this potential problem, and as the parents of generations to come, we must support all efforts to replace the use in industry of substances which are not rapidly broken down and which could present health risks either to humans or to animal life. We have to start to protect our young daughters – the mothers of the future – from contamination and feed them, if possible, less contaminated food. As a pregnant or breastfeeding mother, you should be watchful of the food you eat, since some types of food can be contaminated with pesticides used in agriculture. In many countries, there are public sources of reliable information on health matters such as these, indicating items that are better to avoid and those you can safely consume.

Radioactive Substances

There are astonishingly few studies of radioactivity in breastmilk, perhaps because the quantities present, if any, are too small to be measured with any accuracy, and perhaps because this has not been viewed as a current problem. Many mothers are nevertheless concerned, and the Japanese nuclear plant accident of 2011 shows us that vigilance is indeed called for.

After the accident at the Chernobyl nuclear power station in 1986, there were a few European laboratories that checked possible contamination of breastmilk, and reports from Sweden (Andersson & Nyholm, 1986), Italy (Di Lallo et al., 1987), Norway (Lindemann & Christensen, 1987), and Austria (Haschke, Pietschnig, Karg, Vanura, & Schuster, 1987) were subsequently published in scientific journals. The investigators were particularly interested in radioactive iodine (indicated by the chemical symbol ^{131}I), and two forms of radioactive Caesium (^{134}Cs and ^{137}Cs). It is sufficient to say that the quantities the scientists found in the milk did not exceed the very strict limits that had been set for levels of radioactivity in infant foods. Should any further accident of this type occur, however, mothers will inevitably wonder whether there is not something they can do to protect themselves and their babies. Indeed there is!

As far as radioactive iodine is concerned, this disappears quite rapidly, being converted to its normal non-radioactive form within a few weeks. A mother who already has a sufficient level of iodine in her body will hardly absorb any radioactive iodine when she is exposed to it. You would be exposed if, for example, within the first few days after a nuclear accident you were to go out in the rain, bareheaded, just when a cloud of radioactive iodine dust were to pass over your area. Avoiding that sort of exposure is one sensible step. You can also take a capsule of *potassium iodide,* available in any pharmacy without a prescription and entirely harmless, but it is only needed if another nuclear accident occurs in your part of the world. In such circumstances, the health authorities will certainly keep everyone living in an affected area informed about possible radioactive contamination of foodstuffs, and advise breastfeeding mothers whether there is anything they should avoid (Lawrence, 2011).

WHAT SHOULD A BREASTFEEDING MOTHER AVOID?

There is no reason for you to give up any particular type of food just because you are nursing. Some of the substances in the food you normally eat will pass into the milk, but there is no evidence that this has any harmful effect on the baby.

In principle, no sort of food can be regarded as harmful for a breastfeeding mother, unless, of course, it is contaminated. Where there is serious contamination of the sea, for example, toxic substances may be particularly prone to accumulate in very fatty fish, which are then better avoided. The health authorities are likely to issue advice on any such matter.

Should you have the impression that your baby is prone to nappy/diaper rash or to stomach ache, occurring after you have eaten certain types of food, you should try leaving aside these foods and seeing if things improve. It is not at all certain that your child really is reacting to such a food, but it is not impossible. It does indeed happen that even something as healthy and innocuous as cabbage causes a baby to develop stomach cramps.

Some mothers notice that their babies develop diarrhea or rash if they themselves eat or drink a lot of one particular foodstuff, such as orange juice or various soft drinks, grapes, or candies.

A small piece of good advice: if you really think you have run into a problem of this type, make a written note of what it is you ate and how the baby reacted, recording the date and time, and perhaps the amount of food. One can't always rely completely on memory in matters like this. But over the years, and certainly in our time, there has been an almost exaggerated concern with what a breastfeeding mother should and should not eat. It sometimes looks as if the advisers have taken a perverse pleasure in making life complicated for breastfeeding women. That is why we want to stress the need to use your common sense, and if you think your baby is having problems with your diet, be systematic about tracking down the cause. That is far better than subjecting yourself to a series of rules and restrictions which are justified neither by science nor practical experience.

Serious Food Allergy in the Family

In families where allergies are common, a mother should always bear in mind the possibility that her baby may turn out to be hypersensitive to some of the things she eats. This is more likely to happen if both parents have allergic tendencies. All the same, it is not a common problem, and it can be quite difficult to track down precisely the food components to which the baby is reacting. As always, the mother is most likely to solve the problem by using her common sense, and when necessary, seeking the help of a doctor specializing in allergic disorders.

Nicotine

If a mother smokes or uses snuff or nicotine chewing gum, the nicotine will be concentrated in her milk. It has been shown that nicotine can affect the levels of prolactin (Matheson & Rivrud, 1989). It is well documented that smoking mothers tend to breastfeed for a shorter period, although it is not clear why (Amir, 2001). Colic has been found to be more common in the children of mothers who smoke during pregnancy and afterwards (Canivet, Ostergren, Jakobsson, Dejin-Karlsson, & Hagander, 2008; Søndergaard, Henriksen, Obel, & Wisborg, 2001; Matheson & Rivrud, 1989). In addition to an increased risk of colic, maternal smoking is associated with Sudden Infant Death Syndrome and other adverse effects on the baby (Einarson & Riordan, 2009).

Remember that even passive smoking is a threat to a baby's health. If you don't succeed in giving up tobacco, the best thing is to smoke only *after* a breastfeeding session, so that as much time as possible elapses between your intake of nicotine and the next feed. Try stubbing out your cigarette halfway through to reduce the amount of nicotine getting into your system. But once more: even if you smoke, breastfeeding will still be better than formula for your baby – that is, judged in the light of our current knowledge.

Part 2.

Breastfeeding in Practice:
How to Manage It

Chapter 5.
AFTER DELIVERY: GETTING TO KNOW EACH OTHER

REMEMBER – IT'S *YOUR* BABY!

Never uncritically believe everything you hear about breastfeeding. In the first place, use your own common sense and your own knowledge to decide what you feel is best for your own child. A useful question to ask yourself from time to time is this: *"What would I do if I was cast off with my baby, all alone, on a desert island?"*

Hospital, Mother, Baby

In olden days, women birthed their babies at home, unless they were nomads, in which case, they delivered them wherever they happened to be.

In experienced hands, home birthing has functioned well, and in many countries, it is still common, provided the home offers sufficient space for it. That was and is not always the case. In Europe in the 19th century, for example, industrialization and urbanization drove many families from their country cottages to cramped and unhygienic workers' apartments in the cities, often only one overcrowded room. Understandably then, the poorest mothers were usually the first to accept the opportunity of confinement in a hospital. All the same, many decades passed before a majority of women in industrialized countries chose to have their babies in the hospital.

But You Are Not Ill

You may be one of the many women who have arranged to have their babies delivered in a hospital environment. That may be all to the good – but hospitals, after all, have always been designed primarily with *patients* in mind – people who are ill and seeking a cure or relief of their illness. A pregnant woman arriving for her confinement is different. As a rule, she is not in the least ill – she is not a patient in the usual sense of the word.

Most women coming to a hospital to have their babies are there for the first time. As a very new first-time mother, you are suddenly faced with an environment you have never known before. Surrounded by oversized beds fitted with gears and brakes, packages of sterile bandage, uninviting stainless steel dishes, unfamiliar smells, and so many people hurrying to and fro in overalls, looking fearfully efficient and hygienic – you find yourself in the middle of it all feeling more than a little ill at ease. These are not exactly relaxing surroundings. You may well feel uncertain, perhaps even humbled, and begin to wonder what on earth you (with your little baby into the bargain) are doing there.

And the Baby Is So Tiny...

And then there is the baby – many first-time parents have never even touched a newborn infant before – how vulnerable it seems! Can it not easily be damaged? Can one move its arms without breaking them, or might they simply fall off? And the head seems so large – you have been told to support it, but what is the right way to do that? You admire the nurse as she handles the fragile little body with all the deftness of training, but will you ever manage it yourself? As the moment approaches when you must take over from her, you suddenly feel that your fingers are all thumbs... You may feel that this fragile little treasure is merely being entrusted hesitantly to you by the hospital staff – on loan, as it were. Many mothers are so nervous of rearranging the professional packaging in which the baby is wrapped that they do not see their baby's legs until they arrive home.

NEW ROUTINES – AND NEW ATTITUDES

There has, however, been a massive improvement in practice and attitudes, both in birthing and in nursing units – and in many places things are getting better. A real effort has been made to bring mother and baby closer together and to show in practice that breastmilk is best and breastfeeding is feasible. Much more so today than even a generation ago, staff refer to and respect the mother's judgement when decisions have to be made as to what is best for her baby.

BABY-FRIENDLY HOSPITALS

In many countries, an ever increasing number of maternity units in hospitals are designated "Baby-friendly," a term defined and described by the World Health Organization and UNICEF in 1990 (WHO, 2009a).[4]

One requirement for the designation is that the unit draws up a breastfeeding policy with a set of procedures, which the unit is bound to follow and make known to mothers. The procedures are prominently displayed in the maternity ward, so any mother can see them. The Baby-Friendly hospital must also ensure that all staff who work with mothers take a special training course on breastfeeding support, so their advice to mothers is sound and consistent. Accommodation and procedures are designed so mother and child can spend unlimited time together and get to know each other, while still surrounded by helpful and well-trained staff. The Initiative has proved very successful, and the staff involved have been active in introducing further improvements (Kramer et al., 2001; Merten, Dratva, & Ackermann-Liebrich, 2005; DiGirolamo, Grummer-Strawn, & Fein, 2008). One must add, however, that not everyone on this earth appreciates progress, and one still encounters health workers (and occasionally whole departments) who, over time, have slipped back into the old way of working.

IN A BABY-FRIENDLY HOSPITAL:

- Breastfeeding can and should start in the delivery room:

- The baby is placed against you, skin-to-skin, immediately following birth, and remains there for at least an hour – the longer the better!

- The baby is left with you (the mother) until it has breastfed.

- The baby is allowed to do what it wants – follow its signals – enjoy!

Some of the professionals working with mothers and their babies even today have not had the chance to become familiar with modern teaching

---

4   The name (in English translation) varies between countries, for example: Mother-Baby Friendly (South Africa and Norway), Baby Friendly Health Initiative (Australia), and the Baby-Friendly Initiative (Denmark). See reference to WHO definition at the end of the book.

on breastfeeding or to gain experience with it. So long as that is so, one will have to press ahead, with the backing of the national breastfeeding associations and breastfeeding clinics that are increasingly found in almost every part of the world, to get these principles accepted.

Maternity Homes, Hostels, and The Like

Today, women give birth under all kinds of circumstances. In many countries, there have been good *maternity homes* for a long time – institutions specially devoted to birthing, where a woman can have her healthy baby delivered with expert midwifery and nursing care, and with doctors on call, and she can stay until she is well prepared to return home. A maternity home is designed to take care of mothers who are not experiencing health problems or birth complications. Somewhat simpler is the *maternity hostel* – only a small step away from home, but providing the quiet and space that a busy home may lack. The mother wears her own clothes, and it is possible for her husband or partner or a good woman friend to stay there with her to provide companionship, particularly at night when she may have the most need of it. A problem with the simplest type of hostel is that there may be little in the way of service and expert support – a mother may find herself left to her own devices and obliged to decide for herself when more help is needed. In that situation, a mother who is hesitant to ask for assistance may receive less expert help than she needs. But at least she does not have the problem of dealing with talkative and interfering busybodies, be they patients or certain types of staff, who may occasionally make things difficult in a hospital ward.

Night Feeding

In a hospital that has been designated "Baby-Friendly," it should be clearly explained to every mother that she has the right to have her baby with her 24 hours a day. The baby's natural breastfeeding pattern will be such that – especially at the start – it should have access to the breast at any time, day or night. Very often a mother develops an acute sense of hearing when it comes to picking up signals from her own baby, and immediately recognizes when it is *her* baby's stentorian little lungs that emit a loud call for feeding. This is a particularly good reason for mother and baby to sleep together. The breastfeeding hormone prolactin is particularly active at night, and mother and child soon adapt to one another's sleep pattern. A small night feeding lamp is helpful if she is in a ward with other mothers, so they are not disturbed by a bright light when she wants to feed during the night.

Your hospital bed will hopefully have been fitted with a firm mattress and with side rails, so your baby can lie beside you without risk of falling out. Normally, you don't need to be afraid to take the baby into bed with you for a feed (see Chapter 6).

THE BABY LOSES A LITTLE WEIGHT – AND THAT TOO IS NORMAL

Your milk production comes up to full volume progressively between the second and third day, with some babies having to wait for several days more. During this period, before the milk is produced at full volume, the baby may actually lose a little weight before it begins to grow steadily, as it soon will. This weight loss is, however, not just a consequence of the fact that the baby is feeding relatively little – it also reflects the revolution that is taking place in its body, as it adapts from the sterile and watery environment of the uterus to the dry and airy world in which it now finds itself. To make this change, it has to dispose of any excess water, as a result of which its weight for a time goes down.

WHEN THE MILK ARRIVES – NOAH'S FLOOD OR THE SAHARA DESERT?

The colostrum or pre-milk that has been present in the breast during pregnancy is increasingly mixed with mature milk during the first days of feeding, as the production of this milk slowly builds up. Towards the end of the second week, the baby will generally be getting only mature milk from the breast – the yellow color will have progressively faded, and the color becomes the bluish-white of mature breastmilk, just as it should be.

Quite frequently when the milk appears, it does so in large amounts. Following delivery, the mother's body has developed high levels of the hormone prolactin, one function of which is to stimulate the production of milk. It is as if nature is anxious to be sure the infant receives enough, and that there is sufficient milk for twins if necessary.

Most women have the ability to produce more milk than their babies need. When a baby does not manage to take all the milk that is offered, production will decline over a few days to adjust supply to demand. If, on the other hand, one consistently pumps all the remaining milk after each feed, the breast will get the idea that it is being called on to supply twins, and it will continue to produce just as much as is taken up. One professional breastfeeder was said to have delivered on average 5.7 liters of milk daily – sufficient for seven sizeable children!

Too Much of a Good Thing?

The overproduction of milk during the first few days, during which the blood flow to the breast is greater than at other times (since the breast tissue is still developing), can lead to disagreeable excess. Hard, painful breasts and milk leakage were particularly common in the past when the baby was put to the breast no more than four or five times a day. These days, hospitals and mothers are less often confronted with this problem since the baby is put to the breast much more often.

If you do find that you have an uncomfortably large amount of milk in your breasts at night, and the baby does not wake of its own accord to demand to be fed, you can wake the baby and seek its help. Alternatively, either hand expression or an electric breast pump will provide relief. Do remember, however, that vigorous milking will simply perpetuate the problem by causing more milk to be made, so take out only enough milk at one time to stop the leakage and relieve your discomfort. It may seem contradictory to claim that frequent, small episodes of milking relieve the problems more effectively, but that is truly the case.

When the Let-Down Reflex Is Too Vigorous

Some mothers have an unusually strong milk let-down reflex, and under its influence, milk can spray out of the nipple and several feet into the room. Most children have no problem with this, but there are those who are occasionally upset by it. If this does become difficult for you both, the best solution is to try a little hand milking (see Chapter 10) until the flow of milk has been reduced to a level your baby can handle.

When the Milk Volume Is Disappointing to Begin With...

For some reason, there are mothers who don't manage to get breastfeeding fully established as long as they remain in the hospital or maternity center.

There can be various reasons for this. The most common reason being that the baby is not managing to stimulate the breast efficiently, which may be the case after a cesarean section or when the baby gets off to a slow start. It has also happened that mothers only attain satisfactory lactation after several weeks. Some do not feel at ease as long as they are in the hospital, and others quite simply need more time to discover what it is like being a breastfeeding mother.

Since breastfeeding can be influenced by your feelings (see Chapter 1), there are reasons why it can be difficult for a mother and child to settle down to breastfeeding at first, but that does not mean you will fail – it may just take a little longer. And the delay has nothing to do with your motivation or your desire to breastfeed.

It can be tough to keep up your spirits and avoid losing your self-confidence if you experience such a slow start. Should you need encouragement, go to Chapter 6 and see how well it may go after a while.

Reasons for a Slow Start

Once in a while (this is another *very* rare problem), the milk supply is low because a fragment of the afterbirth (the placenta) has remained in the wall of the uterus. Here it continues to produce estrogen, as it did during pregnancy, in sufficient amounts to prevent the milk-producing hormones from doing their job properly. Such a fragment is easily removed by the midwife or the doctor, and then – presto – the milk flow is suddenly normal. The milk may also be slow in coming in some cases where the baby was delivered by cesarean section or the mother is severely overweight, but that can be corrected by offering the baby the breast more often.

Other reasons for a delay in the milk production during the first days after birth could be diabetes or because you are overtired after an exhaustingly long labor (Powers, 2010).

Weak Feeders

Some children are found to be "weak feeders" at the breast. In some cases, they may have been born prematurely or are ill, but in other instances, it is simply that the baby is finding the process to be oh so difficult to learn. In all these cases, it can take a time before breastfeeding is reasonably well under way (see Chapter 8).

THE ART OF POSITIONING

As we remarked in earlier Chapters, the survival of every species depends on its ability to get food. For a newborn baby, the mouth and chin are the most important parts of the body. For this small individual, these bodily parts are at the origin of everything, they are the site of intensive activity, and it is here that the complex of reflexes the baby has brought with it into the world now come into play.

Reflexes Govern Your Baby's Encounter with the Breast

Nature takes no chances: all the reflexes needed to secure milk from the breast have been put in place during the previous months, neatly packaged, and ready to leap into action at the time of birth. In Chapter 1, we grouped them together as the *milking reflexes,* for that is the process with which they are all concerned, working in harmony as they do. It is helpful to have read what we said about reflexes in Chapter 1 to get a glimpse of the whole fascinating process, but don't try to remember it all. Let the reflexes get on with their work without you thinking about them – that is precisely what they are for.

Nipple Shape and Size - Does It Matter?

For good attachment, it matters very little how the nipples look – they may be large or small, conical or domed – the only thing that matters is that they and the surrounding tissue can be stretched so that it becomes possible for the baby to secure a good mouthful of breast to press against its hard palate.

Breastfeeding Should Not Be Painful - Check Your Position and Your Baby's Attachment

During the first week or two, breastfeeding may feel painful for the first couple of minutes of each session. It is as if the milk passages complain to you about all this unforeseen activity. The pain will usually fade after a few minutes of feeding – after that, breastfeeding should not be painful. If it still hurts, this is a sign that something needs adjusting. Your own positioning and the baby's attachment to the breast are the most important factors ensuring that the reflexes work as they should. Too great a distance between the baby's mouth and the nipple or uncomfortable positioning can be at the root of much trouble. If either of these things is occurring, you will soon know, and then you can correct them and solve the problem. Good positioning is not really difficult, but because bad positioning can raise all sorts of unnecessary problems, it's worth spending a little time here to consider the rights and wrongs of it.

Babies Can Do a Lot with Their Mouths - And They Do It Very Well

We have described here and in earlier chapters what an ingenious little wonder a newborn baby's mouth really is. There is not much empty space in the small mouth (much less than in later life) for it is almost entirely filled by the tongue – an ingenious set of muscles that can move in any direction and comprise what we have called a miniature milking machine. What is more, the tongue is highly sensitive to what is going on around it, and both the senses of smell and taste are already well developed. The mouth is also your baby's loudspeaker, ready to make it known when it approves of what is going on and to raise the roof when protest is called for. During the first year of life, the mouth is also important in exploring the world; very often the first deliberate movement that a baby makes is to put its hand to its mouth.

Learn the Signals!

As you get to know your baby better, you will begin to recognize the small signals it emits, especially as the time for a feed approaches. With many a baby, it is as if at these times it begins to become more aware of the mouth and collects extra energy around it, as if it recalls vaguely that somewhere *around here* a delicious treat could be expected to arrive. Often babies begin to salivate at this moment, and the small fingers find their way to the mouth. It is clear enough what they have in mind – the tongue begins to make milking motions and forms itself into a tiny funnel, while the head moves from side to side *"what does all this remind me of...?"* If it all takes too long, you may hear the first cry, a sign of utter frustration and despair, *"... here I lie, explaining clearly that I need some milk and a warm skin – but where are they?"* Things should not be allowed to go that far. Tiny as one is, one should not be obliged to start screaming when all one is modestly asking for is food and attention.

POSITIONING AND ATTACHMENT: JUST TAKE YOUR TIME

Positioning and attachment (latching on), because they are so important, are things you need to learn properly from the very start, while you are still in the maternity unit with helpers on all sides. But look out: you will not learn very much about it if the staff do it all for you, putting the baby to the breast without you taking the lead. Remember: the good nurses will not be going home with you. The best helper at this time is someone who teaches both mother and baby to be independent of her aid. The first time you do the attachment alone, you may feel a little uncertain about it, so just take your time.

GOOD POSITIONING

Finding the Right Position

However impatient you may be to start feeding, do not forget that you need to be comfortable while you are breastfeeding. Make sure that all the things you may need while you are feeding are within easy reach – a glass of water and pieces of cloth for example (see Chapter 6), so that once you settle down with the baby, the two of you can be still and undisturbed for a while. Find a position in which you can sit or lie down comfortably, cushions, eiderdowns, and rugs may come in useful. You should not find it necessary to move, stretch, or turn for a while. You are going to take a well-deserved rest.

If you prefer to lie down: your head and neck should be well supported on one or more pillows. Now just check: can you see your baby's nose without straining a muscle?

If you find it better to sit: remember that you shouldn't take the baby's whole weight on your arms. If you have enough cushions (preferably in various sizes) for support, you will be able to adjust the baby's position to suit your own, for example, by pulling its body up against your own, so you are both equally comfortable.

You may find that the two of you have your own favorite position. In fact, anything goes, so long as you and your baby are comfortable with it.

Once you feel that you are lying or sitting really well, the next step is to position your baby so that it is well placed for its feed.

Now Position Your Baby...

Your baby should be lying so that it is looking directly at the breast. Try to hold the baby in such a way that it will not need to twist or crane its neck to get to the breast. Imagine how uncomfortable it would be for you to enjoy a good meal with your head askew and looking up at the sky. Remember the baby should come to the breast, not the breast to the baby. Your starting point should be the shape of your breast (Figure 5.1).

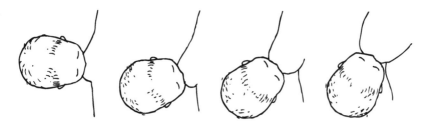

Figure 5.1. *The baby has to be placed according to your breast's shape.*

Source: Drawing by Ingerid Helsing Almaas. Used with permission.

If you have chosen a sitting position, use your arm (the one on the opposite side of the breast you are going to offer) to support the baby's neck and shoulders (see Figure 5.2). In this position, you can, if necessary, shape the breast with your hand, and it is simple to pull the baby closely into place once it has its mouth sufficiently wide open. Once your baby is well latched on or its head clearly doesn't need to be held in place, you can move your hand down and hold the baby's trunk. Some mothers find that this traditional sitting position works well from the start. Others have their own favorite position.

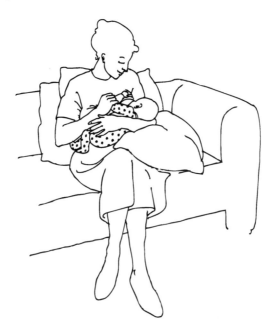

Figure 5.2. *Basic position – sitting up*

Source: Drawing by Ingerid Helsing Almaas. Used with permission.

The simplest way to move the child is to use the other arm – the one on which the baby is lying. Take a gentle hold of the baby's buttocks or hips with your hand and use them to "steer" the trunk – and thereby the head – into place.

Never try to grip the baby's head with your free hand. Many babies will resist, tightening their muscles in protest, angry that they can't move their heads freely while they are busy finding their way to the breast.

And Now, To the Breast!

When you offer the breast, let the baby toy with it for a while, feeling and caressing the nipple with its mouth, just as it likes. This prepares both the breast and the baby for what is next. The nipple becomes more prominent, and undergoes a sort of "erection" to prepare for the job at hand. Once the baby feels the nipple close to its lips, its mouth will soon move into "searching" mode, and then into "funnel" mode – it will open more widely, while the tongue starts its milking movements – and all the while, the baby may wave and wriggle its arms and legs in mounting enthusiasm (see Figures 5.3a, b, c). You may even need to use a finger in order to pull an excited small arm out of the way, so it doesn't come between the baby and yourself, while you wait for the moment that the baby's mouth opens more widely, and the welcoming reflex and the baby's hollowed tongue provide a good link.

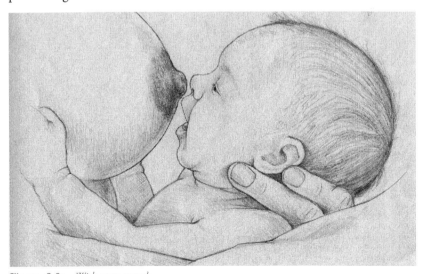

Figure: 5.3a. *Wide open mouth*

Source: Drawing by Pollyanna von Knorring. Used with permission.

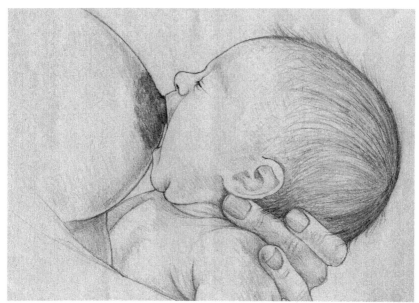

Figure: 5.3b. *Latching on*

Source: Drawing by Pollyanna von Knorring. Used with permission.

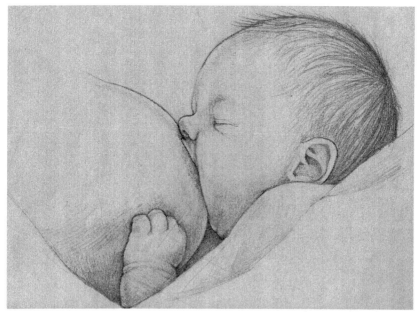

Figure: 5.3c. *Good latch*

Source: Drawing by Pollyanna von Knorring. Used with permission.

A Few Tips That Can Be Useful On the Way

In putting the baby to the breast, you can use its nose as a guide to the right position. The nose should be at the level of the nipple (Figure 5.3a). This will ensure that the part of the breast grasped in the mouth is mostly below the nipple (see Figure 5.3b).

As we have seen earlier (see Chapter 1), the baby uses the tongue and the lower jaw as a small milking machine. The milk is, as you now know, not primarily "sucked" out of the breast. It is *suckling*, the motions of the tongue, greatly helped by the mother's let-down reflex and some negative pressure, which move the milk in the direction of the infant's stomach.

When you can see that the baby's mouth is well opened, with its welcoming tongue pressed down into the lower jaw, the moment has come to pull the baby still closer to you so the breast slips readily into the open mouth, and the miniature milking machine can start working (see Figure 5.3c).

When a baby is really well latched on to the breast, you will see that its lower lip is folded downwards and outwards against the breast; the lower lip is more in contact with the brown area around the nipple (the areola) than is the upper lip. At this moment, feeding should not hurt (see Figure 5.3c). Always remember that to get the whole process started, the baby should be latched on to a good mouthful of breast, and he or she should be held so close to you that there is *no need* for vigorous sucking to keep the breast in place. *A baby can exercise very strong suction and can easily injure the nipple by suction alone – or worse, by biting on it.*

When the baby releases the nipple after feeding, it should still be round and point in the same direction as the breast itself. That is a sign that the baby has been well latched on and the positioning was sound.

Why Can Things Sometimes Be Difficult?

It may be that you will have to try several times before you have mastered this. Even if the baby's reflexes are all in fine shape, it may start off on the wrong foot and find the whole process confusing. A baby that doesn't immediately get milk from the breast can get cross and frustrated. If your baby screams when it takes the breast into its mouth, it is possible that the tongue gets on the upper side of the nipple instead of the lower side. When that happens, it will not be able to get a reasonable hold on the breast.

You can also try a novel approach to attachment/positioning, such as Susan Colson is proposing (Colson, 2010). This approach to supporting the baby at the breast is part of her concept of "biological nurturing." Instead of sitting or lying down, the mother leans back, supported by pillows, and the baby is in a vertical rather than a horizontal position. This is considered to be in line with both a mother's and a baby's instinctive behavior (Colson, Meek, & Hawdon, 2008).

BIOLOGICAL NURTURING ASSUMPTIONS - A SET OF BELIEFS

- Mothers and babies are versatile feeders. There is no single correct way to breastfeed.

- A baby does not need to be awake to latch on and feed.

- Babies often self attach; mothers can help them to do this.

- Babies often have reflex movements called cues that indicate they are ready to feed while asleep.

- Looking for baby reflex feeding cues helps mothers get to know their babies sooner. This increases confidence.

- Crying and hunger cues are late feeding indicators, often making latching difficult. Getting started with breastfeeding is about releasing baby feeding reflexes as stimulants, helping babies find the breast, latch on, and feed... not about interest.

- The breastfeeding position of the baby tends to mimic the baby's position in the womb.

- There is no right or wrong breastfeeding position. The right position is the one that works.

- Babies do not always feed because of hunger; "non nutritive suckling" is hugely beneficial to increase your milk and satisfy your baby's needs (Colsen, 2011).

Friendly Assistance from Those Around You

If you do find yourself faced with one angry baby, calm it down before trying again. For a mother who is frustrated and disappointed that may be easier said than done. There are those moments (especially if it happens at home when there are no helpers around) when one feels that two hands are not enough and that you need at least four.

In a situation like that, there is nothing like asking for a little friendly help – the father, a granny, a friend – any of these may help you to arrange things so that you can breastfeed in comfort. But don't let these kind people run the show, you are still in charge, and only you and your baby can decide what you really need!

A LITTLE HELP MAY BE WELCOME TO:

- Check whether the two of you really are lying comfortably.

- Massage your shoulders lightly now and again.

- Read to you – or perhaps sing to both of you?

- Look after the baby while you take a few deep breaths.

- Take a good look with you at the pictures and the text on the preceding pages of this book and make sure that you have understood them correctly.

Figure 5.4 shows how the baby should be lying close up against you, with its head and body more or less in line with each other. If, when you are feeding in a sitting position, you feel you need to support your breast, cup the baby's lower side in the palm or back of your hand (Figure 5.5). Try to keep your fingers well away from the nipple, so they are not in the baby's way. Don't try to squeeze the breast to make it more prominent, and don't try to nudge it into the baby's mouth as if it were a feeding bottle. The breast should slip into a voluntarily welcoming open mouth if the baby is to get a sufficient hold on it.

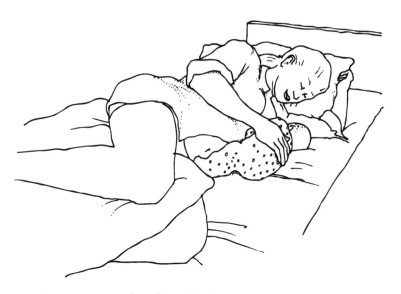

Figure 5.4. *Basic positioning; lying down while breastfeeding*

Source: Drawing by Ingerid Helsing Almaas. Used with permission.

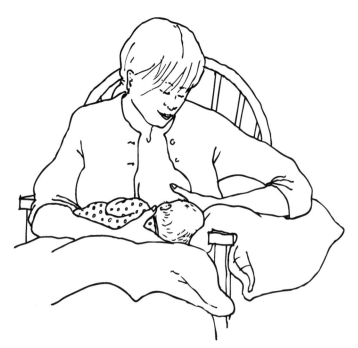

Figure 5.5. *Opposite hand position*

Source: Drawing by Ingerid Helsing Almaas. Used with permission.

If the baby is able to take milk from a breast well placed in its mouth, so it has no need to suck hard to keep it in place, you have a good chance of avoiding sore nipples and making a real success of breastfeeding.

Once more let us stress one of breastfeeding's golden rules:

Golden Rule Number 6

The baby should come to the breast, not the breast to the baby.

It can be useful to try both sitting (Figure 5.2) and lying (Figure 5.4) when finding a preferred position. If you find it difficult to pull yourself up, just ask for a little help. You will soon probably find that, if the baby is having difficulty getting a firm hold on the breast while you are lying down, it will prove easier when sitting up. In a sitting position, you also have a better overview of the situation than when you are lying down.

Can the Baby Breathe Properly During Feeding?

You have *no need* to worry about this; the shape of the nose is, in the case of most babies, such that when it is well positioned at the breast the nostrils are quite close to the breast, but not entirely parallel to it. For that reason, fortunately, most babies have no difficulty at all in feeding and breathing at the same time. Should you feel that there is not much room for the nose, all you need to do is to pull the baby's lower body closer to you, so that the head is tipped back a little; the face and the nose will then be tilted slightly outwards. What you can always be sure of is that if your baby really is not getting sufficient air, it will simply stop breastfeeding. You can try once more with slightly different positioning, so the baby is lying with its head tilted further back as it takes the breast into its mouth. It does happen – but this is very unusual indeed – that a baby is overwhelmed by the breast and truly cannot get sufficient air. In that case, it is sufficient to press the breast away from the baby's nostrils with one of your fingers.

Should You Limit the Baby's Time at the Breast?

If the positioning and attachment are right, you don't need to be afraid of any wear and tear on the nipples! And there is no need at all – even in the early days – to count the passing minutes or to ration feeding time in any way. Just forget the clock: right from the start, let the baby take all the time it needs at the breast to do the job properly. Babies do, of course, differ in their behavior; one will clamp down on the breast joyously and display a voracious appetite, and another will sniff and lick its way around for a while, taking one little taste at a time before getting down to business. One baby may stay at the breast for five minutes, another for 45. Mothers with several children will tell you that these things vary even within the family, probably as early pointers to differences in style and character.

Let the Baby Finish With One Breast First....

Most babies make it quite clear when they have taken enough milk, either by releasing the breast or simply by falling asleep. The majority take as much as they need within a strikingly short time – often they have taken most of their feed within no more than five minutes. So long as one can feel or hear the baby swallowing one portion of milk after another, one can be sure that it is busy feeding and not merely amusing itself. But whether the baby is swallowing or merely toying around, let it go on, just as it likes, until it releases the nipple. When that happens, it may be that the baby is truly satisfied or that it is now getting so little milk for its efforts that it is not worth carrying on any longer. It may also be the case that the baby simply wants to take a pause, or that it feels the game has gone on long enough. You will soon learn to recognize what is going on, and what your baby wants.

It has happened that mothers have moved the baby several times from one breast to the other and back again during a single feed. This can mean that the baby is taking mostly foremilk (which is rich in lactose, but low in fat) from each breast and very little of the high-fat energy-rich after milk or hindmilk that normally follows towards the end of a feed. That in turn *could* mean that the baby will receive too few calories and be less likely to thrive. But...there is no need to worry about such things provided the baby is doing well, putting on weight, and seems to be a happy baby.

Golden Rule Number 8

Let your baby first finish nursing on one breast – don't move it unnecessarily from side to side during a feed!

POSITIONING AT THE BREAST - SOME RIGHTS AND WRONGS

There may be various reasons why a baby and a breast don't seem to match up at first, but every such problem has a solution.

The most common problem when putting the baby to the breast is that he or she may fail to get a good hold on it. There can be several reasons for this.

Situation: An Over-Filled or "Difficult" Breast

During the first few days after birth, the breast, which already has a larger inflow of blood and lymph than at other times, may be so full of milk that it becomes hard and tense, with tightly filled milk passages just under the skin. It can be almost impossible for the newborn to get enough of the breast into its mouth for the nipple to reach the palate and thus trigger the milking reflex.

Solution: Try a Little Milking

It may sound strange, but maybe you are not breastfeeding often enough. Frequent breastfeeding actually reduces the risk of getting "breast bombs." If you still run into this problem with the baby not able to latch on, the first thing to do is to express a little milk out of the breast, either by hand, the best choice in this situation, or by using a pump (electrical or hand-operated). After expressing a little milk, there will be less milk inside the breast, the areola will become softer, and the nipple will be pulled out sufficiently far for the baby to be able to take a grip on the breast again.

You can also try the "bouquet grip" (also known as Reverse Pressure Softening -RPS) that is described at the end of this Chapter (Cotterman, 2004). It involves softening the breast by means of counter-pressure. Ask the nurses if they have experience with this technique. You can decide whether you would like to try it yourself or leave it to the nursing staff.

The Baby That Struggles to Get a Hold on the Breast

If you have tried Reverse Pressure Softening, hand milking, or pumping, and you still feel things should go better, try adjusting the baby's position when you bring it to the breast. Position your baby, for example, as shown in Figure 5.6, so that it is lying under your arm or try the "cross cradle hold" (also known as the opposite hand position) shown in Figure 5.5. If you need to mold the breast a little, try to do it in such a way that it fits the shape of the baby's mouth. When you use the under the arm position, you will find that your breast needs molding into a more horizontal shape, your hands are formed like a "C," whereas with a baby in the cradle position, your breast will be shaped more vertically and your hand will form the letter "U" (see Figure 5.7).

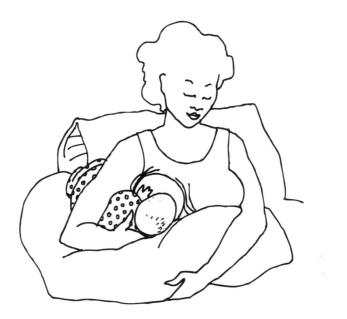

Figure 5.6. *The under-the-arm position*

Source: Drawing by Ingerid Helsing Almaas. Used with permission.

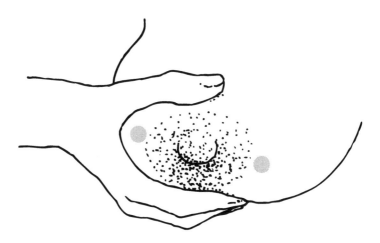

Figure 5.7. *Supporting the breast. The hand is showing horizontal support, the C-grip. The grey circles are vertical support, the U-grip.*

Source: Drawing by Ingerid Helsing Almaas. Used with permission.

Do try to avoid letting the baby get too hungry before it has a chance to come to the breast. Look for those early feeding cues before baby has to yell for dinner. It may be helpful to give it a little milk snack from a cup, using milk you have expressed beforehand (see Chapter 10).

An Obstinate Breast

It can happen that one of your breasts is reluctant to play the game according to the rules; it's simply uncooperative, slipping out of position or just not willing to be gripped. Don't offer a hungry baby such a breast; wait until it has taken a little from the other breast and is less eager. If necessary, you can soften up the difficult breast by milking it by hand or using a pump; it will then be easier for the baby to latch onto it.

Problem: Inverted Nipples?

It is not unusual for a woman to look down at her nipples during pregnancy, conclude that they are inverted, and wonder whether a baby will ever be able to feed from them. The truth is that such nipples, as a rule, are not truly inverted – just a little short. The shape may only be noticeable on one side. Nipples that seem inverted can often be induced to protrude by a little gentle pressure on the breast around them.

Solution: Is The Surrounding Tissue Supple Enough?

What matters much more than the apparent shape of the nipple is that the whole area around it, including the areola, proves to be supple or protractile enough when the baby is put to the breast, so that it can take a decent mouthful of breast and milk it to its heart's content. Around the time of delivery, various changes take place in this tissue, and many mothers who have been told that they have "inverted nipples" go on to breastfeed without any problem at all. If things do get difficult, look for the solution under the heading "The baby that struggles to get a hold on the breast," in the previous section. Should you really have an inverted nipple that truly refuses to come forward when invited, however much the baby tries, you may be encouraged to use a product that is held onto the nipple by suction. If a truly inverted nipple is diagnosed during pregnancy, such a device should only be used under medical supervision since too much suction can cause uterine contractions. The efficacy and safety of this treatment has not been proven.

Problem: The Baby Is Afraid of the Breast or Angry With It

A baby can get upset about the whole process if it has to struggle and strive at the breast to get its milk, or it may have become angry at having had a breast forced into its mouth against its will (especially if a strong hand has been applied to hold its head firmly in place). After one such experience, it may become quite desperate when it finds that same fearful breast advancing upon it yet again, apparently with the same purpose as before.

Solution: Enlist a Little Help, But Go on Trying

Try at least to make it *look* as if you still have oceans of patience in reserve, even if you feel that your baby's impossible behavior is driving you up the wall. If you once betray a sense of irritation, the baby may sense it right away and follow your example to the point of becoming more or less uncontrollable. If you are still in the maternity ward, you should explain to the staff just what you are struggling with, and tell them that it looks as if you are going to need some help. If your partner, friends, or family are close at hand, one of them may be able to pick up the little inconsolable bundle of rage and take a stroll with it, while you close your eyes and lean back to relax for five minutes.

After that, take a deep breath, make it clear to yourself and the little wretch that you have all the time in the world, and that you have not the slightest intention of surrendering. With that, you lie down quietly at your baby's side and try to convince it to have another go. If it still doesn't work, nothing is lost, you simply go through the process once more, and if necessary, once again after that. To give both your baby and yourself something else to think about, you can alter your positioning: try the under the arm position (Figure 5.6), try feeding with the baby lying on your stomach, try everything upside down and back to front – whatever comes into your head. Sit on a chair, sit on a stool, sit down on a settee–be as inventive as you can. If you like, try "biological nurturing" described earlier in the chapter. Try massaging out a few tempting drops of milk if you don't find it too complicated and messy. Could it be that your baby likes to be talked to while you are both trying to make it work? Or sing to it – about it's being the very nicest and cleverest baby in the world, and about the fact that it's all going to go smoothly in the end.

Another possibility is to try and experience again that very first meeting between your baby and yourself after delivery, as we describe a little later in this chapter – just lying together in bed, quietly skin-to-skin for an hour, or two, or three (see Chapter 6 and Chapter 12 on dealing with a baby that doesn't want to come to the breast).

So long as things are still not working out, you will need to empty your breasts regularly, using either a pump or hand milking. What you must *not* for a moment do is to believe that the baby is rejecting you in some way. It is not *you* the baby is objecting to; it is this still unfamiliar and rather scary situation that it finds itself in at the breast.

Problem: A Troublesome Tongue and a Little Ligament

It can happen that the tongue itself gets in the way, blocking contact with the breast. That is more likely to pose a problem if the baby has been frightened at the moment it is put to the breast. Some babies also seem to have amused themselves before birth by sucking on their tongues, so that they tend to hold their tongue in the wrong position when it comes to breastfeeding. Sometimes one encounters a baby whose tongue ligament – the contraption by which the tongue is attached at the bottom of the mouth – is too short. In that case, it can be difficult for the tongue to grasp the breast as it should.

Solution: Get That Tongue into Place

Since it is the tongue that does most of the hard work during breastfeeding, it needs to be in the proper place. That place is low down against the floor of the mouth. From there, it can press the nipple and breast up against the palate and "milk" it like a small milking machine, as we discussed earlier in this chapter. If the tongue is not properly placed, try all over again. See if you can calm your baby before you start afresh (see point 2 in "Now position your baby…"). Try dripping or spreading a little milk directly onto your baby's lips, that may tempt the tongue to come forward as it should.

If necessary, the medical staff can easily clip or incise too short a ligament, so the tongue can move further forwards.

Problem: A Tired, Tired Baby Who Can't Be Bothered to Feed

A baby should never be allowed to become exhausted by its own screaming protests. Babies that don't feed well may get very sleepy because their blood sugar is low. A baby that is making very little effort to feed may be tired or simply getting over that first urgent need to suckle. These things are more likely if you were given a sedative, such as pethidine or a benzodiazepine tranquillizer, during delivery or an epidural anaesthetic; such a drug can be passed on to the baby through the umbilical cord and cause its milking reflexes to be weakened for several days. It can also happen – not so often nowadays, one hopes – that because bad old habits die hard, the baby has been given some unnecessary supplementary feeding. Or, as we said, the baby may be genuinely tired, especially if it is so exhausted by its own screaming protests that it has, for the moment, too little energy to concentrate on the breast. Babies born prematurely or with some inborn defect can also have weak reflexes or simply not be strong enough to get a good hold on the breast. When any of these things happen, breastfeeding sessions can, for a while, be strenuous and far less enjoyable than you have a right to expect.

Solution: Look for the Cause

For your own sake, it is important that you find an *explanation* for the problem you are facing, so you know it is not due to any fault of yours, and you don't lose faith in your ability to breastfeed. Some of the situations we just mentioned will cure themselves, for example, as the baby gets over the effect of supplementary feeding or supplementary medicines. What you need to do is keep faith in yourself and the fact that you can and will succeed. As long as your baby is not managing to handle the milking by itself, you will need to help it by expressing some milk by hand.

Take a look at *"It's never too late"* (at the end of Chapter 6) about repeating the experience of the first feeding session. That trick has helped many disappointed mother-baby couples find their way to happy breastfeeding. Some ways of helping the baby get over the problem are suggested in Chapter 8.

Problem: The Baby Does Not Want to Release the Breast

There are many babies who insist on keeping that wonderful piece of breast in their mouths, even though they seem to have finished feeding and fallen fast asleep. If you try to slip the breast out without the baby noticing, the baby sucks more vigorously than ever, holding on as tightly as an octopus.

Solution: Stealth and Cunning

Don't try brute force—it won't work; you need to be crafty and cunning. Very gently, slip a finger between the breast and the baby's lips until you touch the gums. That is enough to let in a little air, releasing the vacuum and the suction, and when that happens you will be able to slip the breast out without anyone noticing.

IF THE LET-DOWN REFLEX LETS *YOU* DOWN

The milk let-down reflex, also known as the oxytocin reflex, is (as we saw in the first Chapter) something we find in all mammals, and it is as important for successful breastfeeding as it is for the production of milk, and possibly for the process of mothering itself (see also earlier chapters for more about the mechanisms of breastfeeding). If this reflex really were fully automatic, there would be fewer mothers faced with breastfeeding problems, and all animals would be as easy to milk as the obliging cow and goat. But, as we now know, it is not quite as simple as that.

ADRENALINE GETS IN THE WAY

The let-down reflex is governed by oxytocin, but it can also be influenced by another hormone, adrenaline. Any person who is angry, frightened, or excited produces adrenaline that enables him or her to react quickly. Adrenaline causes the small blood vessels throughout the body to contract. It is precisely these small vessels that carry oxytocin to the alveoli and cause *them*, in turn, to contract and eject the milk when the baby sets the let-down reflex in motion. No oxytocin = no milk! The baby lies struggling unsuccessfully at the breast as long as the let-down reflex is blocked. Fortunately, adrenaline persists only for a short while in the body; it is soon broken down and disappears when one is no longer tense or anxious. This explains why the let-down reflex soon returns. Only a little while after a breastfeed has failed, a belated let-down may cause the milk to drip or spurt.

The Blessing of Expert Help

Health workers and breastfeeding counselors have sometimes arrived to find mothers who have been struggling too long alone and in vain to get their babies to take the breast. When at last these mothers get help from someone who understands how the reflexes work and how a baby can get a good latch-on to the breast–a person who radiates knowledge, authority, and calm, they can relax. Once that happens and the baby is put to the breast again, all the milk that has been locked inside the breast can be released, and wonder of wonders, there it comes. It is really no wonder, though, but rather pure physiology: the mother calms down, the adrenaline level drops to normal, the baby's milking wakes up the oxytocin supply to the alveoli, the small muscles spring into action, the milk flows once more, and everyone is happy again.

Being Nice to the Let-Down Reflex

Like other reflexes, the let-down effect is not under the control of the will, but since it is a *conditioned reflex,* it can be affected by your feelings and by events around you. There are several things you can do to encourage the let-down reflex to be co-operative:

- Before a feed, find an opportunity to take five quiet minutes for yourself. Lie with your legs up, close your eyes, and try to think of something enjoyable or of nothing at all.

- Habit and familiarity seem to help. When you prepare for a feeding session, choose the same comfortable spot every time, and take a little drink before you start.

- Try in advance to anticipate and prevent the sort of things that may disturb you. People who annoy or upset you, a telephone that may ring, small siblings who are getting up to mischief should all be kept at a distance for as long as you can manage.

It may take some time before the let-down reflex is operating smoothly. Some people notice exactly when the reflex occurs, others not at all. Once it starts, it will be as reliable as a clock, and you can stop worrying about it.

Problem: Over-Full Breasts - Again

Another reason for problems with the let-down reflex can be that the alveoli are very full of milk. This means that the smooth muscles around the alveoli have difficulty in contracting to expel the milk, and the ensuing discomfort may block the let-down reflex.

Solution: Reduce the Excess Pressure

Here again, the solution is a little milking by hand or with a breast pump. It is usually sufficient to pump just enough so that the breast no longer feels so tense. Alternatively, try the Reverse Pressure Softening maneuver, which is explained below.

The Reverse Pressure Softening Maneuver (The Bouquet Technique)

This is a method described by USA lactation counselor Jean Cotterman (Cotterman, 2004) to soften up the areola to make it easier for the baby to latch on to in spite of the raised internal pressure that can occur in the early weeks of breastfeeding. The cause can be an overfull breast that has become swollen and/or the overuse of a breast pump or suction device to the point where fluid has begun to accumulate in the tissue most exposed to it – something that is most likely to occur when high-powered suction is applied. This inflammatory layer can "bury" the milk passages. When that happens, it becomes impossible to extract the milk – the baby's tongue, hand milking with the fingertips, or the pump are of no avail.

An attempt to soften the area using counter pressure is best undertaken immediately before the baby is put to the breast. It works best when you are reclining or lying down. It involves exerting gentle, even pressure with the fingertips on the area where the areola meets the nipple, directed towards the chest wall (Figure 5.8). If you have very short fingernails, the fingers should be slightly bent, so the nails lie almost at the edge of the nipple. The five fingertips should form a ring around the nipple base. Continue the pressure for a minute or so, but rather than watching the clock, try humming a lullaby (which is likely to be about the right length).

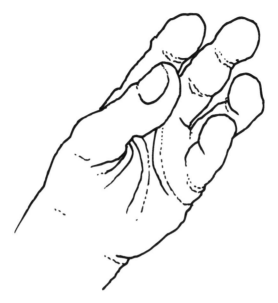

Figure 5.8. *The Reverse Pressure Softening Maneuver: Position of the fingers*

Source: Drawing by Ingerid Helsing Almaas. Used with permission.

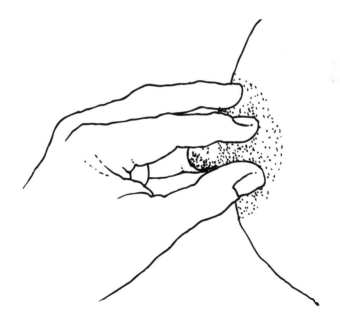

Figure 5.9. *The Reverse Pressure Softening: The maneuver*

Source: Drawing by Ingerid Helsing Almaas. Used with permission.

If the breast is very hard and tense and you are using all your fingertips, you may have more success if you continue to press for two to three minutes. The lullaby won't be long enough, but you can watch the sand pour through an egg-timer!

A slightly different method is to use two thumbs or two fingers and move the pressure points once a minute – this may produce a more even result.

There are several reasons why the maneuver works so miraculously:

- The way in which the pressure is exerted on the distended milk duct pushes the milk to the rear. This lowers the pressure on the distended walls of the ducts and reduces the discomfort when the baby takes the breast. The tissue becomes more elastic, so the baby can pull the nipple and areola more deeply and comfortably into its mouth, and the milking motions of its tongue become more effective.

- The excess of lymphatic fluid in the tissue is moved inwards to the area into which the lymph normally drains.

- With this even stimulation of the nerves that supply the nipple and areola, the milk let-down reflex is automatically set in motion, almost always within five minutes, so the milk begins to flow forward.

Fingertip Milking

After using counter-pressure to soften the whole area, it becomes easier to milk the breast using the fingertips if required; this softens the areola even more. This is more comfortable and more productive than trying to breastfeed or use the pump on an over-filled breast. Where the problem has been very marked, some extra fingertip milking is also helpful in making more room for the baby's chin, so the baby can take a really deep hold of the breast.

When your breast is swollen, it is best not to use a pump, rather let the baby do the work or remove some milk yourself by hand.

OTHER REASONS WHY THE LET-DOWN REFLEX MAY FAIL

It can also happen, once in a while, that a mother who has been breastfeeding successfully suddenly finds herself "holding back" her milk. For some reason, the milk let-down reflex has for the moment gone on strike, and the baby is not getting to the milk that is present in the breast. There can be several reasons for this.

Problem: The Mother Is Embarrassed

Some mothers feel uncomfortable to find themselves with their breast exposed to public view in a room where various people are present.

Solution: A Moveable Screen

The mother needs to get over her embarrassment sufficiently to ask for a screen, so she is not visible to all. Many hospitals have plenty of moveable screens or curtains.

Problem: The Mother Is Upset by After-Pains

In some women, the let-down reflex during the first days after birth is accompanied by after-pains, relatively strong contractions of the uterus when the baby is put to the breast. It seems rather unreasonable of Mother Nature to spring this surprise on a new mother. Just when she thought everything associated with birthing was done, those painful birthing contractions begin. Assurances that with correct positioning the discomfort will soon pass sound awfully hollow to someone who is suffering with them. The pain leads to worry, the worry can upset the milk-let-down reflex, this can cause even more worry, and one is soon in the middle of a vicious circle. If the after-pains are not just disagreeable, but really painful, it may be necessary to ask for painkillers for a few days.

Merely trying to "grin and bear it" can actually make things worse, prolonging the pain. You may find it possible to shorten the painful contractions if – as you learned to do during delivery–you manage to "ride with the tide" (and hope that the tide soon will stop rolling). Apart from that, don't be frightened by the pains. They are a nuisance, but quite harmless. At a given moment, they will go away–as unwelcome guests usually do.

Problem: The Mother Is Afraid of Closeness

A woman, who has been the victim of a sexual assault of some type, either in childhood or as an adult, may have developed a deep aversion to physical intimacy, skin contact, and especially any touching of the very sensitive nipples. Such contact may set the adrenaline gushing out into the bloodstream, eventually making it difficult for the baby to access the milk.

Solution: Some Overcome Their Aversion - And Some Don't

One can point to examples of admirable women who have succeeded in overcoming their fear of physical intimacy and have then managed to express the love they feel for their baby by physical closeness to it. However, there are others who may have had to suppress the conscious memory of a painful event in the past, but still suffer its effects, unable to experience physical closeness without suffering real pain. It may be that in such instances, it is better not to breastfeed, if the conditions for artificial feeding are present. Women who have overcome their aversion, however, say that they have enjoyed the reward. Helping them is not for amateurs, as it is difficult for a counselor or friend who has not experienced such trauma to provide real support. Perhaps the victim will be helped by sharing her experience and concerns with someone who has at some time gone through a similar trauma, especially if she has later tried to breastfeed and perhaps succeeded. You can read more in Chapter 7.

Problem: Mother Is Exhausted, Desperate, Irritated, or Plain Angry

Feelings like this are all too human, yet they can trigger a flood of adrenaline, and with it perhaps a period of trouble when it comes to breastfeeding.

Solution: Massage, Perhaps? Meet an Angel? Or Just Lie Down and Breathe

Unless one happens to have an angel in the vicinity (and there does seem to be a chronic shortage of real angels on this earth), one is going to have to wait for the problem to pass. But do not think that giving vent to your feelings will automatically turn off your milk flow! One person's threshold to trouble, beyond which he or she is likely to react violently in body or spirit, is quite different from another's.

One good remedy for all sorts of troubles, including a thoroughly bad mood, is often skin contact and massage. Both can adjust the level of oxytocin and improve your milk flow. One of us (Anna-Pia) experienced an instance where a mother with only a meager supply of milk was given a shoulder massage, and the milk flow increased fourfold!

If you do find yourself in such a situation, but with no one around to massage you (and still no angel in sight) you can nevertheless help yourself. Try lying down on a carpet on the floor to get a new view of the world. Breathe deeply, using your midriff rather than your ribs to get plenty of air into your lungs. Then get something nice and warm to drink. And after that, read all about the milk let-down reflex once more (Chapter 1 and this chapter).

Ambition and Fear of Failure

Occasionally, one encounters a mother who, on the one hand, is tremendously eager to make a success of breastfeeding, yet who, at the same time, is certain that she isn't going to be able to do it. No sooner is the baby put to the breast than she shrinks back in terror, the adrenaline surges into action, and the baby lets loose of a breast that refuses to provide any milk. It's as if her failure is a self-fulfilling prophecy.

Solution: Talk to Someone and Admit You Have a Problem

A mother finding herself in this situation needs help to calm down and gain the confidence she has never really enjoyed. The very best support of all is that provided by a good friend or relative, or by a health worker or breastfeeding counselor who has successful experience in dealing with situations like this–someone who conveys a sense of trust, who understands the situation, and who truly wants to help put things right. A sensible starting point is to find out why the prospect of breastfeeding has somehow seemed so menacing. Has it something to do with the fear of accepting one's role as a mother? Does the mother need to be reassured that she has the strength and the ability to achieve what she set out to do, and that she is also capable of becoming a good mother? Quite simple solutions may emerge, for example, the assurance that if she has once experienced a good flow of milk she can experience it again. One can also try one of the "lactagogues," preparations that are believed to stimulate milk production. They are not world wonders, but they may help build confidence if one takes them in the firm belief that they really will put things right.

ACUTE FEAR, ANXIETY, UNHAPPINESS, OR DEEP SORROW...

A state of mind like this on the mother's part *can* sometimes lead to oxytocin being blocked in the way we have just discussed. Not that it is inevitable – breastfeeding may prove to go on robustly, however concerned the mother is about breastfeeding or anything else. Over the centuries, mothers have breastfed through flood and famine, crisis and war, without losing a drop of breastmilk. For others, the arrival of a difficult mother-in-law on the doorstep is enough to reduce them to a dried-up state of nervous panic.

There are, however, many mothers who tell of their milk having "vanished," almost as if it dried up on the spot. There is no reason to disbelieve such stories for that is the way these mothers have experienced the situation, yet we know that it is physiologically impossible for the milk supply to stop acutely in this way. What has happened in these instances is that the mother has lost not her milk, but her self-confidence, and she hasn't gotten the help she needed to overcome the effects of the adrenaline shock.

Golden Rule Number 9

The less you worry about your milk the better.

So now that you know how your milk let-down reflex works, just forget about it and concentrate all your attention on your baby.

BACK TO THE BIG WORLD

A little while before you are due to leave for home and while you can still bask in the peace of the maternity ward, you might try drawing up a list of all the things that can be done at home – *by other people!* For now, it is time to set about ruthlessly recruiting all the help you need from your family and friends, including running errands for you and managing the kitchen. And the list you just made? Well, having made it, you can set it aside with a clear conscience. Reality proves to have little to do with checklists, but making one is probably good for you, like your morning exercises.

And then the moment comes when, with hands trembling a little bit, you empty the drawers of your bedside table, measure your skirt around your new waistline, dress your baby in its own small clothes, and step out into a world that will never be the same again; for now you are the mother of one of its newest citizens.

Chapter 6.

HOME AGAIN: A TIME FOR LEARNING

COMING HOME

It is not an unusual story: you lie in the hospital bed, dream of home and family, and look forward to returning to them – and then when you do come home, you somehow find that things are rather different from what you had anticipated. It may be that you feel more tired than you had expected. And if you are alone much of the time, having the responsibility for a tiny new human being may suddenly seem to be a daunting prospect. Small problems can loom as disproportionate challenges, and at times, the tears may not be very far away.

Many new mothers experience this scenario, though fortunately, it is unusual for it to last very long or to become too serious. It is sometimes termed the "baby blues," and it must be distinguished from what the doctors call "post-partum depression," which can be much more serious and for some women lead to real misery (Kendall-Tackett, 2010; see Chapter 9).

Various physiological and biochemical factors can be at the root of the blues. The body's functions have been attuned for months to the state of pregnancy, where the uterus and the placenta are central, and now it has to suddenly adapt to the new state of nursing. The entire machinery of pregnancy is shut down, and the glandular tissue of the breast assumes the responsibility for the baby's growth and well-being until the child reaches the point where it is truly ready to face the world independently, standing on its own two feet.

Don't Overreach Yourself

There is no point in assuming an attitude of stoic invincibility. "After all, I'm not ill, just a little tired…" No, you are certainly not ill, but you have just been through a tremendous physiological change, quite apart from the mental need to rethink your existence. These are not trivial matters, and nowhere in the world have they ever been dismissed as if they were.

A Word about Nursing Mothers

Rightly or wrongly, nursing mothers have always been placed in a very special category. The nursing mother has not been supposed, and in some cases not even permitted, to take up again her accustomed role in society as soon as her baby has been delivered. Whether this represented an attempt to protect her or to subjugate and even humiliate her is perhaps a matter for debate (see Chapter 13), but the overall effect of these admonitions and prohibitions has generally been to relieve her for a time from the heavy, routine work that has commonly been a woman's daily lot. The system might use stern measures to this end; the nursing mother was, for example, often categorized by the Christian church as unclean and a heathen for the first six weeks following delivery, and was therefore strictly forbidden to prepare food that would thus be rendered unclean. For such reasons, instead she had to be waited upon. In some societies, she was forbidden to enter the stalls and stables for fear that her presence would harm the animals. One could well imagine that such extreme measures were deliberately imposed to keep the busybodies away from work for a while—to the benefit of her baby and herself.

For it was, and still is, a fact that the nursing mother needs a period of restitution in order to get over the stresses of pregnancy and delivery and to get breastfeeding properly established. When in a few countries, such as the Scandinavian ones, women have succeeded in winning the right to quite long periods of maternity leave (for instance ten months on full pay); this is not merely to be seen as a gift from a generous community. It reflects a right, based on women's experience with the physiological needs that must be met if the human race is to survive and multiply, or meet the constant need for new worker bees for the hive. So whenever you, with your small baby, are offered the slightest opportunity to play Queen Bee in the hive, seize it with both hands; you have earned and deserved it.

SIMPLIFYING THE HOUSEWORK: SOME HINTS

First, some motherly advice:

This is the right moment, if the finances will allow it, to expand your armory of labor-saving devices that lighten the domestic workload. A *dishwasher* avoids many a grunt and grimace and has saved many a marriage. The time you save on routine work can be bestowed on your baby, yourself, and the remainder of the family, and now is the time to profit from it.

- It is not a bad idea to make a small inventory of what needs to be done in the home and the hands and heads available to do it. The new family member will demand your time, get your time, and steal your time. The question is warranted: are all the family members contributing what they can to keep the labor account healthily in balance?

- If you sit down with pencil and paper and engage in a little advance planning, you can probably cut down on the number of trips to the market or supermarket, especially if you have a deep-freezer and make the best use of it. Whoever is handling the cooking-of-the-day may take the chance to engage in some modest mass catering. Cooking a double-sized meal, and then freezing half of it, will ensure that ready-made food is available later when the kitchen's workload threatens to overflow.

- Finally, it is astonishing to discover how many habitual (and perhaps enjoyable) practices can be set aside for a while. For example: will the family's health and happiness really suffer if you drop your home baking or other charming specialties for a few weeks? They will soon enough be back!

Accept Every Offer of Help - Or Ask for It!

If you are in a position to recruit support from family and friends during these early weeks, don't be embarrassed to do it, and never turn down a spontaneous offer of help. You may well find yourself needing more assistance than you had expected. A willing mother, grandfather, or other relative can be an unbelievable source of support – sometimes by merely being close at hand and doing those small jobs you don't have the time or energy to do at the moment – folding the laundry, vacuum-cleaning, or perhaps just tidying up the kitchen drawers?

In an increasing number of countries, there are valuable arrangements for paternity leave, and one may hope that this is the trend of the future. That gives many fathers an opportunity – maybe the first he ever had – to show what a man is worth when it comes to baby care or housework –

provided that his wife can refrain from commenting on how he does it. Just think – this may be the very chance he has been waiting for.

The Joy of a Little Dust

None of the above means an absolute boycott of all household activities. It simply means that during the first weeks of a baby's life, he or she should have first priority. And in the meantime, you might as well spare a tolerant smile for whatever imperfections you spot in the rest of the housekeeping. As an old saying puts it: *dust makes no noise and cobwebs are splendid flycatchers.* To say nothing of the sort of dust that has rolled itself up into handy bundles ("Bachelor's rabbits") that you may pick up between one finger and thumb and transport to an appropriate place one at a time. And respectable accumulations of this and that produce an interesting sound as the vacuum cleaner gobbles them up (especially the little bits and pieces that are found behind doors and in other places known only to you). Truly: to delay cleaning until it can be put off no longer is a pleasure that, at such times, you really should not deny yourself.

DEALING KINDLY BUT FIRMLY WITH VISITORS

It can be enjoyable to welcome interested friends and relatives, flocking in to share in the general jubilation around your baby. But visitors, however well intentioned, are a burden, and not every mother is quite ready to shoulder that burden at this time. It can be sensible to hint politely that you would prefer visitors to wait to visit for two or three weeks. The telephone answering machine is a perfect firewall: *"We have a boy, 61 cm long and weighing 4 kilos, and we will welcome visitors after September 20th,"* to which one may add for the benefit of very insistent acquaintances *"...and preferably no earlier."* Then turn off your cell phone for a while.

When the multitude does ultimately descend upon you, do remember that it is the *baby* they have come to enjoy and not the house or its gastronomic delights. Visits at this time should be a pleasure and not a burden, as they all too readily become in a family with a wide social circle. In olden times, it was unthinkable to pay a visit to a newly delivered mother without carrying a basket of food, knowing that at this particular time, she was not supposed to be concerned with housekeeping matters...

Therefore: by all means impart the suggestion that you are a little less robust than you really are, and avoid the temptation to hurry around with the coffee jug or the teapot. Let the others do that, and go on bearing in mind that one must never turn down an offer of help.

The Other Children...

Most visitors will be thoughtful enough to spend a little time with the baby's older brothers and sisters. If they don't, it can seed a little jealousy in the home. If you do have friends and relations who have eyes only for the newcomer, drop a little hint that big brother and sister merit a moment's attention as well.

Try Selecting Your Visitors

Be more than a little critical as to which visitors you allow into your home during the first weeks. Try to delay seeing that nervous Uncle Fred, who always contrives to depress you, or dear friend Lisa, blessed with all the optimism of a vulture and an endless stock of hair-raising anecdotes about death and pestilence. The visitors you need are your best and kindest friends. Try inviting them personally; they will be happy if you do.

"...AND ALL THE THINGS I WAS PLANNING TO DO DURING MY MATERNITY LEAVE..."

When you get back home from the maternity ward, don't believe that you can now get seamlessly back to all the things you used to do before the baby arrived. One mother may need much more time than another to recover completely from the whole birthing process. Some women are bustling around after just a few weeks; others need several months to get up steam again. But every woman will find that she gets back into form more rapidly if she takes good care of herself. Cut out for the present (and certainly for the first few weeks) all those things that you are not *obliged* to do. You are most likely to convalesce smoothly if, for the first week or so at home, you spend most of your time close to your bed with the baby within easy reach.

BREASTFEEDING IS AN INVITATION TO RELAX

An ingenious aspect of breastfeeding is that it obliges you to sit or lie down several times a day, and if you can manage it, to relax thoroughly at the same time. You will find that you work much more effectively when you are rested than if you force yourself to go on working because of the notion that it is your duty to remain on your feet.

Relaxation and sleep are not luxuries. During the first three months after delivery, you should try to lie down a few times every day to relax or sleep, perhaps when you are breastfeeding anyway, and preferably not get up until you feel that you are no longer seriously tired. There is no harm in dozing off while you are breastfeeding, provided you first make sure the baby is lying comfortably and securely. Follow the child's own rhythm; when you see that the baby is falling asleep, do the same yourself, rather than tiptoeing away to deal with the dishwasher, the dryer, or the computer. An opportunity to take a nap is all too easily missed, and it may be some time before you find another, whereas the dishwasher and the dirty clothes will go nowhere, but will wait patiently for you.

GOOD - AND LESS GOOD - ADVICE

Nursing mothers attract unsolicited advisers as readily as jam attracts flies. A great many people feel they have valid views about breastfeeding that absolutely need to be expressed; but many are not, in the depths of their soul, primarily concerned with helping the breastfeeding mother. When they see you with your baby at the breast, they may feel inspired to relate their own dreadful nursing experiences. It is not pleasant to be force-fed other people's problems, especially if you have certain difficulties of your own to deal with. It is the same phenomenon that one encounters during pregnancy. Many expectant mothers experience the dubious pleasure of being exposed to horror stories served up by insensitive individuals about their own gruesome deliveries or that of others they have heard about.

You have a perfect right to decide that you do not want to be exposed to such drivel. If a friend launches into a juicy tale of sore nipples, simply stop her in full flight, explaining that you do not appreciate being subjected to such dreadful tales when you are currently in the process of feeding your own baby. If you simply cannot dissuade the storyteller and you are too polite to throw him or her out, take some antidote after she has gone in the form of a more realistic chat with a breastfeeding adviser or a sensible friend, read something encouraging on the subject in a good book, or do something completely different. It's remarkable how one can restore one's self-confidence by turning to a kind and sensible person who knows what she is talking about.

Much of the same applies as regards a perpetual flow of thoughtless remarks and advice. "I think the baby looks *hungry* – are you sure you have enough milk?" or "Do you really think it's *healthy* for her to suckle so often?" Breastfeeding is, as we all learn, an emotionally laden topic, and many have their own baggage of personal experiences on the matter. That is true for lay persons, as well as the learned, and it applies to men, as well as women.

The Old Way: Friends and Acquaintances, Including the Neighbors

It is not unusual for friends and next-door neighbors to assume the role that once upon a time was played by the extended family. That is especially the case if your family lives far away or your relationship with them isn't particularly close. A good friend, a neighbor, or the nice people across the road may be able to provide just the salvation you need in the days after delivery. And who knows, it may well prove to be the starting point for mutual support in either direction when new babies arrive in any of the homes concerned....

The New Way: Birthing Groups

Many health centers today form birthing groups to bring together new mothers or parents for a little teaching or simply to enable them to exchange experiences and ideas. Some groups prove to be so popular and attractive that they continue to meet even after the original purpose of the meeting has been attained. Some survive until the children are far beyond the days of breastfeeding. They may, however, influence breastfeeding either positively or negatively; some mothers who struggle to breastfeed remark that their sense of failure is only enhanced when they are faced with these women showing off their prize infants and describing how liberally their milk is flowing. If you run into this situation, talk it over with your nurse or midwife. The health center may be able to suggest some other forum in which young parents meet each other and where you may feel at home. Some centers have special groups for fathers, open nursery schools, or other forms of get-togethers. In larger towns, you will also find that there are forums where single mothers are welcome – another group who may all too readily feel that they have too little contact with peers. You may even have a La Leche League or other mother-to-mother support group in your vicinity (website: www.llli.org). They provide advice as well as an opportunity to meet other breastfeeding mothers.

HOW DEMAND DETERMINES SUPPLY

Breastfeeding is just about the best imaginable illustration of the well-known marketing principle that demand and supply will always adjust themselves to suit one another. In the case of breastfeeding, the adjustment of supply to meet demand is managed through the mechanisms we have looked at earlier. Just consider them this way:

- When the baby feeds at the breast, this sends a stimulus directly from the breast to two areas in the mother's brain known as the anterior and posterior lobes of the pituitary. These release two central breastfeeding hormones known as prolactin and oxytocin, which cause the milk cells to be activated, so they produce milk.

The extent to which this happens depends on:

- How often the baby is put to the breast.

- The amount of milk taken from the breast.

There is reason to believe that during the first few weeks of life, milk production is largely stimulated by the high levels of milk production hormones released at the time of delivery. After this initial period, the level of hormones is determined by the demand, i.e., the amount of milk produced is adjusted to replace the quantity taken by the baby. All these elements work together to stimulate and adjust the milk production, so that at every moment, it exactly meets the need of the baby (or the babies, where there is more than one).

These needs in practice are not as steady and predictable as it might seem from the curves in a growth chart. A baby grows in fits and starts. When your baby is going through a growth spurt, it suddenly needs more food. You will see it taking the breast eagerly and hungrily, continuing to feed until it falls asleep on the spot. Minutes later, it will be wide awake again and as hungry as ever. That may lead an uncertain mother, health worker, or relative to believe that the baby has not received sufficient milk or that the milk supply has suddenly dried up and things are now going seriously downhill. *But that is just not true!*

As a rule, the milk supply rises to meet the increased demand within 48 hours – sometimes sooner, sometimes later. With the baby assured of getting what it needs, production sometimes increases more than need be, and the baby tends to leave more than usual in the breast at the end of a feed. If that happens, the whole process is soon adjusted to bring the milk production in line with what the baby needs.

Breastfeeding's most basic rule, number ten in our series of Golden Rules of Breastfeeding, is:

Golden Rule Number 10

As long as you set out to meet the demand, the production of milk will automatically be adjusted to provide for the baby's needs.

The enlargement of the breasts during the early days is partly caused by an increase in their blood supply and partly caused by the continuing development of the milk gland tissue at that time (see the description of the anatomy of the breast in Chapter 1.) It is also quite common at this time for there to be some overproduction of milk because of the high levels of prolactin that are circulating shortly after delivery. Once breastfeeding is under way, however, the breasts will no longer be so heavy and tense as they were at the start. The milk glands in which the milk is produced and stored mostly lie quite deeply inside the breast, close to its center, and viewing the breast from the outside hardly provides a clue as to how much milk it contains. As the baby feeds, however, the let-down reflex moves the milk forward and out of the breast.

In the case of some mothers, this system works so seamlessly that they barely notice any variation in the amount of milk they produce. In others, as we have seen, the milk flow oscillates between paucity and plenty. It can be quite tiring to find that you constantly seem to be providing either too much or too little, but you can take comfort from the fact that after a time, the pendulum tends to swing a little less sharply. And it is good to recall that over time your baby usually gets just what it wants and needs.

SOME FREQUENTLY ASKED QUESTIONS DURING THE FIRST DAYS

My Breasts Are Getting Smaller and Softer – Is the Milk Supply Failing?

Right at the start of lactation, many mothers develop large, tense breasts that feel as if they are delightfully full of milk. After a week or so – usually after one has arrived home from the maternity ward – the breasts undergo another change. They become smaller and no longer seem to be so promisingly full. Many mothers find this worrying and become afraid that their milk supply is failing. But again: that truly isn't so.

Some swelling of the breasts occurs during the first few days after delivery. It is simply due to the increased blood flow to the breasts and to the continuing development of the milk glands (see Chapter 1 on the structure of the breast). There is also quite often some overproduction of milk because of the high levels of prolactin circulating directly after birth. Once breastfeeding is well under way, you will find that the breasts are no longer taut or enlarged. The milk glands are found in small clusters throughout the breast. It is not possible to judge by looking at the breast how much milk is present. As the baby feeds, the let-down reflex propels the milk forward and out of the nipple.

Big Breasts, Small Breasts – What Is the Ideal?

The size of your breasts gives no indication as to your ability to breastfeed. Women whose figures hardly show any evidence of breasts at all have breastfed splendidly for months on end. In theory, one might expect that virtually invisible breasts will provide little "storage space," but in practice we have found no difference in the breastfeeding performance of flat-breasted individuals and well-endowed women. One might add that many mammals have barely visible milk gland tissue, but nevertheless lactate and feed their young in blissful ignorance of all the problems that humans, first among the primates, dream up to worry themselves with.

Much Milk, Little Milk - What Is Normal?

Some women find that during the early days of nursing, the quantity of milk they produce varies quite markedly from one day to the next. On one day, there appears to be more than enough, while on the next day, the amount is barely sufficient. After a few days, however, the process usually evens out. After one has been breastfeeding for some months, any difference that may persist is barely noticeable. There are, however, great variations – some women find that their babies virtually empty the breasts, while others find themselves constantly lodged with variable residues of milk as long as they are breastfeeding. Such women simply have a particularly sensitive milk output that gives the impression of disappearing, whereas in reality, it merely hides itself from time to time. They just have to get used to it!

How Often Should a Baby Feed?

A hungry breastfed baby can feed as often as it wants. Mother's milk is easily digested and newborn babies have tiny stomachs, so breastfed babies are likely to be hungry again sooner than those on the formula, at least during the first six months of life or until they begin solid food. You need not worry if your breastfed baby has a feeding pattern that is very different from that of the formula-fed baby down the street. The only thing to watch is whether your baby is putting on weight as it should and overall seems reasonably happy and healthy (see later in this Chapter).

As My Baby Grows Older, Will Its Feeding Pattern Change?

A baby who at all times has unlimited access to the breast will feed eight times or more during the first one or two days of life, but may also spend much of its time asleep. Thereafter, it begins to awaken more completely to life and to seek the breast at ever shorter intervals. Between the third and the seventh day, it may feed 12 or more times a day, exhibiting its true nature as a *continuous breast feeder*. After the 14th day and up to the end of the first month, the feeds will probably be frequent (though there are big differences between one baby and another). A Swedish study of the feeding pattern during the first six months of life in babies who were exclusively breastfed noted very marked differences between individuals and concluded that each mother-baby pair should be judged individually (Hörnell, Aarts, Kylberg, Hofvander, & Gebre-Medhin, 1999). Let us simply say that, as long as you and your baby are both content with the way breastfeeding is going, there is no right or wrong.

Unlimited Breastfeeding - Are There Really No Limits at All?

"Baby-led," "unrestricted," "self-regulated," or "on-demand" breastfeeding are fairly new terms, but they do not represent new ideas. Babies have been self-regulating since the dawn of time. A mother without a clock on the wall will feed her baby when she understands from the signals the baby emits that it is hungry. That does *not* mean waiting to feed until the baby begins to scream for it – a scream is a late and desperate appeal to do something to relieve an intolerable hunger. Much earlier, a baby that begins to sense the need for food will show it in more subtle ways – waving its arms, for example, and toying with its hands in the general direction of the mouth. Probably it will open the mouth, while a welcoming tongue, already folded into the shape of a trough, will start to make the wave-like motions that are typical of its activity as a little milking machine. Often the baby begins to salivate as if it has something tasty in mind – which of course it does.

And as we stated before: don't be alarmed if all this happens very, very often in the course of a day. There really should be a strict prohibition on counting the number of feeds in a day or looking at the clock to find out how much time has passed since the last breastfeed!

Golden Rule Number 11

In these early days, it is the baby, and the baby alone, who should decide when it is time for a feed. Listen to the baby's early hunger signals, and ignore everyone and everything else!

WHAT IS THE BABY SAYING?

It is quite remarkable how clearly young babies can express themselves, in spite of their not using our adult language to do so. You just need to be alert to their signs and symbols and grasp what they mean.

Dreadfully tired little babies will, for example, for no apparent reason, often rub their faces – somewhere around their noses. Or they stare fixedly at nothing in particular as if it is too tiring to move one's focus from one thing to another.

In cold areas, young babies are often too warmly dressed. One often encounters a small child, hot as an oven and desperately unhappy, being wheeled through a supermarket under a stifling collection of quilts and woollies – well packaged against the ravages of the winter outdoors. And hot babies scream, and screaming makes the situation worse – with everything heading for a catastrophe unless or until someone sees the light and rescues the miserable little body from its covers.

Listen to What the Baby Says - And React!

Never allow a small child to lie there screaming without getting any response from you. A scream is a signal – a cry for help in a still un-familiar world. You and the baby's father should immediately react to that signal, for example, by picking the baby up, feeding it, dress-ing it, changing its nappy, or perhaps simply by saying hello to it or rocking it a little. Small signals like this can be enough to build the contact and trust which can provide the foundation for a confident personality for the rest of the child's life.

Is Every Scream a Sign of Hunger?

It is definitely not so that every scream means the baby is crying for food; not every cry comes from the small stomach. You will soon find yourself recognizing the baby's various signals. Love, sensitivity, and a pinch of healthy good sense will all help you to correctly in-terpret what your baby is asking for. It may be a call to change a wet and oppressive nappy, a complaint about *"pain somewhere in the belly,"* an irritated message that *"I'm still much too warm"*... to say nothing of the cry: *"and the more I scream the worse it gets – poor me!"* or a shot into the wilderness: *"I feel lonely – where on earth are those soft arms and that lovely smell...?"*

Does Every Feed Mean a Nappy Change?

That is really an unnecessary question when the baby is left in control of its own feeding schedule. In the days when breastfeeds were arranged by the clock, it seemed fair enough, at least in theory, to precede every meal ritual with a change of nappy (diaper). What this often meant, however, was that mother changed the nappy of a hungry complaining baby, and as soon as it finally got the breast and filled its stomach, it produced a fresh stool, obliging her to do it all over again. It was, therefore, a thoroughly bad idea to routinely combine feeding sessions with a change of nappies. A hungry baby must always receive its food first, after which it can be changed if necessary. You will soon discover how often a change is needed, be it four, five, or more times daily. The same rule applies to nappies as to breastfeeding: do it when it's needed; otherwise, leave it in peace!

Is It Possible-or Necessary-To Empty the Breast of Milk?

Different answers to this question have been given at different times. When I (Elisabet) was breastfeeding back in the 60s, we were firmly instructed to offer only one breast at each meal, since a breast "needed to be emptied thoroughly." No clear explanation was forthcoming as to how one was expected to "empty" a breast that was actively producing milk. The result was that many a mother, after a feeding session, sat trying to express her milk. When she found it impossible to empty the breast that was actively making milk, she became unhappy and lost her self-confidence. The truth is that a breast that is actively making milk cannot be fully "emptied." So it is pointless under normal circumstances to continue expressing a breast, whether by hand or with the aid of a pump, after the baby has taken as much milk as it can.

As we have seen, a baby may leave some of the available milk unused in the breast after a feed. The reasons for removing this milk could be to:

- Increase your milk production.

- Build up a stock for use in situations where you will be away from your baby.

- Offer some of your milk to other children who need breastmilk, but who, for various reasons, cannot get it from their own mothers.

It is necessary to avoid over-filled breasts. They can be uncomfortable or even painful, and can lead to obstruction of the milk passages and eventually to mastitis. But don't express your milk without good reason. As soon as the breast is over-full, the raised pressure in the alveoli will send a message to the body that more milk than necessary is now being made, and the hormonal mechanisms will swing into action to reduce the output.

One Breast or Both?

Back in the early years of the 20th century, mothers were solemnly admonished to give only one breast at each feeding session. By the 1970s, however, the medical pendulum had swung the other way. Now it was equally solemnly ordained that *both breasts* should be given at each session. In some cases, this meant that a baby was taken from one breast before it had had a reasonable feed. Today, as in so many other matters, we are more flexible, understanding that individuals differ. Some mothers will find that it suits them to offer both breasts at every feed, while others prefer to give only one breast at each session. Many women simply vary their practice, following no fixed rule. An Australian study showed that, of a given group of mothers, 30% offered only one breast at each feed, 13% routinely gave both sides, while a majority (57%) had no preference one way or the other (Kent et al., 2006). In other words: you do what you feel is best, and perhaps also let it depend on how much time you have available for a feed. Most small children will fall asleep as soon as the stomach is full, and let go of the breast as they do so.

A baby will often not need to spend as much time nursing on the second breast as on the first. When it is time for a feed, it is usually best to begin on the side where the previous feed ended. Since milk production is only possible if milk is being taken from the breast, it may be practical to ensure that the two breasts each receive and dispatch approximately the same signals as to how much milk it is necessary to produce. This can be assured if the breasts are used alternately as described here.

How Long Should a Breastfeeding Session Last?

A century or so ago, when clocks and watches came into general use in most homes and factory workers began to be paid by the hour, it became customary to accept that a breastfeeding session should last 20 minutes. This is an example of the confusion that arose when recommendations on breastfeeding were mixed up with those on bottle-feeding (see Chapter 13). A bottle of infant formula can be emptied in about 20 minutes, but a breast, with the support of the let-down reflex, can deliver most of the milk it contains in a much shorter period, sometimes as little as five minutes, though some children need much more time. Remember that since milk is both food and drink, it is not only the volume of milk that determines the feeding time, but also the amount of energy (particularly in the form of fat) that the child is ingesting. To say nothing of the time needed for cuddling!

Before you get to know your baby well, you may be fooled by the fact that it may continue to work energetically at a breast from which it has already taken most of the available milk. Even if the baby does not indicate that it is finished by releasing its hold on the breast, you can make out quite easily whether it is still taking milk or not: look for movements of the muscles around the mouth and cheek, and listen for those rhythmic sounds as the milk is swallowed. Is it still feeding or is it merely enjoying itself? Or has it just absent-mindedly forgotten what it was supposed to be doing? Your offer to try the other breast will not always be taken, but occasionally the baby will find that it has a little room left for dessert. All this means is that the whole procedure may be shorter or longer than you expect. It doesn't matter. As always, the best thing is to forget the clock – it really has nothing to do with the matter!

In a Nutshell: The Essential Facts about Feeding Patterns

As we have seen, it is your tiny newborn baby who is responsible for determining the rhythm and frequency of feeding sessions and how long a feed should last. As the baby grows a little older, it will be better able to wait a while for a feed, rather than demanding it at the very moment the idea comes into its head, and you may be able to arrange matters to take into account more of your own interests.

There are, however, some mothers who find that they have a small bohemian at the breast, not at all willing to abide by the rules and routines one would wish to apply. Do not despair! Hungry bohemians must also be fed – even if they are troublesome.

SKIN-TO-SKIN CONTACT

Skin contact and every form of closeness stimulate a mother's brain to produce more prolactin and oxytocin, and many investigators believe that oxytocin, in particular, actually promotes parents' affection for the baby. Oxytocin is produced by men as well as women, so father, too, can reap the biological benefits of skin-to-skin contact (Uvnäs-Moberg, 2003). Skin-to-skin contact with your baby will probably help you to recognize and understand its signals, so you can react to them. Allow your baby plenty of time to get used to your breast and to you as a person. One can't force that process – a baby needs to build up an acquaintance in its own good time. Some babies manage to make it very clear from the start that they want the breast, and they have no doubt about what to do when they get there. Others fiddle and mess around endlessly, and get upset and angry as they do so. Don't get upset if things aren't working out right in the beginning. You can help the process along by offering the baby your skin and all the time it needs for lengthy and repeated skin-to-skin contact. Getting to know each other may just be a matter of a few hours, but for some, it may go on for days or weeks. Put simply: taking your time is one of the most important tools for successful breastfeeding.

We will return to skin-to-skin contact in Chapter 8 because it remains an ongoing need – not simply a means of helping your baby at the start.

ON GROWTH AND WEIGHT

Should I Weigh the Baby?

It is *not* at all necessary to have a set of baby scales at home, unless you are one of those people who actually like to measure things, keep records, and enjoy weighing the baby. In that case, you should use the same scales each time and bear in mind that neither ordinary kitchen scales nor non-professional baby scales are likely to be accurate to the last fraction of an ounce!

How much weight *should* a baby gain every week? To answer that question, you have to take into consideration whether or not you or the baby's father are heavily built. You can hardly expect the baby to develop as a giant if the rest of the family is on the lighter side of normal.

Breastfed Infant as the Standard for Growth: WHO Child Growth Standards

Growth charts are among the principal tools used to assess infant nutritional status, health, and development. In 2006, the World Health Organization launched a growth curve based on a new concept. Many of the traditional *growth references* are based on infants fed on formula, and often on a population with poor nutrition. The WHO Child Growth standards were derived from measurements on mother-baby pairs where the mother had not smoked during pregnancy or after delivery; there had been exclusive breastfeeding for four to six months, with a total duration of breastfeeding of at least 12 months; complementary foods were of good quality; and the socio-economic level was sufficient to avoid any impairment to growth. The sample used was multi-ethnic. It was striking that, other things being equal, these children, though of different ethnic backgrounds, grew at a very similar rate from birth up to at least five years. Since the standard is based on breastfed children, it provides a better tool to manage breastfeeding (de Onis, Onyango, Borghi, Garza, & Yang, 2006; WHO, 2009b).

NORMAL WEIGHT GAIN

The individual growth depends on the baby's:

- Birth weight

- Gender

- Age

For an exclusively breastfed baby, the weight gain for the first weeks of life is high. At around two to three months of age, the weight gain slows down.

There is no point in trying to calculate whether the baby is getting sufficient food by using percentages of body weight or suchlike; you will simply end up with a headache. The important thing is that the baby is lively and happy, and you feel it is thriving. If it has a good skin color and bright eyes, if its nappies are wet, if it is reasonably active at the breast, cries in moderation, and waves its arms and legs, you can be sure that it is being properly fed and doing well.

During the first few weeks of life, passing a stool six times a day or so is a good indication that the baby is doing well on your milk. Later, the frequency of stools may vary from one baby to another, from several times daily to once a week ...

Should You Weigh Your Milk?

Test weighing before and after a feed provides no useful information unless one knows the total daily milk output, which can vary as much 300 ml a day for any normal individual mother. One would also need to know the average calorie content of the milk – and to get information like that, one would need to collect a whole day's production of breastmilk, mix it well, and have it analyzed in a laboratory. And even if we were to have all this information, it is not clear how useful it would be! Your baby's stomach has already performed its own analysis, and the baby's system knows precisely what it must do to get the amount of food it needs. Test weighing is time-consuming and can be stressful; and with stress, the let-down reflex may run into difficulties that reduce your milk flow. And all this weighing will hardly give you a real idea as to how much your baby is taking from the breast, normally or daily.

Every Child Is Different

Give your child the chance to develop in its own way. From the start, it has the right to be different from all others. You may have been blessed with a happy, tame, and plump little cherub or you may find yourself lodged with one of the temperamental babies who cry and scream, and barely lie still for a moment. Take these things as they come. You have to accept the baby you got, just as the baby has to accept the mother with whom it has been saddled.

You can leave it up to your baby whether it chooses to be fed small frequent meals or large occasional ones. Don't be concerned if your baby is gaining less weight than the one next door. In our time and in many western countries, overweight among children is a greater source of concern than underweight. Have you ever stopped to think that the term "average weight" means that half of the babies are likely to be over the "average" line and half will be under it?

A Word about Those Quiet Babies

There is a type of baby that is unusually placid and undemanding. It sleeps as much as four or five hours at a time, rarely cries, and lies quietly, seemingly contented at the breast when feeding. The mother is delighted to have such a quiet and apparently satisfied baby until she takes it to the health center or pediatrician and is told to her horror that the baby has not gained any weight since the last visit. We do not know why it is that some babies hardly seem to experience hunger, though we realize that some adults are very much the same. Occasionally, this is the case in a baby with jaundice or one who has been born prematurely, but often there is no evident cause. Provided you make sure that there is nothing basically wrong, which is usually the case, there is no need to worry. A baby who is tending to spend much of the day asleep can be wakened gently from time to time (for example, by lightly massaging the soles of the feet) and given the breast – for example, approximately every second hour in the early days, and later approximately every three hours, so that your milk flow is stimulated progressively. A little care like this, guiding things in the right direction, may help the baby to become more active and energetic, and it will ensure that it has sufficient food.

Take a look at Chapter 8 where we discuss "weak feeders." You may find some of the advice we give there helpful.

SUPPLEMENTING YOUR MILK?

Even today, there are mothers and advisors who are not aware that there are effective ways for a woman to increase her milk production if it has been falling for a time. Without that knowledge, one may be all too easily persuaded to start supplementary feeding with infant formula. Don't let such advice discourage you. Go home and plan to provide several additional breastfeeds a day – read our suggestions further down on "how to increase your milk production." Try to get some expert advice to make sure that you are positioning and attaching the baby in a good way (see Chapter 5). Think again about how you have arranged your daily program, and see whether you can't cut out some activities and take an occasional rest instead. What would you like to do that might make you feel more energetic?

Milking and Pumping in Practice: An Art to Be Learned Early

Once your milk flow is well established, after you have been breastfeeding for some months and feel confident about how it is going, there is nothing to prevent you from occasionally leaving the baby for a while when other duties or pleasures call. On such occasions, a breastfeeding session will have to be replaced either by your own milk taken from the freezer or a reasonable factory-made substitute. If you are likely to be away for more than four hours, you should for your own sake have mastered the art of hand expression (see Chapter 10 – Hand expression) or using a good pump. Pumps can be rented or borrowed (read more about mechanical aids and accessories in Chapter 10).

If You Think Your Milk Is Disappearing

As we pointed out in Chapter 1, it is physically impossible for your milk supply to disappear from one day to the next. What can happen, as already explained, is that the baby is failing to get access to the milk that is present in the breast. As a rule, that happens because the baby is poorly attached in such a way that it is merely sucking or chewing on the nipple without having a grip on the breast proper. This may also mean that the milk let-down reflex is not being adequately triggered, so the milk is not actively spurting out of the breast, as it should be. What is most likely to persuade a father and mother that the milk is dwindling is when the baby indicates, shortly after completion of a feed, that it wants the breast again. The mother feels her seemingly empty breast, and the fear that her baby is going to go hungry sneaks up on her.

The next time she gives a breastfeed she is likely to be nervous, waiting in fearful anticipation of the baby's letting go of the "empty" breast and crying for more. To be on the safe side, she probably prepares a bottle, and as soon as the baby releases the breast, it is given the bottle – with an apparently "satisfactory" result - her baby sleeps for several hours. In reality, what this means is that the number of breastfeeds does not increase, the hormonal stimulus to the breast is not raised, and there is no increase in her milk production.

Weight Gain Over Time Matters

Before concluding, as you may be tempted to do, that every scream is a sign of hunger, do bear in mind some other possibilities (see elsewhere in this chapter). The best indicator that your baby is getting enough food is that it is putting on weight *over a period of time*, subject to some of the reservations about weight we discussed above.

HOW TO INCREASE YOUR MILK PRODUCTION

If you feel that your baby does need more breastmilk than you are currently providing, you can do something about it – there is no need to panic in the belief that it is suffering and going to starve. Trust in your own ability to breastfeed and remember the point we made above that almost every mother can provide enough breastmilk for her baby.

A RECIPE FOR "STIMULATION DAYS" TO HELP BOOST YOUR MILK SUPPLY:

- Check that the baby has a good and proper grip on the breast (see Chapter 5 – Good Positioning) and put it calmly to the breast as often as you can for a few days in succession.

- Don't be discouraged if this program means that you end up with the baby at the breast most of the time. Think of your ancestor – the continuous breastfeeder! If you are to give the breast sufficient stimulation on these vital days, you should breastfeed at least ten times daily. But once you get anywhere close to that, you can stop counting!

- To prepare for these "stimulation days," it is important that you set aside all other obligations. You need to concentrate purely on what you are trying to do with your milk production. Only arrange for such a day when you are quite sure that you will have the time to breastfeed continuously if need be. For example, wait for a weekend if that is the best time to get the support and help you need from others.

- Realize full well that these special days may not be particularly cozy – you may find yourself faced with a fussy baby at the breast much of the time. You may also miss the satisfaction that goes with a breast full of milk. With such frequent feedings sessions, the breast will have little time to fill itself, even if it produces milk by the gallon!

- Don't feel obliged to stretch out every breastfeeding session interminably – the most important thing is to breastfeed sufficiently often. Experience seems to show that the total time spent at the breast in the course of a day should be more than three hours-but don't watch the clock. And there is naturally no good reason to combine feeding, clothing, and the changing of nappies (diapers) in a single session.

- If you have already started to give your baby a fair amount of infant formula, you may well feel that you cannot stop the bottle too quickly. What you can do is to give the supplements less often over the day, and preferably not after each breastfeed. Begin each feeding session with the breast, and then, only if it is needed, provide the supplementary feed... with a cup or the "nursing supplementer" (see Chapter 10). The latter may prove useful in that it is stimulating your breasts and supplementing the child at the same time.

- Cup feeding is an art that everyone needs to master. For the baby who needs to acquire the complicated art of breastfeeding and the routine needed to milk the breast effectively, it will be easier to develop and retain the reflexes needed for that purpose if the scenario is not made complicated by the presence of a bottle teat which, unlike the breast, has to be sucked in order to obtain the milk and which cannot be adapted to the shape of the mouth cavity as the breast does so well (see Chapter 10 – Cup Feeding).

The Upper and Lower Limits of Milk Production

One of the reasons why women were, at one time, so emphatically advised to give supplements to breastmilk was the belief that a woman was only capable of producing a certain, limited amount of milk, and if her milk production began to fail, there was nothing to be done about it.

We know today that all women can produce milk, and the great majority of mothers will produce enough for at least one baby. It is somewhat difficult to say how much breastmilk the female population would be able to produce if every woman were given sufficient and good advice on positioning the baby and maintaining her own self-confidence. Many mothers are probably capable of feeding twins, which means they are likely, as a maximum, to achieve a milk flow of some two liters a day. There must, however, be quite a range of variation in this maximum – just think of the wet nurse who was found to deliver more than five liters of milk a day! See Chapter 13 on the history of breastfeeding.

On the other hand, it is evident that a small proportion of women have a lower-than-average limit to what they can produce. Despite the best advice and good will, these women find very early on that they have reached the limits of their milk production and their babies need more than they feel able to supply. This is not disastrous. Give as much breastmilk as you can at each feeding session, and then follow it with the substitute. The substitute is best given with a cup, but if supplementation is continuing over a long period, you may ultimately find the bottle to be the less tiring. Generally, one does not need to give very much for the baby to be sated–maybe once or twice daily, provided you continue to breastfeed. **This last point is vital: if you reduce the level of breast stimulation you receive from your baby, the breast will naturally produce less milk.** If you reach your upper limit of milk production when the baby is around six months old, you can, of course, give solid food to provide the calories you cannot deliver.

Before you conclude that you really have reached your milk-producing limit, remember that if you did have sufficient milk at an earlier stage (for example, immediately after delivery), then you are capable of providing it again. Self-confidence is the greatest ally of breastfeeding (Figure 6.1).

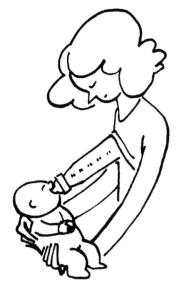

Figure 6.1. *If only the breasts were made of glass…*

Source: Cartoon by Ellen Wilhelmsen. Used with permission.

Perceived Failure of Milk Production - And Real Breastfeeding Crises

As we need to stress again, there are very few mothers who in the early weeks of breastfeeding really do not manage to produce all the milk their babies need. On the other hand, there are far too many mothers who wrongly believe they are experiencing this problem.

In 1983, Charlotte Hillervik in Sweden did a prospective study of 51 well-educated mothers, all of whom stated they wanted to breastfeed. She set out to determine how many of them incorrectly felt at some time that their milk production was failing, why this happened, and what the consequences of perceived breastmilk insufficiency might be (Hillervik-Lindquist, Hofvander, & Sjolin, 1991). She found that nearly half of the women she was studying experienced a crisis at some time that was not real, as their milk production was perfectly adequate. Careful checks on their babies' weight and development showed that most of the mothers in this so-called "crisis group" were, in fact, providing sufficient milk; the flow was not reduced during the perceived crisis or in the following weeks. The babies were putting on weight in a completely normal fashion. When she compared these women with mothers who had not experienced such imaginary crises, she did find that the rate of weight increase in the "crisis" group was slightly less at the ages of two, three, four, and nine months, but that it still lay within the normal range. This group did tend to end breastfeeding earlier than the other participants in the study. What Charlotte Hillervik concluded was that, although the babies whose mothers were experiencing real or imaginary episodes of "milk failure" did put on weight a little more slowly than others, the differences were slight. The crises had no effect on the babies' growth and health; there was no need for supplementary food.

What women with repeated "breastfeeding crises" and a lower level of milk production do need is accessible, sound, and patient professional help, so they can overcome their problems. Without such support, they may remain unhappy and lacking in self-confidence – and that is naturally not characteristic of breastfeeding.

Too Little Milk in the Afternoon?

The majority of women have the most milk in the mornings after a more or less satisfactory night's sleep, and the milk flow falls as evening approaches. This is one of those ups and downs which one encounters throughout life.

If you find that you have very little milk towards the end of the day, try taking a rest for an hour or so, for example, after dinner in the evening or when the other children have been put to bed. Lie down, either with the baby or while another member of the family looks after it. It is remarkable how much good it does to rest completely with your eyes closed. If you like, take a good warming drink before you lie down. Be prepared for the baby to call for the breast more often during the evening.

Too Little Milk - Tried Everything...

If you have tried everything, gotten good support and advice, and your milk production still does not increase, you may be one of the few women with physiological problems. It may be because of a disease (mainly diseases involving hormones and thyroid dysfunction), breast surgery, heavy bleeding after birth, anemia, or in some cases, too little glandular breast tissue. If you experienced only slight or no changes in your breasts during pregnancy and little change after birth, this could be a sign that something is wrong. Contact a competent lactation consultant, or other health staff with special breastfeeding knowledge, and together find out how to cope with this, and if there is a ready solution. A nursing supplementer (Chapter 10) can also be helpful (West & Marasco, 2009).

Feeding at Night

Many a mother will try to give her baby plenty of milk in the late evening in the hope that it will sleep throughout the night. However, it is not so much the size of the evening breastfeed that determines how long the baby is going to sleep, but how far the baby has developed. Here again, individual differences between babies seem to play a role. In many countries, it is customary for the mother and the young baby to sleep together. Studies in many places have shown that when given this opportunity, about a third of the baby's total intake of milk is taken at night. If night feeding doesn't prove difficult for you, let the baby take its night feeds, just as often and as long as it wants to do so.

In the past, it was customary to let a baby lie and scream for half an hour or so before giving it a night feed. Many babies give up the effort to attract attention if they don't soon succeed – but most mothers dislike hearing their babies desperately screaming to no avail, probably wondering why mummy has disappeared into the dark. There is, in fact, no good reason to maintain the old rule, making both baby and mother miserable for the sake of some obscure moral principle. Many people have, as on other matters, expressed strong and divergent views about breastfeeding at night, but only you can decide which approach you prefer.

IS IT DANGEROUS TO SLEEP WITH YOUR BABY?

No baby is likely to thrive as long as its mother is suffering from loss of sleep, struggling to keep herself going throughout the day, and hardly capable of keeping up with everything that needs to be done. A simple solution can be to take the baby into the parental bed at night, arranging it so that both generations can get a proper night's sleep.

In Western countries, there is, however, no shortage of horror stories about mothers who, following this practice, involuntarily smothered their babies in their sleep. Most of these stories arose at a time when contraception and legal abortion were hardly available and infanticide was for some unhappy and unwilling mothers the only means they knew of to limit the size of the family. Officially, of course, infanticide was illegal and mothers found guilty of it were liable to severe penalties. As a result, many such women pleaded that the baby's death was accidental – it had been smothered while the mother slept alongside it.

Some cases have been documented of babies being accidentally smothered at night, but most have been in extreme circumstances where the mother was semi-conscious, drunk, or under the influence of narcotic drugs. Experience shows that both the mother and father, when sleeping normally, will be very alert for any sound or movement by an infant sleeping in the same bed.

All the same, because of reports in recent decades of "Sudden Infant Death Syndrome," various guidelines have been issued for families where there is a wish or need to sleep with a baby (see box below).

We must conclude that there is normally no risk in sharing one's bed with a baby if you feel that it is the solution you prefer. Ensure, however, that the baby is lying securely, where it cannot fall out of the bed.

In cold regions or during a hard winter, it may be difficult to keep the baby sufficiently covered if it has to share a cover with two large adults. The best solution is a warm sleeping suit of the sort used for children who tend to kick away sheets, blankets, and any other form of cover. One other question relates to the parents' sex life – that may prove somewhat tricky with a small child sharing the bed. But puzzles are made to be solved, and this one is surely capable of a solution (Figure 6.2).

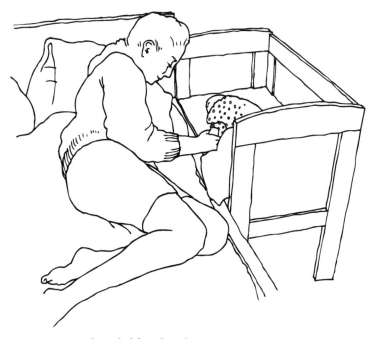

Figure 6.2. *Estonian side-car bed for safe co-sleeping.*

Source: Photo by Ingerid Helsing Almaas. Used with permission.

Apart from that, console yourself with the thought that you are not the only parent to have shared a bed with an impossible little wriggling and kicking specimen of humanity. Fortunately, by the time the child gets into its teens, it will usually return to its own bed.

WARNING

DON'T TAKE THE BABY INTO YOUR WATERBED, SOFA, or collapsible folding bed. It is possible that in this type of bed, with its uneven and varying support and motion, the baby might end up in a position in which it is not able to breathe.

SOME OF THE CONDITIONS FOR A SAFE FAMILY BED:

- THE BABY SLEEPS ON ITS BACK.

- The baby has its own small and light duvet, eiderdown, or other cover.

- The baby does not get too hot.

- None of the co-sleeping parents are smokers.

- None of the co-sleeping parents are under the influence of alcohol or drugs.

- The bed is wide, the mattress is hard and even, and the baby cannot roll out of the bed or into a gap.

FAMILY BED EVIDENCE: FOR OR AGAINST?

WHAT DOES THE EVIDENCE SHOW?

Summary by Professor Helen Ball, Durham University

- Benefits of mother-infant sleep contact to breastfeeding initiation are very clear.

- Evidence is accumulating regarding the benefits of mother-infant sleep contact on breastfeeding duration.

- Risks of bed-sharing to breastfed infants are disputed and no clear evidence is available.

- Known hazards associated with bed-sharing are related to specific dangerous circumstances- alcohol, drugs, smoking, and sofas.

- Breastfeeding is now recommended by SIDS organizations as a means of reducing SIDS risk.

- No 'one size fits all' recommendation is appropriate.

(Ball, 2011)

The Child That Turns Night into Day

A nursing baby with unlimited access to its mother's breast is likely to feed very frequently, but it will tend to take a break of several hours once every 24 hours or so. The parents, understandably, will hope that the pause is taken during the nighttime hours, preferably sometime between midnight and six in the morning. Unfortunately, it is not unlikely that the baby will choose to sleep in the daytime and be active, wide awake, and hungry at night. If, after a while, this becomes intolerable, as it will for many a parent, one can try to persuade the baby to adjust its habits. This is possible if you tackle it the right way. Wait until you notice your baby snatching forty winks in the course of the day, and then try to wake it cautiously, preferably when it is in the phase of light sleep, with its eyes rolled upwards and perhaps all sorts of expressions flitting across its face. In this phase of sleep, it can more easily be wakened than when it is sleeping deeply. Don't be brutal - avoid scratching the soles of the feet or pinching the cheek – it is much better to massage the soles of the feet, change the diaper (nappy), or undress the baby a little and put it to the breast now and again until you are ready to go to bed. After a few days of such treatment, your baby will, one hopes, appreciate what you are trying to do, and will choose to take its rest period at a time which fits the family's schedule better (Figure 6.3).

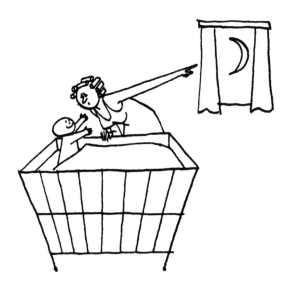

Figure 6.3. *"Isn't it time you went to sleep?"*

Source: Cartoon by Ellen Wilhelmsen. Used with permission.

And then, if you can, keep things quiet at night. Some babies sleep lightly. They are easily awakened by the slightest noise, and after that, they don't easily fall asleep again.

Marianne's Cozy Breastfeeding Corner

Here is a tip that, if you can find room for it in your house, you shouldn't resist. Marianne is an experienced breastfeeding peer supporter who is also the mother of twins. Particularly if you have twins, she recommends that somewhere in a corner, you create a little den of your own, just for yourself and the baby or babies. All you need is a sofa, bed, or large comfortable armchair, with plenty of cushions that no one is allowed to remove, but that you can rearrange as you need them. Within reach, you should have *everything* you could possibly need during long breastfeeding sessions. This might include: a thermos with warm or cold drinks, some small towels or serviettes, a roll of tissue paper, a pencil, the telephone or mobile/cell phone, just a few things to chew on, and anything else you want. If you're feeling bright and lively early in the morning, you can outfit your corner for the whole day, including healthy meals and snacks to keep you going, not forgetting plenty of ready-to-eat fruit. All part of taking good care of yourself – if you have the right food on hand, then you will, hopefully, want to eat, too!

Chapter 7.
SOME RATHER SPECIAL SITUATIONS

From time to time, situations arise that call for a special approach. You may never encounter them, but we must take a look at several of them because they can be important when it comes to breastfeeding.

TWINS – AND MORE!

Some mothers of twins regard breastfeeding as the simplest choice – and entirely straightforward - while others find it a tremendous challenge. What is more, twins are often delivered before term, which means that breastfeeding may get off to a rather unusual start. If it is necessary to stimulate your milk production by pumping, it may be helpful to try "double pumping," which will save you time (Auerbach, 1990; Jones, Dimmock, & Spencer, 2001). We describe the method fully in Chapter 10, but not everyone finds it suitable.

One Breast Each, Or Equal Shares Each Side?

Should each twin have its own particular breast, or should you alternate from time to time? In fact, it doesn't matter – both methods are effective, and you can take your choice. The many animal species that deliver multiple offspring provide no clue as to what might be best – some do it one way, some the other, and yet others change around all the time. The only valid reason for keeping a twin at the same breast could be that the milk glands react individually. If a breast always encounters the same twin, it will produce precisely what that twin needs. Should the two children have markedly different demands, the worst that can happen is that your breasts may look a little lopsided for a while, but that is hardly dramatic. In Chapter 3, we described the case of the sow with her large litter and each piglet jealously occupying its own particular nipple. That makes it possible to arrange things in an orderly manner – one knows precisely who belongs where!

Breastmilk Only or Supplementation for Two or More Babies?

Exclusive breastfeeding is the term used for feeding babies at the breast only, without supplementation (other than vitamins/minerals).

Mixed feeding, on the other hand, means that breastmilk is supplemented, either with solid food or with a breastmilk substitute, depending on how old the baby is. There is no firm rule as to whether a mother of twins or triplets will be able to feed them adequately at the breast alone; much depends on the circumstances. Are the babies providing an efficient stimulus to the breasts? Are you getting enough sleep? How much daytime help do you have in the home? Being motivated is important, but not enough; together with your partner you have to discover what is reasonably possible. Breastfeeding is splendid and time-saving when it runs smoothly, but if you find yourself struggling with it, then it can be exhausting, and with two mouths or more to feed, all the more so.

Do I Feed One Baby at a Time or Both Together?

The answer to this question, too, depends on various factors, such as the babies' personality and feeding habits, and what you and the family find to be the simplest approach. Don't make a problem out of it in advance; there is no need to decide before you start breastfeeding. You will soon find out whether it suits you better to feed the babies at the same time or alternately. You may, for example, discover that it is convenient to feed both at the same time when you are alone in the home, but when your partner or a caregiver is with you, it suits you better to feed the babies in turn. If you feed just one at a time, it will be easier to discover the best positioning, without having to fit the other baby into the available space. You can also devote all your attention to the one baby you have at the breast. In the past, when professional breastfeeders were employed, many of them routinely nursed two babies at a time, finding that this was a sure method to stimulate the milk production to its maximum. The total amount of stimulation received by the breasts will be appreciably more with two babies at the breast at the same time than if you feed only a single baby each time.

If twins have been born prematurely, they may need more help when breastfeeding. In that case, it is sensible to begin by putting only one baby at a time to the breast, so it can receive all the attention, help, and support it needs. If, on the other hand, only one of the two is a weak feeder, it may be better to feed both at the same time: the weaker of the two will benefit from the stimulus to the let-down reflex provided by the stronger. It is true that feeding both babies at once saves time, but it requires that at least one of the two is easy to wake and reasonably flexible about feeding times. On the other hand, some mothers of twins have recalled that they felt they had relatively little contact with their babies when feeding them together, sensing at some moments that they were functioning as little more than a glorified milk bank.

Two Self-Regulating Babies

Like all other young infants, newborn twins will need to come to the breast eight to 12 times a day. However, the exact frequency varies from one baby to another, and it is not likely that two twins, even when identical, will make precisely the same choices as to when they want to feed. Some parents of twins decide to face the challenge of letting each of the two choose its own feeding times, and live in more or less constant chaos; others prefer more planning and discipline and try to get the two to follow a compatible rhythm. As in so many other matters, it is up to you as parents to decide what suits you best. The advantage of self-regulation or on-demand feeding is that the milk production adjusts itself more or less automatically to the child's needs. If you decide to plan the feeds according to the clock, you need to ensure that the breasts are stimulated sufficiently often to provide for the children's constantly increasing need for milk. In any case, it is necessary to feed at least eight times daily, with intermediate feeds when needed. It is of most importance to feed often the first two to three weeks to boost your milk production, after that you can try to feed less frequently if this is what you wish or need to be able to survive breastfeeding twins.

Positioning of Twins

There are various good positions for twins when feeding simultaneously at the breast. Look at Figures 7.1, 7.2, and 7.3 to find out which positioning would suit you and your babies best.

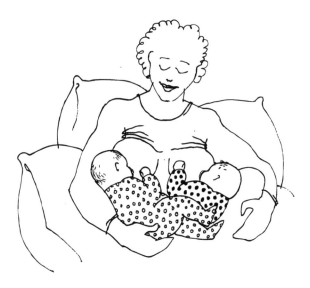

Figure 7.1. *Breastfeeding small twins: Cross-positioning*

Source: Drawing by Ingerid Helsing Almaas. Used with permission.

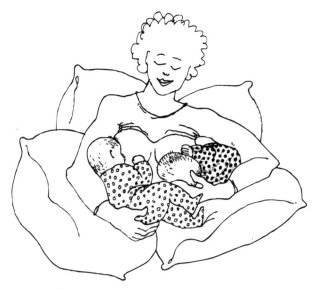

Figure 7.2. *Breastfeeding twins: One in the under the arm position, the other traditionally placed in the Madonna position.*

Source: Drawing by Ingerid Helsing Almaas. Used with permission.

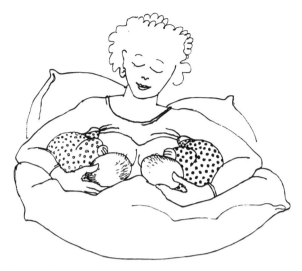

Figure 7.3. *Breastfeeding twins: Both in under the arm position.*

Source: Drawing by Ingerid Helsing Almaas. Used with permission.

BREASTFEEDING MORE THAN TWO BABIES

If you have more than two babies, there are some added complications. With only two breasts, there will still be at least one mouth too many to allow for simultaneous feeding. Exclusive breastfeeding of triplets places very special demands on the mother, and where possible on the father as well. Those who have experienced the situation readily confirm that the entire process of bringing up three offspring – from the time of breastfeeding and onwards – is a great deal easier to manage with strict planning and firm discipline. One common and effective solution is to have two babies at the breast simultaneously, while the third is given expressed breastmilk from a bottle. It may take some agility, but shortage of milk is not usually the problem. Many mothers with triplets and quadruplets breastfeed exclusively for months. What one *must* have is reliable help in the home, so that washing, cooking, changing diapers, and the like do not fall on the breastfeeding mother's shoulders.

Again: Learn From the Experience of Others

We would seriously suggest that if you are among those who have been blessed with a multiple pregnancy, you sit down as early as possible to plan ahead, ideally with another couple who have experienced the same venture. Wherever possible, you will need to rationalize all sorts of necessary activities, ranging from the various tasks involved in running the home to all the aspects of childcare. Quite apart from the breastfeeding support groups, you will find that there are associations for parents of twins and for other multiples, and they will be happy to establish contacts for you and provide sensible advice. Fathers play an essential role. The hospital staff will need to involve the father of twins right from the very first hours, so he will be well prepared to support the mother with positioning and a dozen other essential tasks once the family leaves the hospital On the other hand, one mother bringing up triplets on her own found that breastfeeding was the easiest way to cope with her life as a mother of three.

CESAREAN SECTION

Some women who have been delivered by cesarean section may find that their milk production is a little delayed (Dewey, Nommsen-Rivers, Heinig, & Cohen, 2003; Odent, 2004). This may be because the baby is put to the breast later (after the surgery has been completed), because the baby is tired and those very necessary milking reflexes are a bit confused, or simply because immediately after surgery breastfeeding sessions are likely to be less frequent than usual. If the cesarean has been planned, you can tell the staff in advance that you would like to have the baby at the breast as soon as possible after delivery. Provided you are awake, you should be able to hold the baby in your arms skin-to-skin, while you are still in the operating room (Norwegian Resource Centre for Breastfeeding Rikshospitalet, 2008).

Your baby may be a little drowsy. If that is the case, just be patient with the baby and yourself while the effect of the sedation wears off. Allow plenty of time for the initial skin-to-skin contact to take effect before you start trying to breastfeed; it will help to wake up the baby's milking reflexes. If you are drowsy (or perhaps not yet even awake), it is a good idea for the father to place the baby against his naked chest as soon as it is born (Erlandsson, Dsilna, Fagerberg, & Christensson, 2007).

Positioning After a Cesarean

After you have experienced a cesarean section, you will find that certain breastfeeding positions are much more comfortable for you than others. We have come to recommend the position shown below (see Figure 7.4). This proves to be particularly useful, especially during the first few days after delivery, since it means that there is no need for you to turn your body from one side to the other in bed when changing breasts.

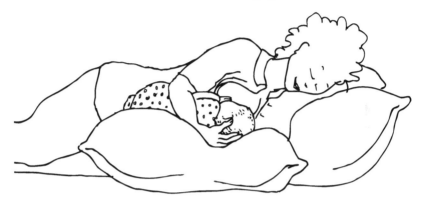

Figure 7.4. *With the help of a pillow, the baby can reach either breast while lying on the same side of you.*

Source: Drawing by Ingerid Helsing Almaas. Used with permission.

After a cesarean, you will certainly need extra help in the home for some time. A helpful and caring partner, if he has the opportunity to spend sufficient time away from work, can manage most of what is needed – otherwise a friend or relative or domestic helper may be able to assist you. Breastfeeding will make life easier for you since there will be no need for all the work and movement involved in bottle-feeding; instead you will be obliged to take that very necessary rest several times a day when you sit or lie down to feed. Better to lie than sit at this time – you need to relax.

WIND, BURPING, AND FLATULENCE

Experienced mothers will assure you that breastfed babies pass less wind than those who have been exposed to the bottle. This could well be true, for the breast (unlike the feeding bottle) contains no air. All the same, a baby will always swallow a certain amount of air that will end up in its stomach. If your baby is often troubled by gas in the stomach, it may be sensible to try holding it upright during feeding, so the air escapes upwards rather than accumulating in the stomach. Whether this is truly effective, however, no one seems to know.

Doctors working in tropical countries have noticed that in those areas where breastfeeding is customary, mothers are rarely concerned about problems of wind and flatulence. They have suggested that this is attributable to breastfeeding positions: the mother, as a rule, lies flat when breastfeeding, and this might be the most "natural" position to adopt (Jelliffe & Jelliffe, 1978).

As you will see, opinions truly differ, and on this, as on so many other matters, you can best choose the solution that with trial and error seems to suit you and your baby best.

Sometimes it happens that a baby regurgitates a certain amount of milk after breastfeeding – it may look as if the whole meal has been thrown up. It may look worrisome, but it is rarely as serious as it appears. If your baby's very small stomach gets too full, it will promptly return the excess. And spilt milk often appears to be much more than it really is: just try pouring half a cupful of milk on the kitchen floor, and you find it looks like a pond. What happens with regurgitation is simply, as we have said, that the few grams of breastmilk that exceeded the stomach's capacity are returned, together with some gastric juice and saliva – it is really not as dramatic as it looks.

VOMITING

All babies vomit now and again, but if your baby is doing it very often and in large amounts, it would be wise to check the weight gain. Provided it is normal, there is no reason for concern. Only if the baby is failing to gain weight should you ask your clinic or your pediatrician to take a look to be sure nothing is wrong.

A PACIFIER (OR DUMMY)?

If you have a baby with a particular need for oral gratification (to put it simply: your baby just enjoys doing something with its mouth, especially sucking) you may want to give it something else to suck on instead of your breast –for example, a pacifier. Another option is that the baby makes its own choice and simply sucks on its fingers. Dentists have contrasting opinions about finger- or thumb-sucking, and the habit should certainly not last for more than a few years. Those small fingers have the advantage over a pacifier that they don't fall on dirty floors and demand constant washing and boiling. Nor are they lodged in the mouth all day because the baby wants to use its hands for other things. Finally, they are always available when the baby seeks a spot of comfort – and a pacifier may not be.

One final problem with the pacifier is that it is readily over-used, which can mean that the breast itself is under-used and receives too little stimulation to perform its task properly. Once breastfeeding is well established (i.e., the first month) and free of problems, you may use a pacifier if you need or want to, but use it in moderation. Using a pacifier has been thought to reduce the risk of Sudden Infant Death Syndrome (Smith & Riordan, 2010), but it is still advisable to avoid using it during the first month, so as not to risk inhibiting milk production.

WHAT IS COLIC?

Some infants develop attacks of violent panic-like screaming, during which they are entirely disconsolate. Some attacks are more serious than others. In the most severe instances, the baby screams piercingly, its face is contorted as if in pain, and its legs are drawn up against its abdomen. After a while, the child falls asleep from sheer exhaustion, only to reawaken a little later and start screaming once more.

These attacks occur most often in the evening between five and ten o'clock. As a rule, they cease when the baby is about three months old, though they can persist until later. For these reasons, the condition is sometimes known as "evening colic" or "three month colic," but this does nothing to explain the cause, that essentially remains unknown. In medicine, the term "infantile colic" is usually applied to cases where an apparently healthy baby suffers these attacks of screaming for three or four hours daily, occurring at least three times a week, with some quiet periods of up to three weeks.

The fact that the attacks vary so much in severity could suggest that the children concerned are reacting to various triggers. Often there is some rumbling in the abdomen, suggesting that the baby is suffering from wind, and if the wind is passed, this seems to give a degree of relief. However, it is quite possible that this accumulation of air in the stomach is a consequence rather than a cause of the screaming - a typical example of the conundrum as to whether the chicken or the egg came first.

Cigarette smoking may give your baby colic (Sondergaard, Henriksen, Obel, & Wisborg, 2001): try to reduce or quit. However, a whole series of other possible causes of colic attacks have been proposed – immaturity of the baby, excessively "strong" (or excessively weak) milk, too long an interval (or too short an interval!) between feeds, nervousness on the mother's part, the baby's feeling of loneliness, an over-active milk let-down reflex – and a great many more. There seem to be as many theories as there are scientists qualified to propound them. In addition: colic is not an issue at all in some cultures, especially in countries where the babies are carried close to the mother most of the time.

So What Can You Do?

There are some things you can do to comfort your colicky little baby, while you count the weeks until the misery passes. Be prepared for the fact that you will need your evenings for carrying and comforting the baby, and plan the rest of your schedule – including your own mealtimes – to take account of that. It may seem odd to take a walk in the evening air with the pram or with the baby in a sling, but that may be just what is needed to enjoy an hour of peace and quiet. Make sure that the baby has plenty of body contact. Above all – do whatever seems to help your baby most - there is no rule that works for every child, but experience shows that there are quite a range of alternatives, each one helping a particular type of individual. Look at the menu of possibilities in the box below.

BREASTFEEDING AND COLIC

It is possible that in some instances colic is due to an over-active milk let-down reflex. In such cases, the baby may seem restless at the breast, fidgeting and releasing its hold on the breast to avoid choking on the fast-flowing milk – sometimes you can hear a sound like the milk hitting the bottom of a steel bucket. If it looks as if this might be your baby's problem, try lying on your back to breastfeed, so the baby feels more in control of the whole process, or alternatively hold the baby in a more upright position against your chest when you are sitting. If none of these things help, try expressing some of your milk before a feed, so it is less inclined to shoot out too forcefully. If you are really letting your baby regulate the rate of feeding, allow it to finish at the first breast before changing to the other (Newman & Pitman, 2000a).

COMFORTING A COLICKY BABY – SOME THINGS YOU CAN DO

- Most children are calmed if they are rocked or carried. Try using one of those shawls that are designed for carrying babies.

- Try some very gentle rocking in a cradle – but don't shake the baby up.

- See if it helps to hold the baby differently – many a child benefits from lying on mother's lap face downwards while she strokes its back calmly.

- With some babies, light massage over the stomach or over the whole body seems to be helpful.

- Most babies calm down when they are taken out in the pram.

- If giving the breast seems to help, do that whenever it is needed.

- Some colicky children seem to be reacting to the fact that so much is going on around them – try a little less light and see what the effect is of leaving the baby undisturbed for longer periods.

- Other babies react well to monotonous, repetitive sounds, like those associated with the vacuum cleaner, the washing machine, or a trip in the car.

- Some mothers have found that things go better if they avoid milk products at this time – we discuss this below.

- **If you smoke, try to reduce or quit smoking.**

- Have a chat with other mothers whose babies have colic – and if they can offer you any help or advice, accept it gratefully.

- But don't expect any medicines to help – unfortunately they won't.

Dairy Milk Protein via Your Breastmilk?

Some mothers say they notice that their babies experience colicky pain when they have been eating or drinking dairy milk products. One Swedish investigator estimates that about 25% of babies with colic prove to be sensitive to the protein in cows' milk (Lindberg, 1999). If you think this might be your baby's problem, you can carry out a little experiment to see if it really is the case. For a whole week, avoid all dairy products in your diet. This will mean cutting out not just milk, skimmed milk, and cheese, but all other foods that contain milk – and they can include sausages, sauces, soups, and many other items – look on the label, where you will find a list of the ingredients. And if, after avoiding all these things for a week, the colic is still there, you at least know that you can safely eat or drink these foods again. If, on the other hand, the baby seems to have less colic, you may recheck everything by cautiously taking a little milk again and seeing if the problem returns. If it does, you have probably found at least a partial cause. It's well worth talking to a nutritionist or a dietician to get reliable advice on a milk-free diet. Finally, although experts still disagree on other possible causes of colic – and how to treat it, we may note that various substances other than milk can cause allergies and possibly colic in a few susceptible individuals – including eggs, nuts, wheat, soya, and fish (Garrison & Christakis, 2000).

It's Not Your Fault!

If you do get the feeling at a given moment that having a baby to care for is just about the worst thing that ever happened to you, *do not feel guilty about that.* You would not be the first mother to be driven to despair and fury at a moment when nothing seems to go right. Just do not let your fury boil over onto your baby or yourself. Give the baby to someone else you can trust for calming and carrying and find something to do that will work off that furious energy. Take a very quick walk, perhaps? Or do something you really enjoy!

It *is* wretched to find yourself dealing with a colicky baby. You will probably feel helpless, humbled, and rejected all at the same time. It can be rough to maintain your parental pride for weeks on end when you are faced with a baby that is clearly not enjoying life, and that you don't seem able to comfort, however hard you try.

You may even find it difficult to imagine that the misery will ever pass – even though you can be assured that it will, generally by the time your baby is 12 weeks old or so.

Breastfeeding associations and health clinics all produce useful materials about colic. But more important than reading brochures, talk to your health visitor, a lactation consultant, or a peer support mother about your struggles and your feelings. You may also find support groups for parents, a help line, or support on the internet.

IF YOUR BREASTFED BABY IS ADMITTED TO A HOSPITAL

If a baby has to be admitted to hospital while it is breastfeeding, you will find that many hospitals allow parents to stay with it, 24 hours a day, living and sleeping together. Article 9 of the U.N. Convention on the Rights of the Child stresses the undesirability of separating a child from its parents where this can be avoided (United Nations, 1990).

In some countries, such as Norway, there is a legal parental right to stay with their sick baby (Ministry of Health and Care Services, 2000). A hospital stay is the worst possible time for weaning – it can be upsetting enough for a small child to find itself in unfamiliar and perhaps forbidding surroundings, and much worse if it is to be deprived of its mother's breast at the same time. Even a somewhat older child, over six months of age, that is already receiving some solid food alongside breastmilk may well benefit from going back to exclusive breastfeeding for as long as it is in the hospital. Once it is well on the road to recovery, it can go back to mixed feeding and receive solid food again.

If a sick child does not manage to feed at the breast, it may be necessary to develop your skill in hand expression or to use a pump. Remember to express your milk as many times in a day as you would normally have given the breast (see Chapter 10). The milk can be given to the baby in various ways – these are described in Chapter 8.

MENSTRUATION

Some women find that their menstrual periods do not return as long as they continue to breastfeed, even for as much as a year, while others see their periods reappear within a few weeks of delivery. Whenever it happens, you are likely to experience a slight drop in your milk production for a few days while you menstruate. This can be frustrating if you are one of those people who tend to feel miserable during a period, and especially if your baby also becomes miserable when the flow of milk weakens for a while. It has been suggested that breastmilk tastes different during menstruation, and certainly some children seem to be reluctant to take the nipple at this time. Take comfort in the fact that it is a very transient problem – after a few days your milk production will be just as plentiful and attractive as it was before. We should add that this is by no means a common problem; many mothers notice no difference at all in breastfeeding during their period.

Can You Become Pregnant Again While Breastfeeding?

Before mechanical and chemical means of contraception were introduced, people had for generations used "natural methods" to prevent unwanted pregnancies. One of those methods was based on the centuries-old observation that women generally did not resume menstruation after pregnancy so long as they continued to breastfeed. Many mothers continued to feed for as long as possible if they wished to have no more children – a fact which, at times, seems to have upset those politicians who wanted to ensure an increase in the population. On occasion, prolonged breastfeeding for this reason was deemed to be illegal (see Chapter 13).

When one looks at the population as a whole, it indeed proves to be the case that women who are breastfeeding are much less likely to become pregnant than those who are not. On a world population basis, it is a fact that breastfeeding prevents a greater number of pregnancies than all the contraceptives currently known to man. That naturally does not prove that the method is an *entirely* reliable form of contraception, and if you are anxious to know how far its reliability extends, you need to know more. This *"lactation amenorrhea method"* (LAM) has been studied scientifically, and what emerges is that it can indeed be reasonably trustworthy (for example, as reliable as a modern intrauterine device) provided certain conditions are met (see below).

Breastfeeding as a Contraceptive Method During the First Six Months

Based on what is now known, various authorities have made official statements about the reliability of breastfeeding as a means of contraception, and they are pretty consistent. We may quote here, as an example, the clear advice that was given by a group of specialists in Norway in October 1996. They concluded, based on global evidence, that breastfeeding could be regarded as a satisfactory form of contraception provided three conditions were met:

1. The baby is not more than six months old.

2. The baby is being breastfed exclusively by its mother, also at night.

3. The mother's menstruation has not yet returned, even though there may have been a little bleeding from the vagina during the first six weeks after delivery, there is no question of monthly periods.

If all these conditions are met, the chance of pregnancy occurring is very low – less than 2%. The mother should be breastfeeding at night to prevent a long interval between feeds. If babies sleep continuously for many hours at night, the interval may be too long between feeds to suppress ovulation. It also seems that the effect is most marked if feeding sessions are frequent; if they are not, the sessions should be fairly long (Ramos, Kennedy, & Visness, 1996; Van Look, 1996; Vekemans, 1997).

What About Hormonal Contraceptives?

A potential difficulty with the contraceptive "pill" is that, as a rule, it contains two female hormones – a gestagen (synthetic progesterone) and an estrogen, and the latter is capable of reducing milk production (see Chapter 1). For this reason, doctors advise breastfeeding mothers not to use these contraceptives while they are feeding if they can possibly be avoided. There is an alternative, the minipill, containing only a gestagen. We could add that all these substances do pass into breastmilk, but only in very tiny amounts that can do no harm to the baby.

PREGNANCY AND BREASTFEEDING

If you should become pregnant again while you are breastfeeding, you will probably notice that your milk production becomes a little less, but there is no reason to hesitate – simply continue to breastfeed as long as you need.

Some mothers find that their breasts become more tender and their nipples become more sensitive when they are pregnant. In some cases, the whole process becomes so uncomfortable that they cannot continue to breastfeed. Oxytocin, the hormone that causes the uterus to contract during birthing, can also cause contractions in pregnancy, especially during breastfeeding. Any mother who from past experience has reason to think that she may deliver prematurely should look out for this sign. If you sense that the pregnant uterus tends to tighten up when you breastfeed, you should talk to your midwife or doctor, since it may be a reason to wean the baby off the breast.

If you have decided to wean your baby in preparation for the arrival of a new sibling, it is wise to do so in good time. One can readily imagine that a baby who has enjoyed its mother's undivided attention at the breast for a long period will find it hard to accept the loss of this unique privilege with the arrival of a younger brother or sister. However, if the two births are not so very far apart, there is much to be said for continuing to feed the first baby after the arrival of a second, breastfeeding the two "in tandem," as it is called. Remember, however, that around the time of the second delivery, the breasts will again start to supply colostrum and "early milk," so be sure to give the younger child priority at the breast.

YOU CAN START BREASTFEEDING ALL OVER AGAIN

You may feel that things are getting hopeless if the milk fails to come in, or your baby hasn't started to feed properly or get on good terms with the breast, so you lie there in hospital with no milk, surrounded by other mothers with more than enough. There is no reason to give up, even if you are sent home with the message that it's time to start giving your baby supplements.

And at this point, we come to yet one more golden – and very important – rule of breastfeeding:

Golden Rule Number 12

It's never too late to start breastfeeding!

Even if weeks have passed since the delivery and you are home, you can perfectly well start breastfeeding all over again, and see whether it might not go much better at the second attempt. You'll need some help from a wise and experienced guide, if possible on the spot, but otherwise at the other end of a telephone line. It should be someone who has been faced with such a situation before. You'll also need some support on the home front from your health visitor or from nursing staff if you're still in the hospital.

In almost every country, you will find mother-to-mother breastfeeding support groups, Lactation Consultants, or the trained staff of Baby-Friendly hospitals who can provide the experienced help you need (see the Appendix at the back of this book). Once you are sitting face to face with one of these helpers, talk to her frankly about how you experienced the birthing process – that may bring all sorts of feelings out into the open that you need to air with someone wise and experienced. It's also good to set some goals, so you can measure your progress as you solve the problem.

The First Time Around, Your Baby Just Didn't Get It...

Half sit in your bed and get *really* comfortable and relaxed, with lots of pillows supporting your back. Make sure you have something to drink within reach, and visit the restroom first, so you don't find a call of nature interrupting a promising breastfeed halfway through. Next, lay your baby down, unclothed, right against your stomach, a little below your exposed breast, just as you ideally lay with him or her immediately after the birth. Now, the baby has a new chance to follow that whole process of seeking around and crawling, ever closer to the breast, and finally latching on to it – just as it should have happened in the delivery room, but for some reason didn't work out. It's not possible to guess how long it might take – anywhere from half an hour to a number of hours, to days, or even longer. You should try at least 45 minutes to begin with.

Never try to force the pace; your baby will need time to discover and recognize on its own all the phases that lead up to successful breastfeeding – crawling, seeking, reaching, focusing, struggling, searching, not quite succeeding, then searching again... It is an exciting process that is prone to elicit strong feelings both in the baby and its mother. Once the baby succeeds and reaches the breast, it will have laid a sound basis for understanding what the process is all about. And if the baby should fall asleep on the way, the road ahead may be clearer once it wakes up. A few babies grow restless, impatient, and angry on the way, and if you sense this is happening, be prepared to provide a little comfort and perhaps a little milk (preferably using a cup) to help the adventure along. You have to remember to stimulate the milk production by hand-milking the breast or using a pump, and collecting the milk for cup feeding. Read, too, the true story in Chapter 8 of the baby that was started on the bottle – and its mother's account of how the baby found its way back to the breast. You may find the website www.biologicalnurturing.com helpful. Suzanne Colson's concept of "biological nurturing" strongly supports these ideas.

Relactation

Relactation means that lactation, which has been "shut down," is opened up again, using the principles and practice mentioned above. A lot of quiet time and a lot of skin-to-skin contact are paramount. Offer the breast as often as possible and avoid the use of a pacifier/dummy (WHO/CAH, 1998).

A very helpful gadget in this situation is a nursing supplementer – see Chapter 10.

When Breastfeeding Has Not Been Anticipated - The Case of Adopted Babies

Mary, though married for several years, had remained childless. She adopted Charlotte, who was two months old. Since Mary had read a great deal about skin-to-skin contact and the fact that both mother and child had a need to be physically close to one another, she took Charlotte to her breast whenever she began to cry, but also after each bottle-feed. Charlotte obviously enjoyed being so close to her new mother's breast and tried to suckle, which Mary encouraged. She had never intended to breastfeed her new baby, simply regarding such closeness as comforting and pleasurable. Imagine her astonishment when after a few weeks, she noticed that "something" was coming from her nipples. Charlotte, for her part, was now taking a third less from her feeding bottle. "Surely I'm not producing milk – or am I?" she asked when she wrote to me (Elisabet) for advice. But it was indeed milk, for that is precisely what the mammary glands deliver. Since she had never in her whole life been pregnant, the glandular tissue had not developed fully, but the milk glands had sprung quietly into action and were producing milk. After eight or nine months, Charlotte weaned herself from the breast. Like many other children, she had lost her fascination for it.

You may prepare even more for breastfeeding an adopted baby by taking tablets to stimulate your hormone production and using a breastpump to stimulate the milk production. Get in touch with a lactation consultant or a mother-to-mother support group to get more information.

EAST, WEST, HOME IS BEST

Some mothers immediately feel better when they return to well-trusted surroundings. You may recall that you have friends or acquaintances nearby who have experience in breastfeeding and whom you can ask for advice. If you don't, ask your local breastfeeding group – check the list at the back of this book to find the address of someone who can help and advise you. These groups of volunteers or professionals know very well what it is like to come home from the maternity ward – most of the requests for help come from mothers in precisely that situation. Lactation consultants, as well as health workers specializing in postnatal problems, know very well how easily little puzzles can develop into big problems, and they are the best possible people to help solve the puzzles – or prevent them from arising in the first place. That is why we quote golden rule number 13 at this point in the Chapter.

Golden Rule Number 13

No breastfeeding problem is so trivial that you cannot ask for help in solving it.

Just bear that in mind!

FEAR OF CLOSENESS - SEXUAL ABUSE OR RAPE

We know something, though not a great deal, about how women who have been exposed to sexual abuse or rape experience breastfeeding, but there is every reason to believe that birth, breastfeeding, and even close contact with the nursing staff can spark strong reactions (Kendall-Tackett, 2007). Sexual abuse of children is still with us, and it shows no signs of disappearing. In recent years, it has been much more openly discussed, but we are still far from understanding what it means to its victims, how we can best provide them with help and support, or how to alleviate feelings of suffering or shame. These words from a mother suffering from sexual abuse gives a little insight into the hard and difficult feelings after her delivery of a baby boy – and how in the end she managed to breastfeed him for eight months. SunnyBoy and his mother have become an invincible team.

The Battle for SunnyBoy

I have just been going through a very painful delivery when the midwife says, "It's a boy!" I feel a flood of happiness, for I already have two girls. I take him in my arms and whisper, "Hello, my little friend."

After a while, the midwife asks me to take my little one to the breast. I know that my fresh milk is his best safeguard against infection, so I do what she says. I feel him suckling and swallowing. He becomes calm.

The next day, everything goes well. But then, when I wake up on the third day, I feel completely out of balance, and I am desperately tired. The nursing staff heard me crying, and they hurry in. 'We'll help you,' they say – so I take off my blouse to try again. And then suddenly, I feel ashamed, ashamed of my nakedness, yet without understanding the reason for my shame. A midwife and a nurse are bending over me, taking hold of my breasts to put my SunnyBoy in place. They can't know what is happening to me—a sudden flashback to something fearful that once happened – people leaning over my bed, taking hold of my body. They try again and again, but there is no milk, and SunnyBoy is screaming for food.

Then, one day, after a battle in the hospital and three weeks at home, SunnyBoy manages to latch on to my breast, and he drinks and drinks until he has had his fill. Now I begin to think the battle is over, but I'm mistaken...

Yes, now I can breastfeed him every day, but that just reawakens those memories of what once happened to me. Every time he cries, he is demanding that I take off my clothes, demanding to lie up against my naked body. In anguish I write a little note:

> *Can it be true that SunnyBoy has the right to demand that I take off my clothes at any hour of the day or night? Does he have the right to lie there and suck at my body? It all feels as if I am being brushed aside...*

I feel a battle going on between my feelings and my intellect. The feelings tell me that he is a boy, but my brain is telling me that he is simply a baby who needs his mother's milk. Now the battle is coming to a climax – every time that he cries because he is hungry, I find myself crying, too. With SunnyBoy up against my breast, I see my violators pressing up against me, and I feel all the fearful things they did to my body.

Now I have been breastfeeding for three months, and all the time I have been experiencing a flood of tears. My violators have been somewhere around me all the time, haunting me like phantoms from a dark past. But I know that I must fight this battle for SunnyBoy. The violators must not get the upper hand, stealing from SunnyBoy the best food he will ever know. They violated me, but they shall not get their hands on the next generation! And suddenly I know that I can win the struggle! I have triumphed, and in my victory, I know that my violators have lost the battle. From then on, I no longer weep as I breastfeed. The feeding sessions become times for cuddling and loving, for both of us. He is putting on more weight, developing so well. My mother-in-law is tremendously proud of him, for it is so long ago that they had a boy in the family. SunnyBoy and I have become an invincible team.

Chapter 8.

IF THE BABY IS OFF TO A SLOW START OR IS ILL

We must take a look at some of the unusual situations in which a mother may find herself confronted if her baby has experienced a difficult start to life – or is perhaps ill. Most of these challenges can be solved, given the necessary understanding, experience, time, and patience. Above all, the wholehearted support and help that can be provided by competent and experienced staff, family, and friends is necessary.

WHEN JOY IS TEMPERED BY CONCERN

In this situation, breastfeeding arrives at a moment in most women's life when a whole series of other changes are likely to be taking place. Not uncommonly, a mother will be unhappy or apprehensive about various things that did not turn out quite as she had expected – unanticipated problems, perhaps at the time of delivery, a sick baby, or a birth that came upon her all too soon. She may feel that she is not experiencing the joy of motherhood as she thinks she has observed it among other women and had expected to encounter herself, or perhaps she will believe she lacks motherly feelings.

Psychologists have taught us how strongly our thoughts can influence our feelings. If your expectations that birthing was going to be a tremendously creative experience haven't been fulfilled, or if the baby has problems at the start of life and needs to be taken to a special care nursery, it is not easy to think positively. But try! Just think about all those things that you already *have* achieved as a new mother. You have provided your baby with the love, the closeness, and the breastmilk that it needs. And even a baby that is ill or has arrived too soon has massive resources of its own to ensure that it will soon be on the right road. Notice every little step ahead and rejoice as you see your baby's personality shining through.

Support and Encouragement

As in so many other situations, it is a great help to share experiences and setbacks. Talk to other parents who have gone through the same things as you have. Any mother who knows that her baby needs special care or whose baby is finding it difficult to get a proper start in life needs someone who can provide encouragement and help in facing these things optimistically. Parents who have experienced a preterm birth or whose baby is not healthy often experience a sense of loneliness. If that is your experience, it can be a great help to talk openly about your feelings – and no one will show more understanding than a mother who has been through the same experience herself. And once you have moved ahead to better times, do remember to share your experiences with still newer mothers who will need *your* support. Take a look at the addresses of parents' associations at the back of this book. Through them or through your local hospital, health center, or breastfeeding association, you can be put in touch with people who have been through the same things that you are now experiencing. In addition, use the nurses. Talk to the staff about your worries and feelings, they will support and help you!

GETTING STARTED WITH BREASTFEEDING

Three Precious Gifts to Your Baby: Your Milk, Your Skin, and Your Time

Most mothers will want to do something important for their babies right away, especially if breastfeeding is somehow delayed. And they can by providing the milk they have expressed from their breasts by hand or with the help of a pump. Skin-to-skin contact with the baby as soon as possible after delivery makes it easier to tackle this new phase in life, as well as giving mother – and father – an opportunity to make contact with the new family member. Many parents have recalled that experience: once you have skin-to-skin contact, you know the baby really belongs to you. The father of one very tiny and ill little girl tells how for a very long time he was not given the chance to hold her. When he finally had the opportunity to do so, he recalls:

Suddenly I realized the truth – I was the father of a little girl! A beautiful, tiny girl. And now I shall never leave you! Never go from you, never let you down... (Skullerud, 1995).

194

Those are strong words about strong feelings, but that is the very point we need to understand – feelings! This is why every baby that, for one reason or another, has to be separated from its mother and father at delivery, must have skin-to-skin contact with them as soon as possible (Figure 8.1). In addition to the "bonding" feelings, skin-to-skin contact has numerous positive effects in both term and preterm babies: longer breastfeeding duration, less crying, more stable temperature and blood sugar values, to mention some of them (Moore, Anderson, & Bergman, 2007; Bystrova et al., 2003; Christensson et al., 1992). And finally – the moment when someone touches you is the moment you know you have arrived in the world.

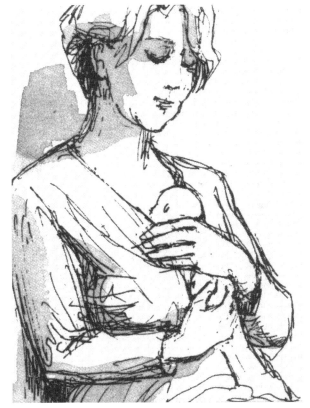

Figure 8.1. *Skin-to-skin contact*

Source: *Drawing by Ingerid Helsing Almaas. Used with permission.*

Skin-to-skin contact is part of the more extensive "Kangaroo mother care" and is an appropriate and useful way to care for babies and their parents in a human and very healthy way, both in industrialized and developing countries (Nyqvist et al., 2010a; Nyqvist et al., 2010b). You can read more about its advantages and how to use the Kangaroo mother care method later in this chapter.

In the Special Care Nursery?

There are many reasons why a baby may need to be transferred to a special care nursery[5] after delivery. The baby may be preterm or show some sign of illness. Difficulties with breathing, problems in maintaining a normal body temperature, a pale or unhealthy skin color, or general weakness – any of these may suggest that things are not entirely as they should be. They are, however, no more than signs – they may be merely transient difficulties in starting independent life. Most babies will soon get over them and be declared fit and free of any serious complication. A father and mother will nevertheless experience the sudden and unexpected separation as something dramatic and painful, even if they soon learn that it was no more than a false alarm. Some of these babies will need to spend time in an incubator, often linked to various tubes, electrical leads, and pieces of equipment. Most of these tools simply serve to keep a constant check on the baby's heart rhythm and breathing – they are not as dismal as they may look! The baby may also need an intravenous drip or feeding by means of a feeding tube to ensure that it has plenty of fluids, and blood samples may need to be taken. Some babies may need the support of a respirator to support their breathing. In a situation like this, it is only natural for parents to feel worried and afraid, and you need to take these feelings seriously and seek support from the staff. It helps a lot if you can see your baby at intervals, touch it, change its diapers, and in other ways care for it, and if the baby is well enough to be moved, have more extensive skin-to-skin contact. If the baby shows interest in the breast, then by all means offer it the chance to feed. Being kept informed, regularly and reliably, about the baby's health situation is also important if one is not to be more concerned than necessary.

---

5   In some hospitals, the special care nursery is known as the neonatal intensive care unit (NICU), or quite simply the neonatal unit or ward.

The Baby-Friendly Hospital's Neonatal Unit - A Breastfeeding Friendly Initiative - Also Friendly To Parents

In 1991, the World Health Organization (WHO) and the United Nations Children's Fund (UNICEF) jointly published 10 steps that should be met if a hospital is to be considered "Baby-friendly" (see Chapters 5 and 15 and the appendix to this book). Those 10 steps were originally intended for healthy neonates in obstetric and maternity units, but in some countries, the 10 steps have been modified and adapted to provide a special standard also for neonatal units or departments dealing with sick neonates. These changes have resulted in higher breastfeeding rates in preterm infants (Dall'Oglio et al., 2007; do Nascimento & Issler, 2005; Merewood, Philipp, Chawla, & Cimo, 2003). Such a unit must also be open and accessible virtually day and night, and the parents should be able to rest, sleep, and eat there – in other words, these units should be parent-friendly, in addition to being breastfeeding-friendly.

When Mother and Baby Are Separated

In those instances where it is necessary to care for the mother and the baby separately, virtually from the time of birth onwards, breastfeeding will not get off to the best possible start. Fortunately, breastfeeding is a flexible process, and it will generally be possible to introduce it as time goes on. Many roads lead to Rome, as the saying goes – some are quick and easy, but others are crooked and stony, and demand a lot of patience. The most important thing to bear in mind in this situation is that one should make sure to get milk production started, while the hormone production that follows delivery is still active and helps you out, and there is, therefore, no time to lose! While you are together with the baby, make sure there is plenty of skin-to-skin contact, and whenever possible, invite the baby to your breasts and give it a chance to try breastfeeding. During the night, see if breastfeeding can be permitted, provided you can manage it, otherwise keep the milk production going by hand-milking or pumping. Expressing milk at night stimulates your level of the breastfeeding hormone prolactin, even if it is not as cozy as your baby... But don't overdo things – your own health is important, and pumping milk at night can become too much of a burden if what you really need is sleep.

There should be at most six hours between two pumping or milking sessions, and it is preferable to stimulate around eight times every 24 hours in the beginning, and by the time the milk production really gets going, not only to stimulate, but also to remove the milk. If the baby is not feeding at the breast, the only stimulus to the milk production will be your own hands or the pump. Read more details about expressing milk in Chapter 10. It is particularly important to keep things in motion during the first few days after birth, or immediately after the baby is taken ill – ensuring a good milk volume in the beginning will help to avoid problems later on, and help you to succeed with breastfeeding.

Many mothers are particularly worried if the sick child is not managing to breastfeed. This, however, will generally solve itself after a while, and most babies will have mastered the breastfeeding technique by the time they go home, even if there are ups and downs. Golden rule number 14 applies here.

Golden Rule Number 14

If you are unavoidably separated from your baby directly after birth, or your baby does not manage breastfeeding, your first priority must be to get your milk production going and to keep it up – and that's urgent!

SUPPORT OF BREASTFEEDING IF MOTHER AND CHILD ARE SEPARATED AFTER DELIVERY:

- Early and frequent stimulation of milk production (around 8 times/24 hours) to ensure good milk production

- Early* and extensive contact between mother and child

- Early and generous skin-to-skin contact

- Early contact with the breast

- Separate mother and baby only if absolutely necessary

- Take every opportunity to breastfeed

- Use an alternative to the bottle (such as cup feeding) if supplementation is needed

* "Early" means as early as possible. In some cases, the baby is so ill you have to wait.

Your Milk: Worth Its Weight in Gold!

If your baby doesn't manage to take the breast after delivery, express the first drops of colostrum by hand directly into the baby's mouth or into a small cup and offer it to the baby. This very early expression works better with hand milking than with a pump, as hand expression is less painful and gives higher volumes (Ohyama, Watabe, & Hayasaka, 2010). At this early stage, the quantity of colostrum is small, but what you are providing is your baby's first "vaccine!"

Too Much Milk?

There are situations in which a mother can find that she has more milk in her breasts than her baby needs. In some cases, it may then be helpful to separate the low-fat early milk from the high-fat, high-energy late milk or hind milk – see Chapter 3 for more about the differences in the composition of the milk. This may be the case if the baby is preterm and does not need much milk in a day, or if the baby has an unusually high need for energy, for example, if it has a congenital heart disorder. When you express your milk, set aside the early lactose-rich milk aside to be used later, and then give the hind milk directly to the baby (Slusher et al., 2003; Griffin, Meier, Bradford, Bigger, & Engstrom, 2000). Ask the nursing staff for help in estimating how much milk the baby will need daily, so you can decide how much to put in the freezer. Some units also measure the fat in the milk. This process is not always necessary, and one should not make things more complicated than absolutely necessary. If you do follow this course, do it in consultation with the staff of the unit. If you have a lot of milk, you may try expressing less – ask the staff for advice.

You may also donate your excess milk to the hospital's milk bank, if it has one, so that it can benefit other babies (see advice on milk banks in the Appendix).

Too Little Milk?

A more common problem is when there seems to be too little milk. If, right at the start, there has been an unavoidable separation of mother and baby and she needs to express milk by hand or by using a pump, or if the mother has been ill during her pregnancy, it may be hard to get breastfeeding started on the right foot. But not impossible! For more advice on what to do when you seem to have too little milk, take a look at Chapter 6. For information on how to use a pump, see Chapter 10.

WHEN THE BABY IS NOT AN EFFICIENT MILKING MACHINE

Why May That Happen?

There are many different reasons why certain babies are what we call "weak feeders," i.e., they are not among the world's most efficient milking machines. The baby may have arrived too early, may be suffering from an infection or from jaundice, or it may have one chromosome too many, as we see in Down syndrome. A difficult delivery or an infection can also knock out a baby's ability to breastfeed for a while. There may also be a mechanical problem, notably with cleft lip and split palate. And sometimes there is simply no obvious cause – one is faced with a baby that seems terribly tired and hardly interested in breastfeeding at all.

Tips and Tactics

Give Skin-To-Skin Contact

We just have to stress it once more – give the baby a lot of skin-to-skin contact. It gives warmth and stabilizes the baby's metabolism, and makes it easier for you as a mother to recognize when your child gives those subtle early signs that it is now getting towards mealtime! For example, you can feel the eyelash like a butterfly on your skin as a sign to wake up. Just ask the baby ...

Stimulate the Let-Down Reflex

You can help a weak breastfeeder get at the milk if you stimulate the milk let-down reflex in advance – see Chapter 5.

The Need for a Soft and Pliable Breast

If a breast is taut and hard, the nipple will be flattened and difficult for the baby to get hold of and latch on to. Ensuring that your breast is sufficiently soft and pliable is the best means of offering the baby a breast to which it can latch on sufficiently. Remember that the baby's various milking reflexes are triggered when the nipple touches the baby's hard palate (see Chapter 1).

You will find that the breast becomes more pliable if you express a little milk by hand before starting a feed. You can use ordinary hand expression or the Reverse Pressure Softening method we explained in Chapter 5. You may also choose to use a pump, but particularly during the first two to four days when milk production is just getting under way, your hands will do the best job.

Strengthen the Milking Reflexes!

It is possible to strengthen the baby's milking reflexes by eliciting some of its other reflexes, for example, the hand-grip reflex. Simply hold your baby's hand or massage your baby on the palms of its hands or the soles of its feet, and you will find that the milk reflex is rendered more active. Or just think about the way in which a healthy mature baby tends to flex its arms, knees, and hip joint, and try to help your baby get its body into a similar position for breastfeeding.

Encourage Your Baby with a Taste of Milk

If you introduce a few drops of your milk into the baby's mouth – either directly from the nipple or using a spoon or a needle-less syringe – the taste of milk will stimulate the baby.

Increase Your Milk Flow

Towards the end of a feeding session, you can help the baby get a little more milk by pressing lightly on your breast – this is known as "breast compression." You should press the breast gently, but rhythmically, following your baby's swallowing rhythm. It can also be used to stimulate your baby to swallow (see Figure 8.2).

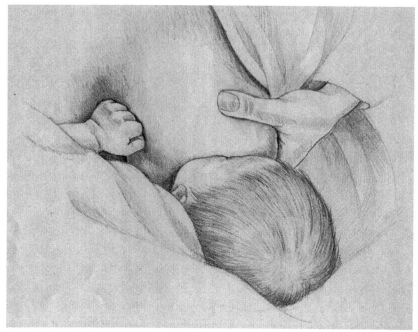

Figure 8.2. *Press the breast rhythmically with one hand.*

Source: Drawing by Pollyanna von Knorring. Used with permission.

Try Different Positions

In Chapter 5, we explained the many ways of holding the baby during breastfeeding, and you may want to refer back to that section. If the baby has arrived too early or needs some help in getting a sufficient hold on the breast, it is well worth trying the "under the arm hold" (Figure 8.3) or the "opposite hand position" (Figure 8.4). Using either of these two positions means that you can free one of your hands to shape and support the breast, so your baby will find it easier to get a good hold. You can then use this hand to support the baby. Many mothers find they can steer the whole process better (and have a better overview) when they are in a sitting position compared with lying down. With preterm infants and those with weak muscle tone (for example, Down syndrome), it may also be necessary to provide some support to the baby's head in order for the baby to maintain a hold on the breast. *Don't* try to hold the head of an ordinarily strong and healthy child who is likely to protest instinctively against having its head held by pushing itself away from the breast.

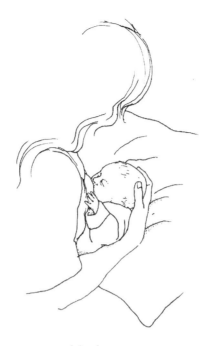

Figure 8.3. *Under arm position with head support*

Source: Drawing by Ingerid Helsing Almaas. Used with permission.

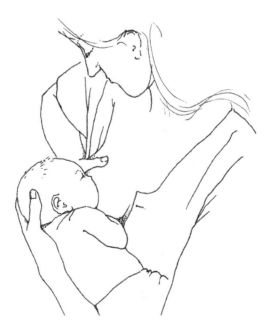

Figure 8.4. *Opposite hand position with head support*

Source: Drawing by Ingerid Helsing Almaas. Used with permission.

Some babies fail to keep their mouths closed because their musculature is too weak. This can be a problem in children with Down syndrome or other neurological conditions. Try to help the baby using the "Dancer hand" as shown in Figures 8.5a-b. This makes it possible to support the baby's weak jaw and chin muscles during feeding.

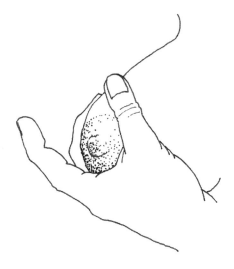

Figure 8.5a. *Dancer hand without baby*

Source: Drawing by Ingerid Helsing Almaas. Used with permission.

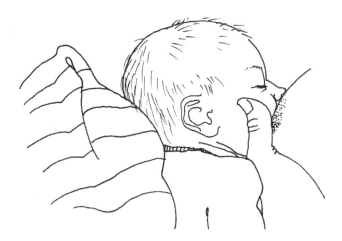

Figure 8.5b. *Dancer hand in practice*

Source: Drawing by Ingerid Helsing Almaas. Used with permission.

If You Need to Wake the Baby

Should you need to wake the baby when it is time for a feed, you can best do this while it is sleeping lightly (so-called REM sleep). You can recognize this phase of sleep because the child lies there with its eyes closed, but is constantly pulling faces, smiling, and waving its arms, and you may be able to see that its eyes are moving rapidly under the eyelids. A taste of breastmilk on the baby's lips can inspire it to wake up. If your baby wakes of its own accord, look for the sort of signals that indicate that he or she deems the moment ripe for a good breastfeed – and when you see those early signals for feeding: *respond right away!* The signals can include pouting, sucking on the fingers, and other movements of the head and mouth typical of the milk reflexes. Make sure the baby is not dressed too warmly – this can make it drowsy and sleepy. Offer skin-to-skin contact to stimulate the reflexes further. Talk to your baby or sing to it, so it knows you are seeking contact. Offer one breast, followed by a change of nappies or of clothes, and then offer the other breast, all help to keep the baby sufficiently awake.

You will probably find there are certain times of the day when your baby tends to be more wide awake. These are good times to put your baby to the breast, so you keep up the frequency of feeding and the volume of milk.

Not Feeding at the Breast This Time? It's Cozy All the Same.

And when the baby just doesn't take the chance to feed very actively, don't be too concerned. Lying at the breast is something he or she enjoys, and why not? Giving the breast is more than just a way of feeding!

SAY NO TO THE BOTTLE - WHY?

Studies designed to compare various groups of preterm infants who were initially breastfed show that those children who had been fed from a bottle were less likely to be breastfeeding successfully when they left hospital than those who had been given milk using a feeding tube or cup (Flint, New, & Davies, 2007; Collins et al., 2004). Using a bottle and teat can lead a child to prefer the bottle to the breast and should be avoided or delayed as long as possible. When cup feeding, the baby uses the musculature for suckling in a manner closer to breastfeeding compared to the technique used with bottles (Gomes, Trezza, Murade, & Padovani, 2006). In addition, the baby's physiological stability is better with cup feeding than with bottle-feeding (Marinelli, Burke, & Dodd, 2001; Rocha, Martinez, & Jorge, 2002). There are some children who are able to alternate effortlessly between the bottle and the breast, but unfortunately, we have no way of knowing in advance which small individual will manage this balancing act!

ALTERNATIVE FEEDING TECHNIQUES

A baby that is ill or has arrived preterm is likely to need a particular volume of fluids that one can estimate on the basis of its age and weight. In some cases, the baby can take part of what it needs from the breast and receive the rest as a supplement, but in other cases, you will have to provide the entire daily intake in the form of supplementary feeding. If you do need to provide food in some alternative way, it's possible to choose from several techniques.

Tube Feeding

This involves using a thin flexible plastic tube, which is introduced into the stomach through the mouth or nose. The tube may be put in place before every feed, or it can be left in position day and night – the routine differs from one hospital to another. During tube feeding, the baby should be close or attached to the breast, have a pacifier in place, or one of mother's fingers to suck on, and a little milk should be dropped into the mouth. If the baby is still in an incubator and unable to come to the breast, simply place your nice warm hands on its body while it is being fed.

Cup

Use of a cup is a very good alternative, and most babies will find it easy to lap up milk using the tongue. Let the baby find its own lapping rhythm. If the baby is healthy enough, feeding from a cup can confidently be used, even with early preterms, e.g., those born at the 29-30th week (Gupta, Khanna, & Chattree, 1999). It is advisable for you as parents to learn to practice cup feeding as early as possible, while the baby is still at the hospital. You will soon become the best qualified experts of all on feeding your own baby! And since skill like that gives confidence you will feel more secure when it's time to take the baby home.

Nursing Supplementer

The nursing supplementer can be a useful alternative to the bottle. It is helpful when the baby needs some supplementation of breastmilk, either for medical reasons or because it is a weak feeder. In the latter case, the baby needs some help to get the milk flowing. The commercially available variant of the nursing supplementer makes it easier for you to ensure that your baby has regular access to milk – all you need to do is to lightly squeeze the attached plastic milk reservoir. You can, however, use a home-made nursing supplementer described in Chapter 10.

What About the Pacifier?

Elsewhere in this book, we recommended that you should not let a baby get used to a pacifier before breastfeeding is well established. The reason for this is that the baby may spend more time working on the pacifier than on the breast, which means that the breast will get too little stimulation and may, therefore, produce too little milk.

However, to the ill baby, a pacifier does offer some degree of benefit. When the baby is fed through a feeding tube, sucking on the pacifier makes the baby less fussy and more relaxed during feeding. Sucking on a pacifier also gives relief of pain during procedures, such as blood sampling, reducing the baby's stress and anxiety (Cignacco et al., 2007; Lago et al., 2009; Pinelli & Symington, 2005). A pacifier can also be used to enable a baby to fall asleep more readily when its parents are absent. So, if you are not available with your breast as consolation for your baby, a pacifier can be offered.

Our conclusion has to be that for preterm or sick infants the advantages of using a pacifier outweigh the possible disadvantages. A study found no association between the use of a pacifier in preterm babies and a reduction in breastfeeding (Collins et al., 2004). But remember: when you return home with the baby, and for a while after that, you should avoid overdoing the use of a pacifier to allow the breast to be stimulated sufficiently to produce enough milk.

THE PRETERM BABY

Some Special Challenges

Breastfeeding confronts the mother of a preterm baby with some special challenges, naturally varying with the degree of prematurity and the baby's general state of health. Some children arrive only a week before term, and in that case, breastfeeding rarely presents any real difficulty. Others arrive much too early, and full breastfeeding directly from the breast may only become possible after weeks of expressing milk, a lengthy hospital stay for the baby, and a period marked by uncertainties and concerns. With the knowledge and resources we have today, however, you are far better placed than ever before in history to make a success of breastfeeding your preterm baby, even though the baby may seem so tiny and the road to success interminably long. Many have traveled this road before you and found that it is possible. All the same, there are mothers who don't contrive to tackle all the twists and obstacles on the way. There are also those preterm children who never quite manage to find out what is expected of them where breastfeeding is concerned. Finally, a family may have other obligations, such as providing care for its older children, and lack the time that is needed for expressing milk to maintain production for the new arrival.

How Many Premature Babies Are Breastfed?

The proportion of preterm babies who are breastfed differs quite markedly from one country to another. The differences could be explained by variations in the gestational ages and weight of the babies studied. However, it is also a fact that breastfeeding in general is influenced by many factors, such as breastfeeding culture in society and education levels. One major factor influencing the situation is the extent to which hospitals support breastfeeding. Babies and mothers are the same all over the world, and it is unlikely that biological variation can explain the marked differences from place to place. In the USA, one study examined the effects of an intervention in accordance with the Baby-Friendly Hospital Initiative (Merewood et al., 2003) – the initiation rate of breastfeeding increased from 35% to 74% at 2 weeks, the "any breastfeeding" rate rose from 28% to 66%, and the "exclusive breastfeeding" rate went from 9% to 39% also at 2 weeks!

A study from various European countries reported breastfeeding rates ranging from 19% to 70% at the time of discharge from a neonatal unit, while the rate of exclusive breastfeeding varied from 6% to 29 %. In Australia, it is reported that 64% of babies were having breastmilk to some extent at the moment of discharge, with 45 % being exclusively breastfed (Bonet et al., 2010). High breastfeeding rates at the time of discharge were also noted in a study from a county in Sweden, where the statistics on 70 babies with a birth weight of less than 2500g were examined – 93% were receiving breastmilk, and of these, 95% were being exclusively breastfed at the time of discharge (Flacking, Nyqvist, Ewald, & Wallin, 2003). In another Swedish study reporting high breastfeeding rates at discharge, 98% of full-term babies were breastfed, as were 92 % of the preterm babies (Åkerström, Asplund, & Norman, 2007). In a Danish study of 478 early pre-term babies, 60% were exclusively breastfed, while 5% received both formula and breastfeeding (Zachariassen et al., 2010). The conclusion, therefore, is that it is indeed possible to breastfeed your premature baby, especially if your breastmilk production is adequate and the hospital is supportive of breastfeeding!

Prematurity is defined as "birth before the 37th week of pregnancy." It is common to categorize preterm birth into three groups:

• Early preterm: < 28 gestational weeks

• Preterm: 28-33 gestational weeks

• Late preterm: 34-36 gestational weeks

In this book, we have chosen not to describe the breastfeeding process very specifically for each of the defined groups of prematurity for one simple reason: a baby's development in breastfeeding varies with the individual; it is influenced by health and illness, and the degree of maturity or age. You will, however, find one part dealing particularly with the late preterm babies – they can be wrongly thought to be more mature than they actually are, and because of that be in trouble.

Preterm infants have a special need for breastmilk to protect them against infections and necrotising enterocolitis, and to provide better development of the nervous system than is attained with formula feeding (WHO, Edmond, & Bahl, 2006). One research study shows that very early administration of breastmilk (from the mother or from a milk bank) can protect early preterm babies from septicemia (Rønnestad et al., 2005).

As we noted in Chapter 3, the milk produced by mothers who have delivered preterm is different during the first weeks of life than that produced following a term delivery (Hurst & Meier, 2010). It is relatively richer in some nutrients (for example, proteins), which means that it offers larger quantities of immunoprotective substances, which the preterm baby particularly needs.

While You Are Still Waiting for "Skin-To-Skin"

Even during the time that your preterm baby is in an incubator and you are obliged to wait for real skin-to-skin contact and breastfeeding, there is much you can do to provide contact. You can put a few drops of breastmilk into the baby's mouth using a syringe without a needle, tempt it with a pacifier, and leave a soft cloth carrying the smell of your own milk. As soon as it becomes possible, you can take over the job of changing the baby's diapers and caring for the baby. In some of these matters, you will need guidance and advice at first, but very soon your hands will be steady and you will have all the confidence you need. Remember: no one is as careful and as competent to look after a baby – even a fragile one – as its parents. Also remember: the baby belongs to you – not to the nurses or the hospital!

The Kangaroo Method: Skin-to-Skin Contact

As we saw in Chapter 2, the kangaroo carries its offspring in a pouch on its abdominal wall. The pouch offers safety and warmth, and the baby has a constant supply of milk within easy reach. In our human world, we have learned the lesson of the kangaroo mother's success. What we now call the "kangaroo method" of caring for preterm babies originated in Colombia at the end of the 1970's. At that time, there was a social crisis in Colombia, with a high rate of infant mortality. Many mothers of preterm infants saw no other way out of the problems facing them than to leave their children behind in the hospital where they had been born. Initially, they would be cared for there in incubators, and later they would be transferred to orphanages. That trend might have become much worse had it not been arrested by the introduction of the kangaroo method of caring for these preterm infants, essentially involving the use of the mother's body as a "human incubator." It helped the mother become attached to her baby, and it ensured that the baby was provided with breastmilk and breastfeeding, endowing it with better health from the start (Whitelaw & Sleath, 1985;

Charpak et al., 2005). The baby was placed, unclothed, against the mother's skin and inside her clothes where it would be warm (Figure 8.6). In those countries where the kangaroo method is practised today, rather than use incubators, the mother's place can be taken by the father, the grandmother, or anyone else able to spend time offering bodily warmth and a modicum of love to the baby when the mother needs a break.

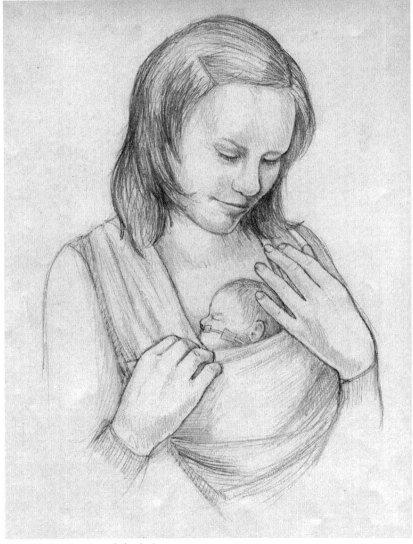

Figure 8.6. *Carrying a baby the kangaroo way*

Source: Drawing by Pollyanna von Knorring. Used with permission.

KANGAROO MOTHER CARE

The Kangaroo Mother Care (KMC) method is intended to provide skin-to-skin contact between the mother and her low birth weight infant, and to do so:

- Early (as soon as possible after birth)

- Continuously (ideally 24 hours/day, 7 days/week)

- For a long time

The method should be used both in the hospital and after discharge. Ideally, there should be exclusive breastfeeding, early discharge from hospital, and adequate follow-up.

Kangaroo Care must continue for the infant's entire hospital stay and for as long as is needed after discharge to prevent hypothermia, which usually means continuing to about term age or beyond (Cattaneo, Davanzo, Uxa, & Tamburlini, 1998).

Many special care units world-wide are using elements of Kangaroo Care, though with considerable variations. In Norway and other Scandinavian countries, for example, all units give babies and parents opportunities for skin-to-skin contact as a routine part of the care they offer, although not all units have facilities for parents to stay day and night at the hospital.

Having the baby close against you for much of the time will also stimulate your milk flow. Studies have shown how this type of contact reduces a mother's stress level and how it contributes to the building of a relationship between mother and baby. Both mothers and fathers describe how it builds their confidence in the parental role (Nyqvist et al, 2010a). What is more, babies make it very clear how fond they are of the Kangaroo approach – infants enjoying such contact cry less than those who lack it, breathe more regularly, are less likely to suffer infections, put on more weight, return home earlier, and breastfeed longer and more intensively (Hurst, Valentine, Renfro, Burns, & Ferlic, 1997; Hake-Brooks & Anderson, 2008; Gathwala, Singh, & Singh, 2010).

Sitting With the Baby – Or Taking a Walk

One can do skin-to-skin with a preterm baby that is supported by a respirator, a positive air pressure device (CPAP), [6] or an oxygen supply, provided some sort of bed is available on the spot. The baby should be held in an upright position, between its mother's breasts or against its father's chest (WHO, 2003). There is hardly a need for clothes, but the very smallest babies may need a cap and perhaps a vest that can be opened in the front, so the baby's chest can have direct contact with that of its parent. And it is obviously sensible to have a diaper in place…

The signals that a preterm baby is able to give (for example, that it would like to be fed) may be very weak, and if they are overlooked or there is no response, the baby may simply fall asleep again. A parent and a young baby together possess a very sensitive and subtle system for giving and receiving such signals, and it works particularly well when there is skin-to-skin contact. Once the baby grows healthier and bigger, and moves from an incubator to an ordinary cradle, there may be less skin-to-skin contact, as the baby is dressed and lies under a quilt. But that is precisely the moment a mother can and should do something to keep this unique form of contact going. Carry your baby around in a skin-to-skin embrace! Simply use a scarf or something similar to hold the baby securely against you, and you will be able to move around the ward instead of sitting on a chair for hours at a time.

The Art of Getting at One's Food

By the time a baby is born, it has already gained some experience in the uterus with such activities as sucking its thumb and swallowing amniotic fluid. When the baby is born preterm, it may not manage to feed, swallow, and breathe – all at the appropriate moments. A baby born normally at term has a fully developed program for these things – the rhythmic movements of its tongue, the process of swallowing, and the process of breathing are all integrated and fit seamlessly together. Nevertheless, an early preterm baby can learn to feed effectively if it is given the chance, even if the breastfeeding pattern is not yet fully developed. One nursing

---

6   CPAP= *Continuous Positive Airways Pressure*. The baby's still immature lungs are kept slightly inflated all the time, which makes breathing easier.

researcher who studied these matters in preterm babies found them able to root, latch on, and suckle as early as the 27th week of gestation, while a baby can breastfeed and take other food from the 29th week. Given early frequent feeds and optimal support, a preterm infant should be able to breastfeed exclusively from the 32nd week. The only reason not to offer a newborn baby the chance to take the breast is when it is unstable or ill (Hedberg & Ewald, 1999; Nyqvist, 2008).

Understanding the Development of Breastfeeding

In a baby born very early, the rooting reflex can take on a very simple form – the baby moves its lips, sticks out its tongue, or tries to suck on its fingers. Mature breastfeeding develops gradually –first there may be one or two hesitant gulps of milk, then several short episodes of real breastfeeding. These short episodes of breastfeeding become progressively longer until a normal pattern has been achieved. In the beginning, one sees how the baby needs to take a feeding pause now and again in order to catch its breath, but then, as the baby matures, it becomes more capable of controlling and coordinating its breathing. A preterm baby born very early may actually seem to be quite out of breath between and after feeding sessions. This is absolutely normal and quite acceptable, provided the oxygen saturation is within normal limits. Swallowing is also something that the baby has to tackle and learn. At first, it will swallow only occasionally, and then pause before trying again. Gradually, a smooth and regular swallowing rhythm is established. The baby will, however, be able to breastfeed – even exclusively – before all these processes of suckling, swallowing, and breathing are perfectly coordinated!

The Development of Breastfeeding in Prematurity: An Overview

The secret is, as always, continuous skin-to-skin contact! Given that, things are likely to happen progressively:

- To begin with, while the baby is in direct contact with the breast, the mother can express a little milk. Even at the start, the baby may take some of the milk and swallow it.

- Soon, the baby will begin to take small amounts of milk more frequently, but swallowing will still be irregular.

- After a time, swallowing will become more rhythmic, and the baby will begin to take ever larger amounts of milk from the breast.

- Ultimately, your baby will be able to take all the milk it needs – the two of you will have succeeded.

Don't Compete

It is important to understand that your baby is developing at his or her own tempo. You should accept that and live with it. The tempo will depend on the child's personality and state of health.

All the same, you may find yourself instinctively comparing your experience with that of others in the ward, both as regards your milk volume and how well your little one is learning to feed at the breast. Naturally, it's good to talk to other new mothers and exchange experiences with them, but concentrate your attention on yourself and your own little world. This is a time to be unashamedly self-centered! Comparisons are quite meaningless, and after a short while, the situation may change. This applies also to the baby's achievements at the breast.

If at First You Don't Succeed...

You cannot know in advance whether a particular baby is going to display interest in the breast right at the start; some babies don't. This is not a matter to be concerned about. Just do skin-to-skin to begin with and offer the breast frequently. You may be able to express a few drops of milk, so the baby is tempted to go on exploring like this. Hold the nipple and use it to stroke the baby's lips – the baby may well feel an irresistible urge to open its mouth widely.

A Little More Each Time...On the Ladder to Success

A baby is better able to handle very small portions of food, given frequently, than a larger amount offered at longer intervals (three hours is definitely a long interval in this situation). For this reason, it is better to give the baby many repeated chances to try its feeding skills on a very small scale than to offer the breast seriously at intervals dictated by a clock – unless there are medical reasons to do things differently. If your baby is born close to term, you may start on the third phase in the scheme summarized below. Try to determine which phase you have reached, but accept that during the early days, the baby will need to have regular feeds because its blood sugar is likely to be low.

One can roughly distinguish four phases in the need for supplementation of breastfeeding, though there is a smooth transition from one to the other:

First phase: Children born too early or in a poor state of health often have small reserves of blood sugar. For this and possibly other medical reasons, it is important that feeds are regular, frequent, and sufficient, so the blood sugar is stabilized at a high enough level. Whether this is necessary (and how long this should continue) depends on various things, such as how healthy the baby is and how early the delivery was. In any case, it is good to offer the baby the breast, if at all possible, right at the beginning, following this up with the prescribed amount of supplement.

Second phase: After a while, the baby may take more milk on one occasion and a little less on the next, but is still not taking a sufficient amount from the breast to cover its needs. Supplement with the help of a cup or feeding tube, preferably using your own expressed milk. It may not be necessary to supplement after every feed, especially if you can manage more frequent breastfeeding sessions. Remember that a baby feeding very frequently – e.g., every hour or two hours – may cover all its needs, even if it only seems to take a little milk at a time.

Third phase: By now, the baby is fully able to get all the food it needs from the breast, but you may find that it still needs to be awakened from time to time as a reminder that a feed is due!

Fourth phase: Here, the baby is able to find out for itself just when it needs to feed and how much milk it needs to take. This is the situation that a baby born at term experiences right from the first few hours of life – a preterm baby just takes longer to get there.

... In the End You'll Probably Succeed!

Most babies are mature enough to master the art of feeding at the breast around the 36th or 37th week of pregnancy, but there is a lot of variation in both directions. What is more, the brain centers that regulate hunger and sleep are not fully developed until about the 38th week of pregnancy.

Therefore, it's only natural that preterm children need a little help in remembering how often and how much they need to eat.

There are, however, babies delivered as early as the 33rd week of pregnancy who have managed to feed themselves exclusively from the breast (Nyqvist, 2008). Even in the case of babies who have been seriously ill or have had long periods of disturbed breathing, it is not unusual to see breastfeeding successfully established, though that may happen later than usual.

When Your Baby Is Born Close to Term - Some Special Challenges

Babies born close to term face some particular challenges – and as a mother, you will have to confront them! They will be looked upon (and treated) as full-term infants, and they may not receive the special treatment they need. A baby born late preterm (34th - 36th week) will run the risk of hypothermia (i.e., a reduced body temperature), low blood sugar levels, and jaundice. Some of these risks can be avoided by ensuring plenty of skin-to-skin contact and by offering the breast frequently. Such a baby may fail to indicate when it is hungry, it may be an inefficient milking machine, and it will readily fall asleep at the breast. If that is the case, you should try hand expression or use the pump to initiate milk production, and offer the baby your milk using a cup once daily or after every breastfeed, depending on how tired your baby seems to be (Meier, Furman, & Degenhardt, 2007). You may find some helpful tips in the section "When the baby is not an efficient milking machine." Remember: your baby is not ill, it is simply immature and in need of a little more support and follow-up during the early weeks if breastfeeding is to be successful!

Should I Weigh the Preterm Baby Before and After a Breastfeed?

If your baby is very small or ill, it may be helpful to weigh it before and after a feed (Hurst, Meier, Engstrom, & Myatt, 2004). If you find that doing this makes you stressed or worried, just admit it. Together with the nursing staff, you will be able to find an alternative for your baby and yourself. It may, for example, be sufficient to try to estimate how much milk the baby has taken – and then if necessary, give more using the cup or the feeding tube. This is not as accurate as putting the baby on the scales, but your impression as to how things are going is just as important! There is always another way of doing things! And remember: your feelings and impressions are often the best guide as to what to do (Funkquist, Tuvemo, Jonsson, Serenius, & Nyqvist, 2010).

When It's Time for Your Preterm Baby to Go Home

Preterm babies are very often discharged before they have arrived at the fourth stage. You may still need to wake your baby to remind it that it's time for a meal, and if it is not yet able to take all the milk it needs from your breast, you may need to resort to a cup, a feeding tube, or even a bottle. It may be that your baby's feeding motions, swallowing, and breathing are not yet coordinated with one another, and it may need to pause now and again. In this phase, a baby may also be more sensitive than usual to light and sounds. It is, therefore, sensible to avoid such disturbances while you are feeding, for example, turn off the TV or the radio. And perhaps you can persuade brothers and sisters, large and small, to keep quiet for a while, although that may not be easy! Feeding sessions are likely to take more time than with a baby born at term. Try to feed often and use techniques to improve milk production. Short but effective breastfeeding sessions are more useful than long sessions, with the baby sleeping rather than suckling. This period can be demanding, and you may feel that it is going to last forever! Remember, however, that it is just these few early weeks that are so tiring, and that as every day goes by, the baby will progress! These are what are sometimes known as "the lost weeks of pregnancy," and you simply need to slow down and relax (see Chapter 6). We will have more to say about the return home later in this Chapter.

In Summary: Tackling and Supporting Feeding of Preterm Babies

Here again, in summary form, are some straightforward tips about the management of preterm or sick babies. The tips will need to be adapted to your baby's situation as it develops from one week to another.

TIPS FOR THE MANAGEMENT OF PRETERM OR SICK BABIES

- The measures that we discussed for dealing with "weak feeders" earlier in this Chapter also apply to a preterm baby, *except* as regards massage and other forms of active stimulation. Take another look at what we said in Chapter 5 about good positioning and various feeding positions.

- Remember that a preterm baby may be very sensitive to touch. During breastfeeding or supplementary feeds, keep your hands as still as you can – a child can be distracted and disturbed, even by a well-meant caress.

- The baby should not be exposed to strong light or loud noises.

- Make sure you give your baby a feed *before* it is due to have a change of diapers, a bath, or any other procedure that will cost it energy. You can change a diaper while the baby is asleep – but breastfeeding a sleeping baby will be more difficult!

- Be alert for those small signs of hunger – and respond quickly and appropriately.

- Help the baby find the best posture, with its arms drawn in and legs drawn up – just as they were when lying in the womb before it was born.

- As parents, get some guidance on understanding the baby's behavior at the breast – and in particular, get used to seeing and hearing its swallowing motions, so you have an idea about when the baby is getting milk.

- Let the baby grasp your finger with its hand while it works on the breast – that can strengthen the milking reflex.

- If you notice that there are long pauses between each cycle of milking and swallowing, try breast compression – pressing gently on the breast to encourage the flow of milk (see Figure 8.2).

- If you have tried everything and the baby is still not feeding actively, see whether a nipple shield will help (see Chapter 10).

SPECIAL NEEDS OF BABIES WITH CLEFT LIP AND/OR PALATE

Breastfeeding babies with a cleft lip and/or a cleft palate presents a real challenge. How well you succeed will depend on how much milk you have, how readily it flows, how well your baby manages the whole feeding process, what sort of help and support you enjoy from family and friends, and how accustomed the nursing staff are to such a situation. The anti-infective properties of breastmilk play an even more vital role in babies with cleft palate because of their increased risk of inflammation of the middle ear. Breastfeeding reduces the risk of inflammation in the ear (Ip, Chung, Raman, Trikalinos, & Lau, 2009).

Your own ability and determination to overcome the difficulties are important, but motivation is not everything – many other factors may play a role. If you have learned *before delivery* that your baby has a cleft lip and palate, you can seek advice on getting expert help – someone with the necessary experience and competence will surely be able to guide you and work out a sensible plan of action. A video about breastfeeding in these situations can also be a great help, both before and after birth.

THREE IMPORTANT STAGES
(National Resource Center for Breastfeeding at Rikshospitalet, 2008)

During the first few days, the mother should:

- Concentrate on developing her milk supply.

- Feed her baby with a cup.

- Put the baby frequently in skin-to-skin contact and in contact with the breasts, even if for a while, there seems to be no prospect of breastfeeding.

After that, mother and baby can begin to practice breastfeeding.

To succeed at this time, the most important thing is to maintain a vacuum in the baby's mouth. Air can very easily enter through the split lip and cleft palate, but you can use the breast to block these openings. Introduce plenty of breast tissue into the mouth to prevent air from getting through; this will be easiest if your breast is soft and supple. It will also help if you stimulate the let-down reflex beforehand (see "tips and tactics" earlier in this Chapter) to ensure the baby gets as much milk as it can take, and it will also make milking the breast easier. See if you can mold the breast, so it fits the baby's mouth. If, for example, the baby is lying flat in the under-arm position (see Chapter 5), the breast will need to be pressed together from side to side, so it becomes taller and narrower. If the baby is sitting on your lap or both of you are lying down, the breast will need to be pressed from top to bottom to fit the shape of the baby's mouth. Breast compression during feeding is a very valuable technique for these babies (see Figure 8.2). Because of the cleft in the upper lip and perhaps in the palate as well, good positioning is especially important, so the baby lies tightly against its mother's body and can secure a good mouthful of soft and supple breast tissue. Mothers who have faced these problems stress that one of the most important elements in ensuring a good latch on the breast is getting as much breast tissue as possible into the baby's mouth. The breast needs to be properly supported throughout the feeding session. As far as positioning goes, you can be as creative as you like in finding out what works best for the two of you. You may well find that things go best when you choose different positions for the right breast and the left. You may find that it is easier for the baby to feed when it is held upright. Some mothers have more success when they turn the baby around and hold it under their arm, with the baby's stomach against the side of their chest and its feet behind the mother's back, i.e., essentially the "under the arm position" we discussed in Chapter 5.

Babies with cleft lip and palate often need to spend more time at the breast than others when they are feeding –it may be as much as an hour. It is also the question whether, with breastfeeding apparently going well, these children get all the milk they need and whether the time spent in feeding creates an excessive burden. Most of these babies are likely to need some supplementation with expressed breastmilk or a substitute. Cup feeding is advisable as the first choice, but if the feeding sessions with a cup turn out to be time-consuming, you may need to use a bottle. Sometimes, the best choice is to give the baby expressed milk with a bottle, rather than directly breastfeeding. If your child has difficulty maintaining a vacuum, you may benefit from using a flexible plastic feeding bottle with a teat. By cautiously squeezing the bottle, you can help the milk on its way.

BABIES WITH DOWN SYNDROME AND OTHER NEUROLOGICAL DISORDERS

Much of what we have said already is equally applicable to babies with neurological problems. The baby may have brain damage, it may have a congenital defect other than Down syndrome, or it may simply have had a tough delivery and difficult start in life. A baby with Down syndrome may prove to be clumsy at the breast, but in some other cases of the disorder, breastfeeding may go splendidly from the start. The most usual problems relate to weakness of the reflexes and poor muscular tone. The mother may need to use the "Dancer hand" position (Figures 8.5 a, b) to enable the baby to obtain a decent hold on the breast. This technique supports the lower jaw, so there is less chance of the baby losing its grip. Alternatively, you can use the "cross-cradle hold" or the "under the arm position," perhaps with some support of the head, methods we explained and illustrated in Chapter 5 and earlier in this Chapter.

Some of these children are easily tired and tend to fall asleep during breastfeeding. They may need some help to stay awake if they are to feed adequately. Feeding sessions may be longer than usual. Certain babies need to spend quite a lot of time searching for the breast and getting their milking reflexes into motion. Fortunately, experience shows that even where a child has at first seemed fatigued and uninterested in feeding, these things may improve in the course of a few weeks. Holding the child in a sitting position and talking to it during the feed can help it to do better. Take another look at our "tips and tactics" for weak feeders, earlier in this Chapter.

Breastfeeding also stimulates the muscles of the mouth and tongue, which may be important for the child's facial expression and speech. At the end of this Chapter, you can read the story of how one mother-and-child couple managed breastfeeding successfully, in spite of Down syndrome, after setting aside the feeding tube and the feeding bottle.

THE SPECIAL CASE OF BABIES WITH HEART PROBLEMS

Where a baby born with a heart defect shows only slight symptoms of heart failure or none at all, breastfeeding need not encounter any difficulties. On the other hand, a baby with a heart defect who is struggling to breathe and readily gets tired or exhausted is also likely to be a weak feeder. Some babies with heart defects soon learn to breathe through the mouth as a way of getting more oxygen. That, naturally, can create a problem with breastfeeding since such a baby cannot keep its mouth shut, which is necessary for feeding at the breast! If the baby does not manage to breastfeed completely, it will need supplementary feeding with a cup, tube, or bottle. The bottle should really be the last resort, but there are several things to bear in mind before going that far. Babies like this are happiest with frequent, very small, meals – an over-filled stomach puts an extra load on the heart. Children affected by a heart problem may need more calories than healthy children, since both the heart and the lungs have more work to do, and therefore consume more energy. The responsible doctor will prescribe the necessary fortification and provide you with the best solution. Look back at the section "Too much milk?" earlier in this chapter if you are expressing milk in very large amounts. A "nursing supplementer" (described in Chapter 10) may be very helpful for a weak feeder, who has heart problems and doesn't manage to feed sufficiently, or as a means of providing a sufficient intake of energy. If the baby needs fluid restriction, a reliable pair of scales will come in useful, so the child can be weighed before and after each feed. You may feel very uncertain if you do not know just how much milk the baby has taken. It can also happen that once the heart defect has been corrected by an operation, the baby gets back to breastfeeding, now being able to breathe easily and take in all the calories it needs.

GOING HOME – STANDING ON YOUR OWN FEET AND TRUSTING IN YOURSELF

Leaving the pediatric or neonatal ward to go home brings a mixture of joyful anticipation and concern for many a mother – joy at getting back home to the family and concern that one is now left to one's own devices, both as a mother and a provider of milk.

SOME WORDS FROM A MOTHER OF A PRETERM BABY

"I remember the trip home as a sort of triumphal parade. The first day, we were simply allowed out provisionally, on 24 hours leave. There were two of us to look after the baby, and that made us feel confident. But the next day, she was really discharged, and after spending a few hours at home alone with her, I hurried back along my parade route, right back to the hospital, quite determined to trade her in again. The baby had simply slept and slept, we were experiencing a midsummer heat wave, and I was desperate that she was not getting any fluid" (Baalsrud, 1992).

Baalsrud's description says it all – it is precisely the same mixture of joy and alarm that so many have experienced on returning home.

FORGETTING GRAMS AND MILLILITERS AND TRUSTING YOUR OWN JUDGEMENT

The length of time that babies are kept in the hospital has been getting shorter during recent years, and as a result, they are in ever greater need of care when they are discharged home. During their stay in the hospital, their feeding has commonly been governed by the clock, concern about milliliters, and the ever-present scales. One of the main challenges that parents encounter is the need to rely on one's own judgement, setting aside the regime of clocks and scales. True, there are babies who need to be reminded now and again that it is time for a meal and have to be awakened for that purpose about every three hours – since they should be fed at least eight times a day. If, of course, the baby is wide awake and in charge of its own program, it will probably be eager to get to the breast much more often.

As a rule of thumb, you can say that a baby is taking enough food if:

- It is having five or six wet diapers a day.

- You can hear or see the baby swallowing during a feed.

- It seems contented and is quiet after a breastfeed.

- You can feel the difference in your breast before and after a feed.

Not all these rules hold true for every child. In the case of preterm babies, the swallowing act may be difficult to hear. What is more, both preterm infants and babies who are ill when born at term have a tendency to seem sated and fall asleep, even before they have taken sufficient milk. In that case, however, you can fall back on the other rules of thumb – those five or six full diapers a day and your own sensation in your breasts.

But, a progressive weight gain is the most reliable and sure sign that breastfeeding is going well. During the first few weeks after coming home, you *may* feel more confident about things if you weigh your baby once a week or so, but ask in the well-baby clinic.

WHERE CAN YOU GET HELP?

If you are uncertain about anything or have questions, don't hesitate to contact a lactation consultant, the hospital, local health center, or well-baby clinic. If there is a mother-to-mother support group in your district, it may be able to put you in touch with someone who has all the experience and knowledge you need to help you (see the address list at the back of this book).

GOING HOME EARLY?

As already mentioned, quite a number of hospitals now discharge mothers and their babies early, even when the baby is preterm or unwell. In some cases, this can mean that the baby will need continuing care at home from the hospital's team for domestic care if such a team exists. Ideally, the team will call frequently during the first few days, but less often after that. So long as no particular problems are present, the emphasis will be on the baby's nutrition, its weight, the way breastfeeding is going, and ideally on building the parents' confidence, so they feel sure of themselves in caring for their baby. Early discharge from the hospital has a lot to be said for it: the parents may be together with the baby 24 hours a day; the baby will be in calm surroundings; you will have no need for trips to the hospital; and if there are brothers and sisters at home, they will be together with their parents again! It is also ideal for the progress of breastfeeding: mother and baby will be together day and night, with plenty of opportunity to see how things go at the breast. Some hospitals discharge babies with a feeding tube fitted, so the parents can give feeds that way, others arrange for the baby to go home with a cup or bottle supplementing what the breast provides. Several studies have made it quite clear that if breastfeeding is a priority, it will not be deranged by the move home, especially if the use of the bottle is avoided (Flint et al., 2007). If your hospital does not have a domestic care team, or you live too far away to make use of it, it may be possible to arrange for you to have a 24 hour stay in the hospital before discharge. Throughout the world, there are already a plethora of arrangements – some good and some less so.

FROM THE BOTTLE TO THE BREAST

Although one really ought to avoid the feeding bottle entirely, it is a fact that some babies arrive home from the hospital on mixed feeding, receiving expressed breastmilk in a bottle or through a feeding tube as a supplement to direct breastfeeding.

If you want to move to exclusive breastfeeding, you will need to plan the changeover. It may be best for both parties to tackle this gradually, reducing the number of supplementary feeds one at a time over a period. The whole process may take a few days or extend to some weeks, depending on your baby and on how confident you feel about things. It may prove most practical to begin by dropping the morning bottle-feed, then one of the afternoon feeds, after that the evening bottle, and finally the night feed. But if you are in any doubt about how to manage it, get some advice from the hospital, the well-baby clinic, a lactation consultant, other parents who have been through the process, or the local mother-to-mother support group. If the baby seems content to have larger supplementary feeds now and again, you can go along with that approach – better for your breastfeeding than providing supplementary feeds after each session at the breast. Try to breastfeed frequently between the supplementary feeds. Try to think about the total 24 hour volume instead of feeding every third or fourth hour as usual, when bottle-feeding with scheduled feedings. And for inspiration take a look at the story "Achieving the impossible" further down in this Chapter.

WHEN BREASTFEEDING AND PUMPING JUST DON'T WORK

In some cases, it is not possible to breastfeed a sick baby. After pumping her milk valiantly for weeks on end, a disillusioned mother may push the pump aside and give up. In other cases, it is the baby that never truly discovers how to use the breast, so its mother is obliged to pump endlessly and give her milk to the baby indirectly. This may be a very good solution for many mothers. In yet other cases and despite many, many weary hours spent pumping, the milk volume slowly fades and fails. Many mothers devote a truly massive effort to it all, with no guarantee that one will succeed in breastfeeding in the end. Not every mother manages it all. If you find yourself in that situation, apparently having tried in vain, don't simply conclude that you have failed your baby. On the contrary, you have tackled a difficult situation heroically! What you have achieved, even if it was not everything you would have wished, is still an achievement – the milk you did provide for days or weeks was the very best you could do, and it was valuable for your baby. Look ahead, if you like, to what we say in Chapter 11 about expectations and disappointments in breastfeeding.

ACHIEVING THE IMPOSSIBLE

We must end this Chapter with the story of a mother and daughter who, with valiant support on every side, just refused to give up. It reminds us that, even where things look impossible, there may be hope.

The Baby Who Didn't Manage to Breastfeed from the Beginning

This story is about a mother and a baby with Down syndrome, but the experience is valid for all mothers whose babies have a troublesome start to breastfeeding.

It sometimes happens that lactation consultants get phone calls from mothers who have what seem to be insoluble problems with breastfeeding. This is the story of such a call to one of us (Anna-Pia).

She rang me about her daughter – let us call her Emily – who was just seven weeks old. Emily was the family's first child, and she had been born with Down syndrome. Mother and daughter had come home from the clinic when Emily was six days old. By that time, the baby had gained 10 grams, and the staff considered that she was breastfeeding well. The mother, however, was concerned – Emily didn't seem to take the breast properly, but the mother had still wanted to return home, to get away from the maternity ward, away from all the other mothers with "normal" babies and trouble-free breastfeeding. This was how she described her daughter:

> *Emily was just like a little doll. She was tremendously passive and didn't cry at all when she was delivered. She was only awake when she was deliberately wakened. She fed very hesitantly at the breast, and tended to fall asleep unless her hands and feet were massaged all the time.*

The worries and thoughts of the future that one experiences when one's child is handicapped can be hard to bear, and each of us tackles them differently. Emily's mother writes:

> *I took care of Emily as best I could. My little "doll" received the (very little) milk she wanted, clean clothes, and dry diapers. It seemed as if I had no affection to bestow on her, but instinctively I felt that if I were to love her, I needed to have her close to me – I needed to learn to know her. It was frightening to realize that I lacked feelings for her,*

my very own child. I felt a sense of guilt: imagine how it must be to be born and to find that there is no one who loves you; sometimes I sat down and wept at the very thought. I became unbelievably sensitive to what people were saying about her. At the slightest sign that anyone in the family had not accepted her, I grew afraid and angry. All I wanted was congratulations, assurances that nothing was really wrong. I declared to anyone who was willing to listen to me that she would pull through and that children with Down syndrome develop remarkably well nowadays. All this to reassure myself that these people would learn to be fond of her – even though I wasn't managing it myself.

And so this mother returned home with her feelings in chaos. Fortunately, her husband gave her every backing and was a priceless source of strength – and yet she had a daughter who was not feeding. Two days later, Emily was almost constantly asleep and was hardly wetting her diapers; she was rushed back to hospital. After a further week in the hospital, with feeding through a feeding tube and numerous unsuccessful attempts to breastfeed, the mother was homesick and deeply miserable, and she asked whether the baby could not be given expressed breastmilk using a feeding bottle, so they could at least return home.

All the same, the mother could not give up entirely the idea of true breastfeeding, and she rang me when Emily was seven weeks old.

She had gone on pumping for all that time and was producing just enough milk, but no more than that. Emily was feeding every four hours; she still seemed tired, but as the days and weeks went by she was increasingly awake. The problem with breastfeeding her, by and large, was that on some occasions she would be too tired and want to sleep, whereas on other occasions, she was ravenously hungry and angry. The mother was finding it difficult to give up the trusted idea of giving a set amount of milk at fixed intervals. Nor was Emily putting on sufficient weight. I suggested that the mother needed to decide what course she really wanted to follow. I couldn't promise her that breastfeeding was going to be a success, but it certainly didn't seem to be impossible. Putting the whole situation right would demand a real effort, and she would need plenty of support from those around her, not only from her husband, but also from the nurse at the well-baby clinic in whom she clearly had a lot of faith. I recalled with her how she could determine whether the baby had a good hold on the breast and what she could do to stimulate Emily's mouth to open wide. A wide open mouth would mean that more of the breast could enter it and that the nipple could press up against the baby's palate, which would strengthen the milking reflex. Putting a plan like this into motion demands planning, and I suggested that she allow herself a week to succeed. To succeed with breastfeeding, one needs to put one's heart and soul into it, pausing now and again to take stock of progress and of the effort that it is demanding. At this point, the mother can take up the story herself:

> *I took the baby to bed with me, shut myself off from the outside world, and just concentrated on what I was doing. Emily received no bottles at all, but I tried to put her to the breast every hour. At first I seemed to be getting nowhere. Emily protested violently, screaming every time the breast entered her mouth. Between these attempts to feed her, she simply slept. But by the evening of the first day, she had latched on several times, and I felt that the worst was over...*

But in this flash of enthusiasm about the improvement that Emily was showing, the use of the breast pump was neglected for a time. As a result, the mother got plugged milk ducts. For a whole night, she suffered from fever, while Emily had to be fed expressed milk in a bottle. Happily, the dawning of the next day brought fresh optimism with it! In the course of one further day, the mother was noticing that if Emily was given the chance to search on her own and was allowed all the time she needed to prepare her mouth and take the breast, she secured a much better grip than before. All this naturally demanded more time – ten to 20 minutes at each feeding session. On the third day, Emily was feeding splendidly, and a proud and satisfied mother hurried off to the well- baby clinic to have her weighed. But then it proved that her weight had actually gone down – and hope seemed to ebb away again. The nurse was reassuring, "Just take her home and carry on – this will solve itself." And sure enough, a few days later, her weight began to rise again. When Emily was eight weeks old, she was breastfeeding normally, and with that, there was an end to pumping and sterilizing feeding bottles. The milk volume was also fine. Far from having to pump in order to have sufficient milk, the mother was now having to change the bed linen after a night's sleep because the breasts overflowed!

Looking back, the mother feels that Emily never, at any time, managed to breastfeed as well as another child would have done. She spent a long time at the breast, often lost her hold on it, fell asleep from time to time, and was dependent on her mother to hold the breast in place if she was to maintain a sufficient grip on it. Emily went on being breastfed until she was six months old. Today, Emily is the big sister of another baby. But her mother reminds us that at no time in her breastfeeding career did Emily match the excellent feeding latch-on which her little sister proved capable – at the very first attempt.

This story tells how one mother-child pair solved their breastfeeding problem. Others may find different ways of tackling such a situation.

Many factors played a part in Emily's and her mother's success. Among them were:

- A mother who did not give up, who actively went in search of expert advice and found it.

- A mother who was able to set herself and her baby apart from the rest of the world for a week, canceling all the appointments in her diary.

- A mother who turned back the clock and started all over again – just as if she was beginning once more from the moment of delivery.

- A mother who enjoyed the full support of her husband and of a competent and sympathetic nurse at the well-baby clinic.

As that mother puts it in her own words:

I believe that breastfeeding was so important for me because I had felt rejected by my baby. There was nothing I wanted more than to give and receive the closeness and contact that I knew about from the books.

And that mother indeed found the closeness and contact with her daughter that she had seen described in the books – perhaps just because of her breastfeeding.

Chapter 9.
WHEN MOTHER IS ILL OR HAS SORE NIPPLES

MOTHER IS ILL - CAN SHE AND SHOULD SHE BREASTFEED?

There are really very few illnesses that make it impossible – or inadvisable – to breastfeed; and even in these situations, breastfeeding may be feasible once the illness is being treated. If your family doctor is unsure as to the right course to follow, he or she may contact health staff with special competence and interest in breastfeeding, a lactation consultant, a breastfeeding resource center, or a Baby-Friendly hospital where the staff may have wisdom or experience to share.

In the case of some minor everyday illnesses, such as influenza, a bad cold, or diarrhea, your baby may pick up your infection – that is difficult to avoid. Breastfed babies are, as a rule, well protected and unlikely to become seriously ill in such cases, thanks to the antibodies passed on in the milk, as we saw in Chapter 3. Remember: breastfeeding is a shield against infection. Often one sees that a breastfed baby is the only member of the family able to shake off a virus infection that lays low everyone else in the house.

And vice-versa: if your baby acquires an infection from someone other than yourself, you may be infected in turn. But you will be able to produce antibodies to combat such an infection, something that your baby may not yet be able to do. These antibodies will then be passed on in the milk and provide the baby with the defenses he or she needs. Clever, isn't it?

The Seriously Ill Mother

A mother who is taken seriously ill is likely to need all the energy she can summon if she is to recover quickly. A chronic illness or a serious acute condition can be a reason why a mother is unable to breastfeed, doesn't feel up to it, or is well advised not to try. Every case needs to be assessed individually. It may, for example, be that a mother has been prescribed a medicine that is not compatible with breastfeeding, as we shall see later in this chapter. Again, there are various autoimmune disorders that may be affected by the hormonal changes that take place during pregnancy or breastfeeding. This group of illnesses includes various forms of rheumatism or certain inflammatory conditions of the intestine; these *can* flare up after delivery, or they may simply appear to do so because they have been moderated for a time by the hormones circulating during pregnancy.

Keep A Sense Of Balance - Don't Look on Breastfeeding as a Holy Cow!

If your state of health raises the question as to whether you should go on breastfeeding or not, you should, as a mother, try to view things in perspective. Breastfeeding is ideal for your baby's health, but that mustn't always weigh more heavily than other interests. If breastfeeding is going to put an impossible burden on your own health, and thereby on your family's overall situation, it is obviously not the right course to follow. Should you find the choice difficult or feel terribly disappointed about the idea of abandoning breastfeeding, turn to someone whom you know and trust and with whom you can talk it all through. When it comes to making a decision, the view of the parents matters a great deal. You may feel that carrying on with breastfeeding will make things better – or perhaps worse. Sometimes partial breastfeeding may be the best solution.

On other occasions, the best approach may be to delay further breastfeeding for a while, pumping your milk and, if necessary, discarding it. Discarding the milk will be advisable if you are taking medicines that are not compatible with breastfeeding.

Stopping Breastfeeding - And Then Perhaps Starting Once More?

If you are to stop breastfeeding, you need to do so progressively, rather than all at once, to avoid a blockage of the milk ducts. Now and again, you should take the baby to the breast (if that is possible) or pump your milk, but the intervals should get progressively longer until you can stop completely. If your illness is acute, but short-lasting, and after you recover, you feel like breastfeeding again, you should be able to get your milk flowing in the course of a few days or a week. You will find some advice in Chapter

6 on how to stimulate the milk production at such times, and in Chapter 7, you can learn how to return to breastfeeding. A nursing supplementer will be an excellent aid in both cases, see Chapter 10.

Are You Going Into the Hospital?

If you have to be admitted to hospital you can, if you have decided to continue to breastfeed, probably arrange to take the baby with you. That will make it possible to avoid the monotonous pumping routine, and it is quite possible that having your baby with you and caring for it will help you get better more quickly.

WHEN YOU ARE ONLY MILDLY ILL

If nothing is seriously wrong and you simply need to stay in bed for a while, the best thing for you is to be relieved of housework and baby care (except, of course, breastfeeding) for a few days. These things take a lot more energy than simply producing milk.

Do You Have a High Temperature?

A rise in temperature may, among other things, slow down your flow of milk for a few days. Don't worry about it – the milk will be back. Go on putting your baby to the breast as usual and make sure that you get plenty to drink. It may happen that (as if having a fever was not trouble enough) the baby becomes obstinate, refusing to take the unusually warm breast or to drink your warm milk! In that case, you will simply have to pump your milk to ensure that it goes on flowing as normal and that the milk ducts don't become blocked, which would only add to the misery. Medicines to bring down your temperature may also help.

BREASTFEEDING AND DIABETES

Breastfeeding can actually be a very good thing for a mother with diabetes. Producing milk has a favorable effect on her energy balance. She is likely to find that, at this time, she needs less insulin than usual. Like all other mothers, a woman with diabetes will need to increase her food intake. She may well discover that in spite of the extra calories she does not need a higher dose of insulin. To make whatever adjustments to her treatment are necessary when she starts breastfeeding or at the time of weaning, she should talk to her physician. With his or her help, she will need to adapt her energy intake and her insulin dose, since her energy needs will rise when breastfeeding starts and will fall again when it ends. A breastfeeding diabetic mother, who doesn't need insulin, should simply follow a healthy diet, as she did during pregnancy, and make sure that her blood sugar level stays steady.

Mothers with type 1 diabetes may have a delayed onset of lactation due to a lower level of prolactin, but they should not give up – their milk will come in sooner or later (Riordan & Wambach, 2010).

Babies of diabetic mothers may have problems with low blood sugar levels and often need supplementation. On the other hand, exclusive breastfeeding is associated with a reduced risk of diabetes, both type 1 and 2, and the use of formula for supplementation should therefore be avoided if possible (Ip, Chung, Raman, Trikalinos, & Lau, 2009). Jack Newman, a pediatrician working with breastfeeding for a lifetime, suggests that these mothers could instead express colostrum during the last weeks before birth, freeze it, and give it to the baby as supplementation during the first few days of life if needed (Newman & Pitman, 2000b).

BREASTFEEDING AND DEPRESSION

Almost every mother goes through a period when the whole birthing venture leads her to despair. There will probably be days when her feelings about life swing up and down, tears are not very far away, and everything seems tough and challenging. These things pass, and they are quite different from a true depression, which is longer lasting. Anyone suffering from real depression is likely to feel that everything is hopeless, that she is a failure and completely unsuited to motherhood. Symptoms like anxiety, deep uneasiness, difficulty in sleeping, and loss of energy are typical of depression. Whatever you do: get help! Ring your district nurse; make an appointment with your family doctor or whoever else in the health service you know you can rely on. Your local mother-to-mother breastfeeding support group may also be able to put you in touch with other mothers who have been through the same wretched experience. You may need proper medical treatment, such as psychotherapy or a prescribed medicine. There are many medicines that can be used without the need to stop breastfeeding. Depression is sometimes coupled with breastfeeding problems, but in such situations, it can be difficult to know what the basic problem is – did the breastfeeding difficulties lead to the depression or did the depression lead the mother to believe that breastfeeding was an impossible task? Whatever the reason, your breastfeeding problem needs to be taken seriously, and with good advice, it will probably soon be solved. Just occasionally, a true depression may look like a reason to give up breastfeeding completely or to cut it down. Your feelings about the matter are important – what do you see as the best solution for yourself? Setting a more modest goal may be the sensible approach to breastfeeding at these times; worrying less about what you think you are *supposed* to achieve and setting out to do something that seems more within your reach may be the right way to go about it.

What You Can Do

Try not to put ambitious demands on yourself. Decide what you can realistically hope to do every day, and what is right for you. What really matters is just the well-being of your baby and yourself; whether the house has been cleaned or not is much less important. Accept help gladly, and try to spend time with your family and friends, even when you feel tempted to hide away. Get out into the fresh air – take a walk. If you manage to open up, admitting how you feel to someone you trust, you will soon find that a lot of people have at times felt just as you do now. Do it, even though you may be tempted, as we all often are, to show only the sunnier side of your thoughts. Various people have found how helpful it can be to have your baby with you in a carrier pouch – the baby is calmed, experiencing the closeness that it needs so much, even from an exhausted mother.

MEDICINES AND BREASTMILK

All the medicines you take pass into your milk to some extent, but the great majority do not have any effect on your baby. There are just a certain number that you should not be taking while breastfeeding, and they can usually be replaced by something else at this time. Just how much of a medicine gets into the milk depends on various complicated factors: how strongly the medicine is bound to your blood, the drug's pH value (i.e., its acidity), its solubility in body fat, and its so-called "distribution volume," which reflects how widely it is spread around your body. The amount of medicine getting into the milk also differs with time – it can be quite different shortly after birth than during the later phases of breastfeeding. Obviously, an average mother can't assess these things for herself. So if you need to take medicine, ask the advice of your pharmacist or consult a doctor who can tell you what is known. For that matter: if a doctor does prescribe any medicine for you, always say that you are breastfeeding before he or she starts writing a prescription. Should your own doctor not have all the facts at hand, he or she can get advice on the matter from a drug information center, the national breastfeeding association, or a website, such as: www. infantrisk.com. There are also various dependable "drug compendia" and specialized books that provide independent information and advice on the use of medicines during breastfeeding (Hale, 2010).

POSSIBLE PROBLEMS WITH THE BREASTS

Sore Nipples

As we saw in Chapter 5, breastfeeding should, in principle, never be a painful process. Provided you get sound guidance at the outset, you should really not have to expect any problems, like sore nipples. All the same, as in other walks of life, things don't always go quite as smoothly as they should.

We recognize three main sorts of sore nipples:

- Sore nipples caused by sucking that can lead to a bacterial infection or a yeast infection/fungus (thrush).

- Sore nipples caused by a fungal infection, where there has been no damage caused by sucking.

- Sore nipples as part of a skin disorder (for example dermatitis).

Sore Nipples - Some Basic Facts

Sore nipples are quite simply a misery. Anyone who has not experienced them can hardly comprehend that something that looks so insignificant to a bystander can be so excessively painful. The fact is, however, a nipple has the same sort of nerves as those found on the front of the eye, in other words, little nerves that are very sensitive and that react strongly, even to a friendly touch, let alone a painful stimulus. Nipple soreness can and should be avoided primarily by good positioning and proper attachment (see Chapter 5). Above all, the baby should not be held in such a way that it is obliged to suck on the nipple, chew on it, or maybe even bite it in order to keep a hold on it.

A lot has been said and written about sore nipples. Some of the advice dates back thousands of years, illustrating clearly how poorly society through the ages has contrived to help mothers and children to breastfeed properly. The oddest solutions have been recommended and used both by responsible physicians and wise women. Some of these "remedies" do provide relief for soreness of the skin, others only make it worse.

But no remedy was or is likely to work with sore nipples unless one understands and applies the principles of sound breastfeeding, and in particular, good positioning and proper attachment.

Problem: Sore Nipples Caused by Sucking

If, while a baby is valiantly trying to feed at the breast, it is held too far away from the mother's body, it will be obliged to use strong suction (in other words, to suck for all it is worth) to keep the nipple and a sufficient amount of breast in its mouth. So the baby sucks on the breast and pulls at the nipple, and it is hardly surprising that the nipple gets sore. One can often see quite clearly where and how the small mouth has been at work on the breast, sucking on it vigorously, for the suction is likely to have left a telltale crescent-shaped trail of small hemorrhages, often stretching from one side of the nipple to the other. A baby may also have a bad latch on the breast if the mouth was not sufficiently wide open during attachment. Just compare Figure 9.1, showing a baby grasping the breast too narrowly, with Figure 9.2, where the baby has latched on with its mouth wide open, ready to take in a good portion of breast.

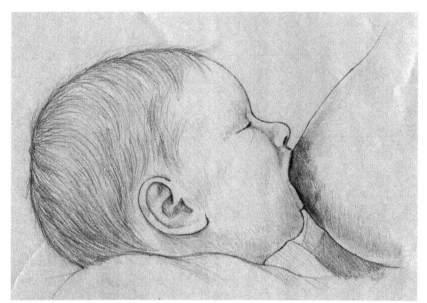

Figure 9.1. *Poor attachment*

Source: *Drawing by Pollyanna von Knorring. Used with permission.*

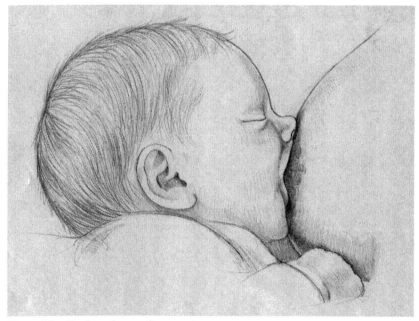

Figure 9.2. *Good attachment after correction*

Source: *Drawing by Pollyanna von Knorring. Used with permission.*

Solution: Wait for the Wide Open Mouth

When you put the baby to the breast, its mouth must be open wide – if it isn't, that little milking machine won't be able to take in a decent amount of breast. Stimulate the baby's lips by brushing them with the nipple, ideally with a drop of milk temptingly in place, until the mouth opens up, all ready to take in a good mouthful of breast without difficulty. The tongue will then be nicely in place, folded neatly on itself and ready to work on the breast. Pull the baby close against you, still making sure that it has a good mouthful of breast.

If you find it difficult to understand how best to position the baby, ask someone with experience to guide you. If need be, take another close look at the section on good positioning in Chapter 5. If the baby is positioned as it should be, you may well find that even nipples that have been sore no longer hurt during feeding, or at least the pain is less. If the baby's movements during feeding are still causing you much pain, try positioning again. It can happen that a baby becomes impatient, but you'll do yourself a poor service by putting up with more than incidental pain for a while. Should it all become too much, try offering some milk in a cup just to assuage your baby's real pangs of hunger – and then try breastfeeding once more!

Solution: Vary Your Positioning – Or Alternate Between Two Different Positions

Sometimes a change of position is all you need. For example, if you try the under the arm position (see Figure 5.6 in Chapter 5), the pull on the nipple will be different, and that may well be sufficient to overcome the pain and promote rapid healing. You can also change things by moving your baby from one breast to the other, or you can try sitting or lying down. Moving around like this changes the shape of the breast, and this can be enough to enable the baby to get a better grip.

Solution: Help the Let-Down Reflex Along

If you find that it takes a while before your milk begins to flow (in other words before the let-down reflex comes into play), you may want to try getting it moving *before* the baby is positioned at the breast. After washing your hands, try rolling the nipple between your fingers, preferably without a bra or other clothing in the way, and making sure that you are only pressing on the least painful side of the nipple. Or use the Reverse Pressure Softening method described in Chapter 5. You can read more about this in Chapter 10.

Solution: Soften up that Breast

Now and again, a baby may find it difficult to get a sufficient grip because the breast is so tightly filled with milk. If it is already sore, the resulting struggle will only make it more so. By a little hand milking (see Chapter 10) or using the Reverse Pressure Softening method (Chapter 5), you can soften up the breast and make it easier for your baby to get a decent mouthful without the need to engage in a tug-of-war to reach the goodies.

Problem: Sore Nipples That Just Won't Get Better

If the nipples remain sore even after you have improved the positioning and in spite of your having tried all the other solutions we suggest, it may be that the soreness is due to a bacterial infection, infestation with a fungus (thrush), a skin disorder, an allergic reaction, or a short frenulum (tongue tie). The last three possibilities are rare, but not unknown, so we will take a look at each of them.

Problem: Sore Nipples Because of a Bacterial Infection

If the skin that covers the nipple has been damaged, it becomes a ready entry point for bacteria. That doesn't necessarily mean visible pus or an obviously open wound – the area may be quite dry and the entry point can well be no more than a small split in the skin. The result may be persistent pain, tenderness, or further splitting of the skin. The pain may be felt in the breast itself, rather than just in the nipple, and may be present even when you are not breastfeeding.

You should wash the breast daily in the shower. Use a slightly acid soap (i.e., one with a low pH – your pharmacy can show you the sort you need). Allow the breasts plenty of air – avoid packing them inside a bra all day. Change the nursing pads often to keep dry. A woolen inlay has to tolerate washing in quite hot water (60°C).

Solution: Call in the Health Team

Contact your doctor to find out if you have a bacterial infection. Some doctors, common in Scandinavia, will do bacteriological testing of the milk, as well as the infected area, to diagnose just what sort of bugs are causing the trouble and make it possible to treat you with the correct antibiotics. It may be necessary to use an antibiotic, either immediately or after the bacteriological report arrives, depending on how the health team assesses your infection.

Problem: Fungal Infection ("Thrush")

This is an infection caused by the fungus or yeast known as *Candida albicans*. It may have come from your own body, the baby, or your partner. In a typical case of candida infection, the nipple (and sometimes the areola around it as well) is persistently red, irritable, sometimes itching, but smooth and glistening. Breastfeeding can be very painful indeed, even with the best possible positioning, and the pain usually continues right through the feeding session. Although the pain is concentrated in the nipple, it can radiate out through the whole breast, and it can continue or recur, even when not breastfeeding. You may see small white specks on the nipple, while the skin around it reddens and may tend to flake off. The small white specks on the nipple may look like traces of milk or there may be a whitish film, but one can't wipe them away. Your baby may or may not have thrush in the mouth. Many babies have thrush in the mouth, but rarely with symptoms of candida infection, i.e., with red areas and pain. A yeast infection can occur without any obvious reason at any time during breastfeeding. It is most common after you have been breastfeeding for a while, but you have a greater chance of contracting it if your nipples have been damaged by faulty sucking, if you are receiving antibiotics for any reason, or if you have a yeast infection in your vagina.

Solution: Treat All Possible Sources of Thrush at the Same Time

The aim of treatment cannot be to banish the fungus completely, since it is one of the microorganisms that are normally present on the skin and the mucous membranes where they live quite peacefully, causing no trouble at all. In treating a troublesome infestation, the goal must simply be to re-establish this peaceful co-existence. To break what may well become a vicious circle of infection affecting both mother and baby, one will need to treat the nipples and the baby's mouth simultaneously, and one should do this even if the baby currently shows no sign of thrush.

It is necessary to treat your own vaginal thrush and any sign of thrush around the baby's buttocks, also.

Solution: Contact Your Health Services

The health service will probably prescribe an anti-fungus cream that has to be applied locally. You should replace the nursing pad every time you apply the medicine – a new one can be cut out of an old towel or bed sheet. If you use woolen pads that can be washed and re-used, they must be able to tolerate really hot water (60°C); the same goes for your bras, bed linen, and towels. During the fortnight or more that treatment continues, you will need to keep everything scrupulously clean to avoid leaving any surviving fungus here or there – for example, on a pacifier, a teething ring, toys, or parts of a breast pump. All these things need to be washed well in soapy water every day, and then boiled for five to ten minutes. Wash your hands thoroughly, especially after a feed, after changing a diaper, or after visiting the toilet. If you have expressed milk while thrush is around, you can give it to the baby right away, but don't add it to milk you plan to keep in the freezer for future use – the fungus can survive freezing. In some instances, it may not be sufficient to treat the infection locally with cream, and the doctor may give you tablets to take as well. Don't worry – there are several effective remedies that can be safely used while you are breastfeeding.

Solution: Plenty of Air and Light

A fungus thrives wherever it is damp and dark, so exposing your breasts to plenty of air and light is always a good thing. You can also try taking acidophilus with bifidus – probiotica in the form of capsules, or drinking milk or eating yogurt enriched with these bacteria – it will all help to support the normal population of healthy bacteria in your gastrointestinal tract.

Problem: Soreness Because of a Skin Disorder

If the skin around your nipples is sore and it is not because of faulty latching on or positioning and not caused by a fungus or microorganism, you will need to look for some other cause. You may be having a reaction to the detergent or textile softener you use or even to some chemical in the clothes you are wearing or have worn recently. Some people's skin can react badly to the paper used in commercial nursing pads. Certain people react to the woolen inlays or lanolin ointment. If you suffer from eczema or psoriasis, these conditions are just as likely to affect the breast or nipple as any other part of the body.

Solution: Get Rid of the Cause or Seek Medical Help

If you can track down the cause and get rid of it, the soreness should very soon be over. If it persists or if you have psoriasis or anything that looks like a skin problem, go and see a doctor – ideally a dermatologist.

Problem: Relieving Soreness – Whatever the Cause

Solution: Give the Breast Plenty of Air and Keep It Dry!

Go on breastfeeding, but after each feed, leave your breast uncovered for a while, so that the last drops of milk have a chance to dry on the nipple. Thanks to the fact that the milk provides protection against infection, it is the best medicine imaginable for sore nipples! Try going without a bra in the daytime and sleeping without a bra at night, unless you have a problem with leakage. If you find your breasts need some support, take an old bra and cut out holes for the nipples. A breast shell (see Chapter 10) can also provide relief and ensure there is plenty of air around the nipples.

Keep your breasts as dry as possible. You may find that a larger cotton bra (a so-called breastfeeding model) or a standard elastic bra is helpful, keeping the nursing pads nicely in place. And take another look at the solutions we suggested above under the heading "Sore nipples caused by sucking."

Creams

In principle, breastfeeding mothers should try to avoid applying any sort of cream or ointment to the nipple. Some mothers do, however, find that it helps to put on a very thin layer of lanolin ointment to keep the skin soft. If you see that a crust has developed over the sore area, it is wise to soften it up with a lanolin ointment or a neutral fatty cream. If you keep the crust soft, it won't so readily crack when you take off your bra or during a feed, and the area will heal more quickly.

Problem: A Short Frenulum ("Tongue Tie")

Occasionally, a baby will have an unusually short frenulum (the ligament that holds the tongue to the floor of the mouth), and this may cause soreness of the nipples. Ask your nurse to see if that is your problem. If so, it is very simple for a doctor to cut the frenulum, and that will, as a rule, solve the problem.

Problem: "White" Nipples

Some mothers with painful breastfeeding may feel severe pain and have an unusual whiteness of the nipples – as if they are bloodless – after a breastfeed, also called vasospasm. Sometimes the color turns to red or blue before going back to normal. The change may occur within seconds or minutes of the baby leaving the breast. The phenomenon also occurs occasionally in women who have experienced no pain when breastfeeding. Some women get ischemia in toes and fingers (Raynaud's phenomenon).

Solution: Do Not Touch

If the nipples are sore, first find the cause and treat it. Avoid as much as possible directly touching the nipple. It may be helpful to apply heat to the breast or drink a large cup of tea before a breastfeed; tea contains theophylline, which causes the blood vessels to relax. If the pain is severe and shows no sign of improvement, contact your health team for advice and possible medical treatment.

Blocked Milk Ducts

Not uncommonly, milk may fail to appear from one or more milk passages or one or more segments of the breast. The affected area is likely to be hard to the touch and very often tender. The body temperature may be slightly raised. Blocked milk ducts are more likely to occur in cold climates, if you have been thinly clad in very cold weather, or if the breast has been exposed to cold air or water. They can also occur if the breast has been overfilled. Sometimes a tight bra can cause the problem, or it may simply be a sign that you are tired and stressed.

Another form of blockage is called "milk stasis," where both breasts are tender, taut, and painful. This tends to happen after a baby has slept through the night without feeding. You need to get some milk out of the breast to relieve the pressure, and you should do it right away!

How to Get the Milk Moving Again

Your baby is likely to be best able to help you. To get the milk moving, you should first try positioning the baby in different ways – you may find a position in which the milk flow starts up again. A baby's jaw, as we have seen, is the most effective milking device of all. Try positioning it so the baby's chin points directly to the area where the milk flow seems to be blocked. Continue to do this while you try different positions, including some less common varieties like the "under the arm position" (Figure 5.6, Chapter 5), the "wolf" position, where you are on all fours over your baby (remember the story of Romulus and Remus), or let the baby "stand" in your lap. Every position that is not painful or too uncomfortable is worth trying. If that doesn't seem to work, you will have to express the milk by hand (or, as a last resort, with a breast pump). Once the milk begins to flow again, you can try "stroking" it out – lightly massaging that segment of the breast in the direction of the nipple to keep the milk flowing – use the flat of your hand rather than your fingers. But don't be rough with yourself – remember that the alveoli are delicate little structures. Sometimes the blockage is right up front in the nipple. In that case, apply heat on the nipple, and at the same time, press gently on the areola behind the nipple. You may have to try this several times before the milk begins to flow again. When you are faced with a milk blockage in the outermost part of the breast, you can try lying down on your side with the problem breast uppermost, and lay the baby in front of you, ideally on a flat cushion. Next roll slightly forward so the baby is directly in front of the breast that needs help. In this position, the force of gravity will help to direct the milk forward and downward. Once you hear the baby swallowing regularly, try massaging the breast towards the nipple as we described above. Incidentally, this position can also be very suitable for breastfeeding after a Cesarean section – see Figure 7.4 in Chapter 7.

Help the Let-Down Reflex

It can be helpful to apply a warm towel, take a warm shower or bath, or apply some other warming appliance to a breast with blocked milk passages. All these things may help the let-down reflex to perform as it should, and they may also relax the small muscles around the nipple, so the milk can flow more readily.

The Virtues of Frequent Milking

Where you have a milk blockage, it is always good to offer the breast frequently – for example, hourly during the day and every three hours at night (set the alarm clock) until the symptoms have completely disappeared. As we always say, your baby is the best milker of all, but if you don't want to offer both breasts so often, you can feed your baby mainly from the breast that has the problem to ensure it doesn't recur. On the other breast, you can express the milk by hand or resort to the breast pump.

Relax...

Take things as easy as you can until your problems with milk production are completely resolved. In that way, you will avoid the risk of the blockage developing into mastitis. If you have a raised temperature, you should stay in bed. If possible, call on your support troops to take care of the rest of the family and run the kitchen.

Mastitis - Inflammation of the Breast

Mastitis, popularly known as inflammation of the breast, is most common the first weeks after birth, but can happen at any time during the whole breastfeeding period. With mastitis, you are likely to feel as if you are ill in every inch of your body – rather as if you are developing a nasty bout of influenza. You may begin to feel generally ill, even before you actually develop symptoms in the breast, but more commonly the first sign is when the breast becomes hot, tender, and reddened, and the general bodily symptoms follow. You are at increased risk if you have cracked nipples; are stressed or fatigued; have untreated plugged ducts, engorgement, or too much milk; or if your baby sleeps through a feeding. The breast condition can, as a rule, be treated successfully without interrupting feeding, but it is important to tackle the problem properly.

It is important to realize that flu-like symptoms *can* develop without any bacterial infection being present.

When Should You Call on Medical Advice?

If you don't experience any improvement or your symptoms are getting worse after you have spent 24 hours having the baby suckle the affected breast and doing everything else that is needed (see suggestions for treatment in "blocked ducts" below), contact your health support team or a physician with experience in breastfeeding problems. In some instances, bacteria will prove to be at the root of the problem, for example, if you have already been suffering from sore nipples. Before starting you on antibiotics, it is a good idea to carry out a bacteriological test of your milk. Yellow Staphylococci are the most common cause of bacterial mastitis, so the first choice of treatment is likely to be an antibiotic that is capable of tackling these particular microorganisms. Take the full course of antibiotics that has been prescribed for you – don't stop the treatment without consulting your doctor. Go on emptying the breast often during the course of treatment. There is no reason to stop giving your baby the milk it needs.

Pain Associated with Mastitis

It can be very unpleasant to breastfeed with a tender breast, but you have to try. If necessary, you can take something to relieve pain. The first choice when you have mastitis is ibuprofen, which will reduce both pain and inflammation. The second choice is acetaminophen (known outside the USA as paracetamol). Remember, too, that warmth can give relief from pain.

Breast Abscess

Occasionally, but not very often, mastitis may develop into an abscess. If that happens, the breast will be swollen and reddish, and you may feel a persistent lump or perhaps something like a balloon filled with fluid. The affected breast may produce less milk than usual. You may have a high fever, but it is also possible that your temperature will be only slightly raised or even normal. You will need an ultrasound examination, and if it shows that pus has accumulated in the breast, it may need to be released through a small incision or with aspiration by a needle. In most cases, you will be able to continue breastfeeding.

Lumps Which Do Not Disappear

One last point: if you do find that you have one or more lumps which either do not change in size or which grow in size in the breast, whether they are painful or not, you should *always* ask your physician to examine you!

Chapter 10.
BEING PRACTICAL ABOUT THINGS

CARRYING THE BABY

Women have been carrying their babies close to their bodies for thousands of years; being carried around like that is quite simply something that most babies thoroughly enjoy. Colic and thumb sucking are rare in places where babies are traditionally carried. Put the baby in the pram (stroller), on the other hand, and just about as soon as it gets wise as to what's going on, a shrill protest breaks loose. We tend to overlook these signals of indignation because we are so convinced that this is the way things should be (everyone uses a pram, don't they?). That is what we have been told so often and by so many people who are supposed to know (especially by people who sell prams), that we take it to be true. But perhaps we ought to show just a little more respect for baby's own views and preferences on the matter – at least if we have a healthy pair of shoulders to carry our baby around.

Some cultures have been more ingenious than others in devising various ways to carry a baby – look around the world if you have the opportunity and see the differences for yourself. Carrying a baby in a mother's shawl has come back into fashion, and mothers – and babies – who are trying it are enthusiastic. Look them up on the Internet addresses at the back of this book.

CARRYING - AND BREASTFEEDING

If you carry your baby in a shawl, cloth, or sling, the breast will be conveniently close at hand when it is time for a feed. What's more, it will be easy to hide what you are up to when it's time for breastfeeding if you feel that too much openness may be embarrassing or when it may not be appreciated by the people around you! Slightly older babies, especially those aged six to nine months or so, may be able to concentrate better on feeding if they are shielded from prying eyes, so they don't get distracted.

A very young baby (less than six weeks old) can best be carried in front of you, using a cloth of a suitable size or a sling. In that way, you are always in touch with how your baby is faring, and its head and body will be well supported. You may, of course, buy a commercial baby carrier, but it is not necessary. A piece of cloth is very flexible. By using it in various ways, you can start making use of it just after birth and continue until the baby is about three years old. A shawl, cloth, or sling should be fairly taut, so the baby is resting against your body, rather than hanging in front of you. This puts the least strain on your baby's body. Preterm or low birth weight babies can be carried skin-to-skin using a shawl or a variety of other methods (see more in Chapter 8). An older baby can be carried in a sitting position on your back – something that is a familiar sight all over the world. Whichever method you use, you will find that as you carry your baby, you will have at least one hand free to do other things, while your baby remains close to you. And you'll probably soon find that it's at least as convenient as pushing a pram around – or more so!

TRAVELING WITH A BREASTFEEDING BABY

Whether you're traveling by plane or car, going camping, or leaving for a safari abroad, breastfeeding is best – especially in the tropics. In warm climates, breastfeeding has tremendous advantages over anything else – it's the most hygienic way of feeding, the simplest, the coziest, and the safest. Also, your breastmilk is always ready when you need it – nothing to mix or warm up. Breastmilk is also an ideal way for a baby to quench its thirst on a hot day. You don't need to give your breastfed baby water – in fact, it's better not to.

A mother traveling to a foreign country soon builds up her immunity to unfamiliar microorganisms, and the antibodies that protect her are passed on to the baby in her milk. It is much better not to confront a fully breastfed baby with local water of unknown quality or with unfamiliar foods – either may be spiced with untrustworthy bacteria. And if your baby is upset by strange and changing surroundings, offer it something that is comfortingly familiar – your own breast.

All the same, even breastfeeding under these conditions brings some simple rules of hygiene with it – try to wash your hands before putting your baby to the breast, and if you can't do that, then clean them with wet wipes. Should your older baby experience diarrhea because of all those unfamiliar bacteria, just give it all the breastmilk it wants. This is WHO's advice for such occasions.

Flying with Babies

A little child can't manage to yawn or swallow to get rid of those uncomfortable sensations in the ears that are caused by changing air pressure when a plane goes up or down.

Breastfeeding mothers have found the solution: just put the baby to the breast. As the baby swallows the milk, the pressure differences in and around the ears are evened out. Once again, the best advice to a breastfeeding mother is the simplest: you have breasts – use them!

The most suitable clothes for a traveling breastfeeding mother will always be the sort that enables the breast to be within easy reach at all times. Few things are less enjoyable than to find yourself in a crowded railway compartment with a hungry baby and discover that you have to do a striptease in order to breastfeed. All the same, people tend to be friendly to a mother who needs to breastfeed her baby. Divans and secluded corners are willingly offered, and the occasion may be the time to make new friends.

Breastfeeding and Strenuous Physical Training

Some years back, international medical journals reported prominently that breastfeeding mothers who had taken up hard physical training were finding that their children preferred the milk they produced before a strenuous session to the milk they produced immediately afterwards. Further research showed there was indeed a difference in the milk – after a training session, it contained more lactic acid than before (Wallace, Inbar, & Ernsthausen, 1992). This milk, however, is not harmful in any way for the baby; the difference is only evident after very tough exercise indeed, and in some women, there is no difference at all. If your baby should turn up its nose at your milk after a sports session, simply give the baby expressed milk. Try to exercise right after a feeding, so your milk has time to return to normal before the next feeding. Plus it is easier to exercise with empty breasts than with full ones!

The most important thing is the general agreement, which now exists that even strenuous training by a breastfeeding mother has no harmful consequences for the baby. Physical exercise to keep in good condition has everything going for it; just make sure to drink enough fluids whenever you feel at all thirsty, try some warming up exercises before things get really tough, and increase your exercise level gradually.

Breastfeeding on the Job

For a mother who has her daily work outside the home, and who can arrange for others to look after the baby for much of the day, breastfeeding can be a thoroughly enjoyable experience. By continuing to breastfeed, the mother feels that she has something unique to offer her baby, and perhaps she experiences with particular intensity those hours of the day when she is with her child. Quite apart from breastfeeding offering her the chance for close and intimate contact with her child; for the baby, these hours of the day may make up for the physical absence of the mother at other times.

Laws and regulations about leave from work for pregnancy and nursing depend very much on where you live. The Nordic countries are good examples of what can be achieved – leave for pregnancy and nursing in Norway runs to 33 weeks on full salary or as much as 42 weeks on 80% of salary. The Norwegian rules for State employees also state that once the mother returns to work, she can claim two half-hourly breaks every day to breastfeed, or alternatively, she can have a reduction in working time of one hour daily, as well as sufficient time to get to her home and back. It is also common for a mother to use these times to express her milk, so it can be given to her child later. There are somewhat different rules for women in public service jobs, but these, too, make ample provision for a long period of breastfeeding.

Still Some Way to Go....

As we have said, the rules about leave for breastfeeding differ with the country where you live, and they may also vary with your place of work. Your health center can advise you well in advance what your rights are. In many parts of the world, those rights are increasing, but we still have some way to go. For example, one would like to see everywhere:

- Crèches or day care centers provided by large employers so that, as long as necessary, a mother and father can be with the baby several times during the working day.

- Shorter working hours for parents with small children. A woman who gladly seizes the opportunity to get out of the house after confinement will probably work all the more enthusiastically for that reason, perhaps achieving as much in four hours as she would if she were obliged by law to work for eight and spent much of that time wondering how the baby is getting on and worrying that she is not able to find more time for the family.

Investigations show that, with proper and far-sighted rules in place, breastfeeding women are able to play a full part in society, and that breastfeeding is more common among women going out to work than among those working at home.

Striking also, though not entirely fair, is the fact that working women with a higher level of education seem to enjoy better labor conditions than others, as regards breastfeeding, and are more likely to go on breastfeeding and working at the same time. A woman with a more senior post may be in a stronger bargaining position with her employer on such matters than a woman in a less powerful position. This is truly an area calling for solidarity among women! These matters are as important for the children as they are for the parents. It is particularly during the first year of life that lasting relationships within the family are developed, and parents can more easily bring up children whom they feel they know, and when they feel confident about the relationship.

Some Practical Tips

To make the best of a situation where one is going to be breastfeeding while working outside the home, you need to make a deliberate effort – and perhaps have a little luck as well. Here are some practical tips you may find helpful.

Before You Start

Try to establish a regular feeding rhythm before you return to work.

If You Start Work or Study Before the Baby Is Six Months Old

Since a baby of this age will probably still be getting only milk, expression or pumping are going to be a prominent part of your life. Try to make arrangements for the baby to stay at a day care center or with a responsible person close to your place of work. Take a look at the labor regulations, which will apply to you as regards taking time off for feeding. If possible, you should be able to feed the child once or twice in the course of a working day. You should avoid an interval of more than four hours between feeds. This should be enough to keep your milk production going, and after you get home in the afternoon, you may be able to provide slightly more frequent feeds. This sort of arrangement may, however, prove fairly costly, especially if you are not allowed to take time off with pay for the feeding sessions, but it is certainly the most enjoyable solution.

You can also pump your milk at home, and then leave it to others to give it to the baby while you are at work. Many women find it simplest to express milk by hand. Some mothers manage to pump milk from one breast, while the baby is feeding at the other – something that can work quite well if the baby is not easily distracted or too interested in the mechanics of what is going on.

If you cannot manage full breastfeeding, you can, of course, try to combine breastfeeding with bottle-feeding.

If Your Working Day Is Very Long

If you have a working day of eight hours or so, you may well find your breasts getting very tense from all the milk they contain, and if this happens too often, there is a chance that your milk supply will begin to decline, or even that you will develop a blockage of some milk ducts. For that reason, it is advisable to express your milk by hand or using a pump several times during the working day, preferably at the times you would have given breastfeeds, and at intervals of not more than three to four hours. Should you notice that your milk production is declining more than you like, express your milk more often or try breastfeeding a little more often when you get home from work, and take a rest whenever you can.

A Room of One's Own

The least you can reasonably expect from your employers, in the interest of a strong and healthy nation in the future, is a decent, nice room where you can carry out your pumping and other breast hygiene matters. To show their appreciation of what you are doing for their future work force, they can also see to it that you have a refrigerator and a water heater in the room. Banishing you to the toilet, as has frequently happened, just will not do!

If possible, try going to bed with the baby for an hour or so after you return home, and let it do just what it wants–taking milk or simply relaxing very close to you. At night, the baby should have ready access to the breast. If you prefer not to have the baby in bed with you, put the cradle close to your bed so that you can pick up the baby without getting up – take another look at the picture of the Estonian baby bed.

If You Begin to Work Again After Ten to 12 Months

There is no good reason to end breastfeeding when you return to a job outside the home after you have been nursing for ten to 12 months. By that time, most women are giving their babies a fair amount of other food, and breastmilk is a smaller part of the total diet. By this time, most women will manage to get through a normal working day (preferably with a little time off for breastfeeding) without the need for expressing milk, and the baby can have unrestricted access to the breast during the hours you are together. The stimulation you get from suckling is hopefully enough to keep the milk flowing for as long as you want. Many women have managed to combine breastfeeding with employment outside the home, and most of them will tell you that they would not gladly have missed either!

Hand Expression

It's very useful to teach yourself how to express your milk by hand. You will be independent of an electric pump and electricity, and all sorts of breastfeeding problems can be avoided by a little hand milking. Many mothers find that expressing milk by hand is better and quicker than using a pump. One mother described in an interview how she was able, after a little training, to empty each breast by hand in as little as seven minutes. Others find they need 20-30 minutes each time. Some mothers show a stroke of genius in contriving to milk both breasts at the same time. This has the advantage that the let-down reflex is used to maximal effect, acting as it does on both breasts at once, so the whole process is completed in half the usual time.

Don't despair if you are in doubt about how to do it. The milk may not begin to flow right away, depending on whether or not you have managed to elicit the let-down reflex at the outset. *Hand expression should never be painful.* If it does hurt, it is because you have not yet got the technique right. Try again a little differently, or ask for help from someone who can show you how to do it Again: don't be rough with yourself, and try to keep calm, even if you get no milk at all flowing the first few times you try – you will soon pick up the art.

Preparing For Action – Stimulate the Let-Down Reflex

Before you can begin actual milking, you should try to get the milk let-down reflex to work. There are several ways to approach it:

- Take a deep breath. Enjoy the bright side of things, such as the fact that you can now sit down and relax for a while.

- Have a warm cup of tea, music according to your taste, something warm around the shoulders and the breasts – any or all of these things help.

- Relax and think a little about the baby -look at its picture, fondle or sniff some of its clothes – and you may find the milk promptly comes spouting out.

- Elicit the let-down reflex by taking the nipple between the thumb and forefinger, and rolling or stroking it just enough for it to become erect. You can do this through your clothes. In this way, the many sensitive nerve endings in the nipple, especially those at the tip, are stimulated and signals are sent to the pituitary gland to release oxytocin. If you are using a pump on one breast, you can massage the other nipple through the clothing. Try massaging the breasts very gently. Any form of stimulation is likely to help – just do what you find most agreeable.

- Go back to Chapter 1 to review the physiology of the let-down reflex and to Chapter 5 for greater detail in how to elicit it. You may find it more helpful to look at a video. You will find plenty of videos explaining the expression of breastmilk on the internet. Ask a breastfeeding support group if they have one you can borrow – several have been made.

In the next section, we will show you in some detail how you are likely to experience hand milking.

Find Something to Collect the Milk In

Take a teacup, a bowl, or a small pan. A pan has the advantage that it's easily sterilized; just fill it with water, bring it to the boil, and let it boil for three minutes, and presto, you have a sterile container for the milk. Sit at a high table (or on a low chair pulled up to an ordinary table), so the container is the right height to catch the milk. Make sure that you're sitting comfortably. You may or may not get a little help from the force of gravity by leaning forwards (Figure 10.1).

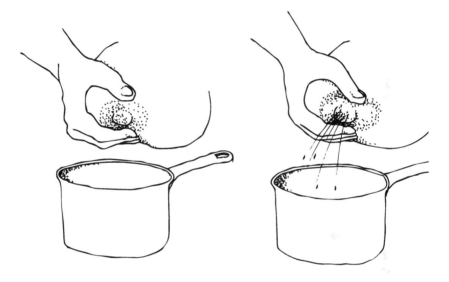

Figure 10.1. *Hand milking*

Source: Drawing by Ingerid Helsing Almaas. Used with permission.

TEN STEPS FOR EXPRESSING MILK BY HAND

1. Wash your hands thoroughly.

2. Elicit the milk let-down reflex in the way we have described.

3. Place your thumb on the upper surface of the nipple, just on the edge of the areola or where you feel the milk ducts; put your forefinger in a similar position on the underside of the nipple. Your other fingers should support the breast without exerting pressure on the milk ducts or the alveoli (see Figures 1.1 and 1.2 in Chapter 1).

4. Press the thumb and forefinger inwards towards the chest, but not hard enough to be uncomfortable. Then press the thumb and forefinger together, and concentrate your thoughts on the milk, which is about to flow out of the nipple. Try to ensure that you are holding the milk ducts where the milk is flowing – close your eyes and experience the sensation.

5. Press the thumb and forefinger together, and then release your hold. Press inwards towards the chest, then press thumb and forefinger together once more. Release your hold... and so the cycle continues...

6. Roll your fingers on the skin, do not slide them.

7. Change your grip after a little while, putting the thumb on the left side of the nipple and the forefinger on the right, then proceed as before. A little later you can change position again, holding the nipple diagonally. Continue in the same way, changing the angle of your grip each time. You will, within a short time, have worked on all the milk ducts and taken milk from all the various segments of the breast.

8. Continue for three to five minutes on one breast, then do the same on the other breast, and then repeat the whole process. If one hand gets tired, use the other. It often takes 20-30 minutes to complete the milking session.

9. Once the milk is flowing, continue without pausing. If you pause, it may be difficult to start the milk flowing again. Continue expressing milk until you have taken out all the milk you need.

10. Divide the milk into suitably sized portions for feeding and put in the refrigerator or the freezer.

Why and How to Use a Pump

There are many reasons why you may need to pump your milk. Perhaps you are starting a new job or taking up a course of study. Or maybe your baby has never quite grasped the idea of taking milk directly from the breast or has some problem that makes breastfeeding difficult. Now and again, a mother may have found breastfeeding so complicated and strenuous that she chooses to pump her milk and give it to the baby in a bottle. Whatever the reason, there are a lot of different views on pumping. Some mothers find it simple, all part of a day's work, while others find it problematical – a daily challenge. There are even mothers who feel that pumping reduces them to the status of a dairy cow.

One thing that is too readily forgotten is the need to set the let-down reflex in motion before you start pumping. Even if that may seem rather stupid, not to say boring, it is incredibly important, so don't forget it! For women who find themselves having to rely on a breast pump, one practical problem may be the lack of time to sit down and use it. If you have support troops on hand, such as the baby's father, a friend, or some member of your family, try to recruit them to take on part of your job, such as washing the pumping equipment between sessions. Here are some tips on how you can best tackle the pumping issue.

Various Pumps

A wide range of pumps have been marketed, and new varieties appear all the time. It is impossible to describe them all here. They range from sizeable machines to miniature pumps about the size of a toaster. They are supplied with tubing and collecting flasks, and the instructions for use generally follow from the organization that is loaning or renting them. You will probably have to buy an extra set of flasks and tubing for your own use, so that one set can be used, while the other set is sterilized. The producers really try to get you to believe that you cannot survive breastfeeding without a pump – do not believe it! If you feel you need one, seek the advice of your health center or a breastfeeding support group, or find out what experience your friends and acquaintances have with the different models.

THE MINIMUM TO EXPECT OF A DECENT BREAST PUMP IS THAT IT:

- Is easy to keep clean and not messy to use.

- Is well designed, so that one can sit comfortably while using it without undue strain to the wrist, shoulder, or neck.

- Can be operated with one hand.

- Provides an adjustable degree of suction.

- Is possible to express milk from both breasts at the same time (in the case of electric pumps).

Some Views on Hand-Held Pumps

If you need a pump for occasional use, you can buy a hand-held pump. The market is crowded with them, so they are fairly inexpensive. Buy one that is easy to clean and make sure you understand how to do it. Some are so complicated that it takes an expert to fit the parts together again if you have been incautious enough to take them apart.

When You Have to Start Breastfeeding Without the Help of a Baby

If a baby is unable to feed at the breast right at the start of life, the mother will need to get milk production under way using hand expression or pumping. The two can perfectly well be used together. Ideally, you should begin very soon after birth, preferably while you are still in the delivery room. In this way, you can benefit from the high levels of the milk hormones, especially oxytocin, which are found in the body during the first few hours and days after birth. It is preferable to begin with hand expression on the first day or during the first few days. The breasts should be stimulated around eight times a day, whichever method is used. It can be helpful to use the pump during the night, if you don't find it too tiring. Particularly in the early period of milk production, some stimulation of the milk production at night raises levels of the hormone prolactin. If you don't feel like doing it every night, you may find that a few night sessions spread over the week are sufficient. By spreading the sessions over 24 hours, you reduce the number needed in the daytime. You can use a double pump to save time. The double pump is especially useful if you need to increase the flow of milk, if you have twins, or if you find that pumping has to continue for some months.

After two or three weeks, you may be able to reduce the number of daily milking sessions depending on how much milk is being produced and is needed. When the premature baby is hospitalized, a good indicator as to how much milk you should ideally be producing at this time is the volume that the baby was supposed to get when discharged from the hospital, plus an extra 100 ml (3.4 oz) to be on the safe side. Talk with the nurses; they will help you figure it out.

We have sketched a sort of ideal picture, and there are bound to be differences between mothers. The milk production begins around the third day after birth, whether the breasts are stimulated or not, but if you do not stimulate, you will get too little milk. Premature delivery, cesarean section, maternal illness – all these, singly or in combination, may affect the milk production. Such things may also mean that you are less active than you would like to be during these first few hours or days. A little extra support from the nursing staff can mean a lot – you shouldn't be using your time and energy on getting hold of a breast pump or cleaning the attachments when you don't feel up to it.

Ask for help. Demand a little extra service. And never forget – if it is possible, have plenty of skin-to-skin contact with your baby.

It's a wretched fact of life that all these demands may be made on you at a time when you least feel able to meet them and while you are still getting used to the pump, but the more you can achieve during these very early days, the fewer problems you will experience during the weeks that follow.

Pumping Over a Longer Period

If your baby is not an enthusiastic breastfeeder – which may be the case if it has been born prematurely or has a persistent health problem – you may face the prospect of having to pump your milk over a period of months – but that will at least render you quite a pumping expert. Should the baby be hospitalized, you will probably find that you can borrow a pump from the hospital's milk bank or rent one through a rental firm with which the hospital has a working arrangement. Once your baby is discharged, you will probably have to pay to rent a pump, if you still need one, though some health insurance systems do cover expenses like this. Some mothers do conclude in the long run that milking by hand is simplest – quite apart from the fact that your fingers stimulate the nipple in a way that the breast pump does not, thereby firing off the let-down reflex. Another advantage is that your fingers are a tool you always have with you! Combined use of the electric pump and manual stimulation is, as we have seen, quite feasible and for some people ideal.

Getting Friendly with the Pump

It's well worthwhile trying to build up a friendly relationship with your breastpump, developing your routines, and getting to a point where you feel quite content to keep things going for as long as necessary with the pump as your only partner. You may find that it is easier to pump (or milk your breasts by hand) if you maintain contact with your baby – for example, holding it close to you and perhaps continuing to hold the baby as you express, or at least having it close by. Try to regard these pumping sessions as times to rest and relax! Not that it's always quite so easy, but self-persuasion in matters like this often does work. Look at a magazine, read a book, listen to music or to a story on tape or CD – anything that will help you relax as the milk flows. TV? A film? It's your choice. And if the baby isn't close at hand, look at its picture or savor the scent of its clothes, just to remind yourself why you are doing all this...

Expressing with an Electric Pump

Preparations:

- Wash your hands thoroughly.

- Choose a good chair or sofa where you will be comfortable.

Check that the shield is the right size – if not, get another one or put an inlay into the one you have. If the shield doesn't fit snugly over the nipple and areola, it may be difficult to create the suction you need to get the milk flowing, or you may find that it is painful or even causes the skin to crack. You should choose the size according to the size of the nipple, not the size of the breast. The nipple should move freely back and forth, and the nipple should be in the center of the breast shield. To begin with, use the strongest suction that is not painful, but after that try to adjust to a lower suction level if possible.

Stimulate the Let-Down Reflex

There are several ways to do this, see Hand Expression earlier in this Chapter. A few mothers need to use oxytocin in the form of nasal spray when they are pumping – talk to the hospital staff or your doctor if you think you may need this kind of assistance; see also the section on oxytocin sprays later in this Chapter.

How often?

If you are not feeding your baby at the breast at all, use the pump six to eight times a day, the frequency depending on the milk production. It is better to have short pumping sessions fairly often than fewer sessions farther apart.

How Long Should You Pump Each Time?

Continue to pump until the flow of milk slows down and you have the impression that there are no segments full of milk in the breast. As a rule, 15-30 minutes are sufficient.

During Pumping:

• Massage the breast gently, stroking it towards the nipple with your fingers.

• Try leaning forward a little during pumping – with the milk moving downward rather than forward, the force of gravity helps to keep it flowing.

As we said before: try to make a pumping session a time to relax! Music? Something good to drink? Have you tried reading?

Pumping When the Milk Is Scarce

If you are dependent on pumping, but you are producing very little milk, you may need to change your routines in some way. Can you manage to use the pump more often? Don't get discouraged – do the best you can, taking a little time to find out what works best in your particular case. Also think about your life situation as a whole – do you have the time and opportunity to pump more often? Perhaps you should accept and be happy for the milk you have. Also look at the tips below.

PUMPING WHEN THERE'S TOO LITTLE MILK - TIPS AND TRICKS

- If you can, spend more time in skin-to-skin contact with your baby.

- Shift from one breast to the other during a pumping session. Try pumping a little more often than usual for two or three days, e.g., eight to 12 times a day.

- Frequent, short pumping sessions are better than fewer and longer ones.

- Try night pumping for just a few nights, or several times a week.

- Try double pumping.

- Try acupuncture to improve the flow of milk. Some mothers claim this works, but it hasn't been proven.

- Use medication to increase the milk production if nothing else seems to work.

Storing Your Breastmilk: Refrigerator or Freezer?

If you plan to keep the expressed milk for some time, you may wish to begin by milking out the very first drops of milk – a teaspoonful or so – into a cup and throwing them away. This is because the milk that comes first has been close to the nipple with its openings, where it will have picked up some of the microorganisms found on the skin. They are not at all likely to be harmful, but it may be sensible to reduce their number.

Because milk contains so many antibacterial factors, especially when it has just come from your body, there will be no risky growth of microorganisms in it during the first eight hours or so after milking, even if it is kept at room temperature, and you can safely use it for your baby. It is, however, better to put it in the refrigerator or freezer as soon as you finish pumping. In an ordinary kitchen, refrigerated milk will remain in good condition for three to five days. Remember, however, that human milk is not homogenized – an industrial dairy process which keeps the cream mixed evenly with the remainder of the milk. Consequently, after a while the high fat cream in human milk floats up to the surface, just as one sees with fresh, untreated cow's milk.

If the milk is destined for the freezer, it is better to freeze it as soon as it has been collected. You can pour it into a container which already holds frozen milk, provided the volume of milk you add is not greater than the amount already frozen; otherwise the latter will begin to thaw. You may also refrigerate the milk to cool it down before adding it to frozen milk. Breastmilk can be kept in the freezer for three to six months; the temperature should be between minus 18 and 20 degrees Celsius (0 to -4°F). Use a freezer thermometer. Store the milk as far down or as far back in the freezer as possible, so that it is not exposed to changes of temperature when the door or the lid of the freezer is opened. The milk can be kept in ordinary (new) freezer cartons or in bottles that have been boiled beforehand. You can also use small glass containers, each containing just about the right amount of milk for a feed. Many of the components of breastmilk survive freezing.

Thawing

When it is time to use the frozen milk for the baby, the best way to thaw it is in a water bath, which is no warmer than 40°C (104°F). *Never use the microwave oven!* There is a real risk that in a microwave oven the milk will be warmed up unevenly, creating "hot spots," which make it difficult to know what its temperature is. The uneven heating means that some parts of the milk will reach an excessively high temperature, sufficient to destroy the milk's invaluable protective proteins and cells. There is also a risk that some part of the milk will be so hot that it is dangerous for the baby to drink it.

Milk that has been thawed should be used as soon as possible, or it should be discarded – never return it to the freezer.

Other Mechanical Aids

Modern medical science for many years provided very little in the way of practical aids to the breastfeeding mother.

Once women made it clear that they had every intention of continuing to breastfeed, a market did spring up for all sorts of breastfeeding "aids" - breastfeeding pillows, bra pads, special nursing bras, to say nothing of glassware and a true proliferation of pumps. One has to look on them all skeptically: are they really necessary? The truth is that one needs virtually no equipment in order to breastfeed successfully, and many of the "aids" that have been marketed hardly deserve the name – they are downright useless. Here we will look briefly at some which do have their uses, and warn against others which are pointless.

In principle, there are two sorts of "breastfeeding aids" – those that are supposed to be helpful in getting the milk out of the breast and those that are claimed to be useful in getting the milk to the baby.

Breast Shells or Milk Collectors

Breast shells, also called milk cups, breast cups, breast shields, Woolwich shields, or milk collectors, basically come in two varieties: those with holes and those without (Figures 10.2, 10.3). Those with holes are meant to give air and protect sore nipples, or to help nipples protrude. Others are holeless and used to collect dripping or running milk from the other breast when breastfeeding. They must not be confused with nipple shields (see later in this chapter). If you use these aids because of overproduction, be aware that they may actually maintain your overproduction. The milk collector exerts a constant small pressure on the breast, and the continuous milk leakage may lead to increased production of milk.

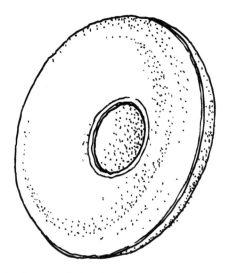

Figure 10.2. *Example of breast shell & milk collector*

Source: Drawing by Ingerid Helsing Almaas. Used with permission.

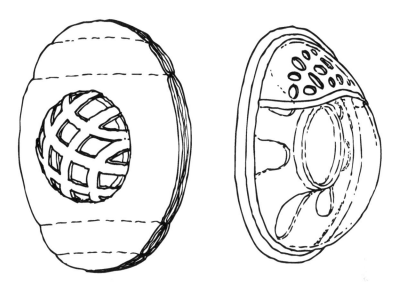

Figure 10.3. *Examples of breast shells*

Source: Drawing by Ingerid Helsing Almaas. Used with permission.

The Nursing Supplementer–An Auxiliary Breast?

The nursing supplementer can be helpful when breastfeeding an adopted child, as a means of dealing with inadequate production of milk, or when your baby needs supplementation and you do not want to use a bottle. A supplementer can also be useful to encourage a baby who is not willing to take the breast to return to it.

If you have insufficient milk, the nursing supplementer both stimulates production and ensures that the baby is adequately fed. Let the baby suckle just as long as it is patient enough to continue before you release the flow of milk from the supplementer. The longer the baby remains at the breast, the more your production of milk will be stimulated. Many mothers find that after a while the baby is taking less from the supplementer, a sign that her production of milk is increasing. You will probably find a ready-made nursing supplementer at your local pharmacy, or the pharmacist can order one for you (Figure 10.4). The complete device consists of a bottle more or less in the form of flat flask, a set of narrow silicon tubes, and an adjustable stopper, which regulates the flow of milk. One of the tubes is fixed to each nipple with a suitable adhesive tape of a type that will not irritate the skin. The tube conveys the milk to the baby; the baby regulates the amount of milk received through the tube by sucking. You can also make a nursing supplementer at home – it is quite simple, though you may need a little help from someone with the necessary experience (Figure 10.5). If you don't know anyone who is familiar with the method, just have a go on your own. When you first try feeding the baby this way, you need to have someone to support you – it may be that you need four hands. Have a look on the internet – there are several videos that show you how it is done.

A HOME-MADE NURSING SUPPLEMENTER

You will need a thin plastic feeding tube or a surgical catheter, a bottle or a cup, a nipple teat if using a bottle, and some surgical tape. The right sort of tubing can be found in the hospital, or you can buy it from a pharmacy or a surgical goods store. If you don't find it, ring your nearest breastfeeding support center and ask for advice. A catheter has the advantage in that it is longer than a feeding tube, but it is a little less flexible. Either type may have holes towards one end. If these holes allow air to enter the tube before the milk reaches the baby's mouth, you will need to cut off and discard this part of the tube.

If using a bottle, cut a very small hole in the nipple teat on the bottle, pass the tubing through this hole, and tape it into place. With this arrangement, no milk will be lost, even if the bottle is accidentally tipped over (Figure 10.5). You can also tie a string under the bottle cap to secure the bottle, and then tie the string around your neck, so the bottle is upright and laying against your chest, similar to the commercial nursing supplementer (Figure 10.4).

If using a cup, have a helper place the tube in the cup of milk and hold it in place throughout the feeding.

Tape the other end of the tube to the mother's breast and nipple.

Put the baby to the breast that has the tube attached. As the baby begins to suckle, this will create a vacuum in the tube, causing the milk to flow into baby's mouth. The rate at which the milk flows can be adjusted by raising or lowering the bottle or cup.

A bottle is preferable to a cup if you are going to need to use the supplementer more than once, since a cup may all too easily be overturned and the milk lost, especially if you don't have a helper.

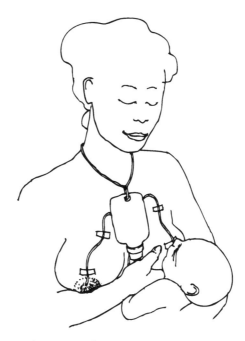

Figure 10.4. *Commercial nursing supplementer*

Source: Drawing by Ingerid Helsing Almaas. Used with permission.

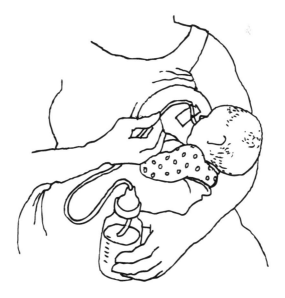

Figure 10.5. *Homemade nursing supplementer*

Source: Drawing by Ingerid Helsing Almaas. Used with permission.

Weak Feeders and the Nursing Supplementer

If your baby is a weak feeder, it may not manage to create the vacuum in the tubing that is needed to draw the milk from the supplementer. In that case, you can attach a syringe that fits the tubing attached to the nipple. When you press down the plunger on the syringe, milk will flow to the baby. If you are using a commercially made supplementer, you can get the same effect by squeezing the flask.

Do realize, however, that this is only a method to ease the *start* of real breastfeeding, and you should not continue with it longer than necessary; the more milk the baby gets through the tube the less it will take from the breast.

Cup Feeding

Cup feeding is a very acceptable alternative to bottle-feeding in cases where the baby needs more than the breast can provide, where the baby is not an efficient feeder, or where the mother has to be absent for a while. A baby who has difficulty in starting to breastfeed after birth can also better be fed from a cup than from a bottle. Using a cup ensures that the baby can enjoy taking milk without experiencing the confusion that can easily arise between bottle and breast – the way the baby uses the tongue and cheek muscles in drinking from a cup is much more similar to taking milk from the breast than is the process of sucking on a rubber teat! The "cup" can be a plastic beaker, preferably one that is fairly pliable and has a soft rounded edge. It should be rigid enough to stand scrubbing with a soapy brush and should withstand boiling. Look around your house to see what you have that might fill the bill – an egg cup, for example, or perhaps a medicine glass, a small mortar, or one of the small beakers that are often used to close feeding bottles. One can also look around the local drugstore, which may have special baby feeding cups in stock or can obtain one to order. A somewhat older infant, for example, aged five or six months, can also be fed from a plastic feeding cup fitted with a spout.

Cup Feeding in Six Steps

The cup feeding routine described below can be used equally well for healthy, preterm, or sick babies:

1. Wrap the baby in a towel so that it not likely to wrestle with its arms and legs to take hold of the cup. If the baby tends to struggle, a

folded towel or shawl can be wrapped around the body at the start of the feed so the arms are more or less immobilized alongside the chest. Once it has begun to drink, it will calm down and the arms can then be freed. But do put a serviette (bib) under the baby's chin – it is bound to dribble a little.

2. Support the baby in a more or less upright position (Figure 10.6). No one can drink properly from a cup when lying down. Watch carefully what the baby is doing as it feeds, and allow for it. And make sure that you are sitting comfortably – pillows can be a great help.

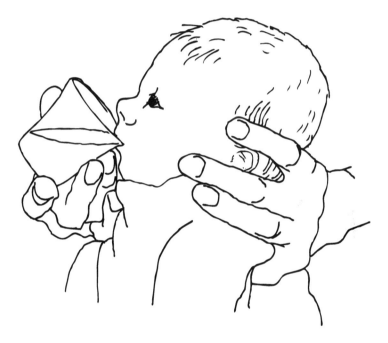

Figure 10.6. *Cup feeding*

Source: Drawing by Ingerid Helsing Almaas. Used with permission.

3. If possible, fill the cup to just over the halfway mark.

4. Tip the cup towards the baby's mouth, so the milk nearly comes up to the edge of the cup, without being spilt.

5. Bring the edge of the cup to your baby's upper lip and upper gums. Then lower it slightly to rest on the lower lip, without pressing on it.

6. Continue like this throughout the feed. Don't take the cup away, even if the baby stops drinking for a while. It is your baby who decides the tempo.

It is important for every baby to find out for itself how it wants to drink. One baby may drink like an adult, another may lap up the milk like a cat, and a third may suck up the milk. Cup feeding does not suit every baby. Some children never seem to master it, others constantly slobber and spill the precious milk, and yet others find it much too slow a proceeding. But do give the baby a chance with cup feeding before deciding to give up. Both the baby and whoever is holding the cup need practice, and, as always, practice makes perfect. Cup feeding should, as a rule, supplement breastfeeding, and not take its place. If the need for supplementary feeding is very prolonged, one may ultimately need to use the bottle.

Nipple Shields

The nipple shield is made of silicone and shaped like a nipple, since it is meant to be placed on the nipple itself. The most common reasons for using a shield are nipple soreness or the failure of the baby to get a good grip on the breast. The idea is that the shield will make it easier for the baby to latch on to the breast, while protecting the nipple. As a rule, it is simply a temporary aid to be used in the short term. The problem is that it can disrupt breastfeeding rather than help it, unless it is used cautiously and with competent guidance. Why are nipple shields not so ideal? Although they may relieve the problem, they usually do not tackle the underlying cause. Plus, the nipple shield prevents direct contact between the baby and the mother's skin. This lack of direct contact can lead to inadequate stimulation of the let-down reflex, an impaired grip on the breast, and ultimately to a reduction in the milk production or to problems with obstructed milk ducts.

For these reasons, it is important to try all other means before resorting to the use of a nipple shield. If everything else has been attempted without success and a nipple shield seems to be worth trying, you should bear the following in mind:

- Stimulate the let-down reflex by rolling the nipple between your fingers before putting the baby to the breast.

- Before applying it to the breast, turn the nipple shield inside out (Figure 10.7).

- Apply a little fatty cream so that it adheres better if the nipple shield does not remain firmly in place.

- Stimulate the baby's lips by touching them with the nipple, and wait until the mouth opens wide.

- Try putting the baby to the breast without using a nipple shield from time to time.

- Take away the shield when a feeding session has lasted for a while, and see if you can continue without it. This may be possible because during the feed the nipple has been stretched and it is easier for the baby to get a good grip on it.

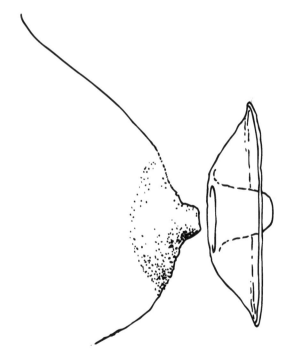

Figure 10.7. *Nipple shield*

Source: Drawing by Ingerid Helsing Almaas. Used with permission.

These same steps can be followed when you want to stop using the nipple shield. It can happen that as a result of using a nipple shield there is an insufficient stimulus to the milk production. You can prevent this if you:

- Keep a close eye on the baby's increase in weight, e.g., weighing it at weekly intervals during the first weeks after the shield has been started.

- Use a breast pump once or twice daily to stimulate the milk production if the weight is not increasing sufficiently.

- If you use a nipple shield only on the one breast, and feeding is going well on the other side, there is not likely to be any problem with the milk production as a whole.

In some instances, the use of the much criticized nipple shield saves breastfeeding since it may prove to be the only way of ensuring that the baby gets a grip on the breast. If you are getting good guidance and continue to check your milk production, there is no reason why your baby should not go on being breastfed in this way for a long time. There are also reports of babies who have been breastfed with the help of a nipple shield for several months, and then quite suddenly succeed in taking the breast properly without the need for a shield at all.

Oxytocin Nasal Spray

You may take extra oxytocin, when needed, in the form of a nasal spray. This will hardly be necessary if a baby is well placed at the breast, since good positioning will elicit the milk let-down reflex and mobilize the body's own oxytocin. Mothers who are pumping may experience some benefit from using it. Very, very few women truly need it. If you should be one of those few, do at least read the instructions for use carefully!

Keep Things Clean

Various objects made of hard or soft plastic or silicone (nipple shields, bottles, pump attachments, feeding utensils, etc.) which come into contact with the skin or with milk need to be rinsed in cold or tepid water immediately after use. They should next be cleaned with soapy water and brushed with a sink brush, then rinsed again in warm water, and finally boiled for three or four minutes. After that, lay them on a clean kitchen cloth or paper towel and leave them to dry naturally. As the baby gets bigger (for example, once it is several weeks old), it becomes less necessary to boil everything; you can now wash most things by hand or in the dishwasher, but it is still sensible to boil a rubber nipple after every use. Should you have problems with sore nipples and you suspect (or know) that you have a bacterial or fungal infection, *everything* that comes into contact with your breast or with the baby should be cleaned thoroughly, even if the baby is older. The temperature in a dishwasher is not high enough to destroy fungi and bacteria. The thin plastic tubes used with a home-made nursing supplementer should be rinsed after use, and then thrown away and replaced once or twice daily. If you buy a ready-made nursing supplementer, see what the instructions for use say about cleaning it.

When you need to boil things, be careful to avoid any risk of fire! Many a kitchen has been burned because nipple shields or bottles were put on the stove to boil and then forgotten. Using an alarm clock or an egg timer will remind you to switch off the heat. You can also buy small sterilizers that are safe to use - ask your pharmacy about them. And whenever you buy an appliance of any sort to help in baby care, take the necessary time to read the instructions – it will generally explain how best to keep everything clean.

Chapter 11.
WHAT PARENTS EXPECT

In the first little book about breastfeeding to be published in Norway, which appeared some 40 years ago, there was no mention at all of the father's role. The omission was quite deliberate. In part, it was a reaction to the romanticized portrayal of idyllic families and doting fathers that one tended to find in books on the subject in various parts of the world, a picture that sometimes contrasted pitifully with reality. We also needed to make it quite clear that a single mother could successfully breastfeed without any need to have a knight in shining armor at her side.

As the years have gone by, however, we have learned from both fathers and mothers that there is a proper place for this topic in a book about breastfeeding. There have also been a series of studies in the meantime showing that a father's attitude about breastfeeding – be it positive or negative – can actually swing the balance between success and failure (Dennis, 2002). In this Chapter, we will take a look at a number of family issues that arise – the social side of breastfeeding, and at some simple ways of handling the problems with which one may be confronted.

THE NUCLEAR FAMILY

The idea of the nuclear family was built around the traditional western notion that just two generations – parents and children – normally live together. But, especially in our time, the "normal" family can be rather different. You may, for example, be living alone with your baby. Or you may have a partner of the same sex. In writing this book, we have often had fathers in mind; we hope that if you are a single mother or have a partner of the same sex, you will be tolerant of our approach, and perhaps look on your partner or a close friend as filling the role that we have accorded to a father. If we examine the breastfeeding statistics, we find that breastfeeding tends to be maintained for a shorter period when a mother is living alone (Lande et al., 2003). One reason for this may be that a single mother does not enjoy the same degree of support at home. A study from Northern

Norway found that a mother who lived with her child's father and a mother having no partner but living in her parents' home were equally likely to be breastfeeding at the third month. By contrast, single mothers living alone were much less likely to be breastfeeding at this time (Bærug, Solberg, & Kjærnes, 1991). The essential factors in all this are the availability or lack thereof of practical help and support. Therefore, if you are living alone with your baby and are anxious to breastfeed, make it clear to family and friends that this is what you want, but that you will need support and practical help if you are to manage it. Just having a chance to take a nap in the middle of the day, while someone else looks after the miracle in the cradle, is worth a fortune!

A Mother's Expectations

Many mothers experience something of a shock when they realize fully for the first time that having a baby is a lifetime project. They may react in various ways – one may sense a welling up of real joy and gladness, whereas another may experience alarm and even depression at the magnitude of the project.

As we have emphasized, babies do cry, and sometimes it is simply not possible to discover why. A baby can certainly express its feelings in this and other ways, but they may be feelings that are difficult for an adult to understand. In public places, people are not particularly tolerant of crying babies. Many a mother has quietly slipped out of a meeting with the feeling that a glare of irritation from every direction is following her as she heads for the exit, along with whispers of reproach that there goes a mother who doesn't even know how to keep her child quiet.

And What Does Father Expect?

Many fathers are immeasurably proud of everything that their partners contrive to do, be it during pregnancy, birthing, or breastfeeding. They are delighted to see their offspring feeding enthusiastically and contentedly at the breast, and they are happy to see mother and baby breastfeeding in partnership.

Many such fathers are their partners' greatest source of support if breastfeeding problems need to be solved. They provide encouragement, read aloud from books on the subject, ring the support services, and hurry forwards and backwards with root beer, herbal tea, or whatever else they think may help the milk to flow liberally. Some take themselves to the underwear shop and ask unblushingly for breastfeeding bras, size D, preferably one that can be boiled, discussing the available models as if they are quite familiar with the subject. Some rouse themselves patiently in the small hours to calm their crying offspring, or find a good way to support a baby while mother positions it for feeding. And each of them glows with pride all the while at the sight of his baby, which is just as it should be.

Animals and Humans Do Differ...

Earlier in this book, we have pointed to the many parallels between various mammals where the biological side of breastfeeding is concerned. When on the other hand, one turns to consider the social aspect of birthing and breastfeeding, the differences are more evident. Nature has devised numerous strategies, ranging from father penguin who sits on the eggs until they hatch or father silk monkey who carries his offspring around all day (handing it to mother only at feeding times), to the shrimp which thinks nothing of changing its sex when necessary.

But one needs to bear in mind how much people differ from one another as well. What is striking when one considers human breastfeeding behavior is that, unlike that of the animals, it is not exclusively directed towards survival.

Essentially, in this book we want to advance a plea for common sense and a sympathetic approach when thinking about the social side of human breastfeeding. Birth is, when all is said and done, an event that concerns both man and woman in equal measure, at least in western culture, and it is followed by a period during which there is a great need for loving care. The baby, after all, belongs to both of you.

When Fathers Have Problems with Breastfeeding

There are indeed those fathers who find breastfeeding problematical. A father may actually find that he is jealous of the baby at the breast. Jealousy like this is more likely to arise when a mother doesn't seem overly anxious to share her baby with the father. She may feel that she has enough on her mind in learning to play her part as a mother, forgetting that there is someone else in the home who is also feeling his way towards performing his role as a father. The result may be that father feels he is an outsider in the whole process, he feels miserable and even wronged – and all this may be felt most acutely when the baby is being breastfed and the closeness between mother and child is so very apparent. His feelings may well lead him to indicate that he would prefer bottle-feeding; at least in that way, he will be just as close as his partner to the baby.

Another source of jealousy can be that a father has come to view the breasts simply as an integral part of the sex play between himself and his partner, and it may come as a shock to see them functioning as milk containers.

Even if thoughts and reactions like these may not reach the level of consciousness, they can lead a father to take a negative view of breastfeeding. By dropping little hints here and there, he may convey the message to his partner that he is less than appreciative of what she is doing. A situation like this can be difficult to solve. In the first place, you both need to put into clear words how you feel and what you want to do about it. Your starting point could well be the ideas we have put forward here. If you simply manage to talk a little about your feelings, you will have made a big step in the right direction. Thoughts that you have put into words are much less dangerous than those that remain buried.

The opposite situation can also arise: father may feel that mother should breastfeed, since only the best is good enough for *his* baby. All this despite the fact that mother may not be in the least happy about breastfeeding or has already experienced more than enough problems with it. She may well feel that it is completely unnatural for one person to try to decide what another person chooses to do with her body. But as we have stated before: breastfeeding is a matter of free will. Fortunately, nobody can be forced to breastfeed.

If a mother is indeed experiencing breastfeeding problems, perhaps painful ones, and she is reduced in her despair to tears, a man who is truly fond of his partner may propose that she should stop breastfeeding forthwith! But this may not be considered by the mother the right and proper way to settle the matter. A father who really wants to help must choose his words carefully, seeking the best way of supporting mother in the way she needs most.

When Mother Has Problems with Father's Role

We need to live and learn. A new father, too, must have the right to make mistakes. This is not the right time, mother, for you to try and show that you are better at baby changing than he is. Remember: you struggled at first to figure out which way you put on your baby's clothes, didn't you? When father starts complaining about your umpteenth remark that he does it so slowly or that the colors of the baby's clothes don't match - beware! He may be on the point of throwing up his hands in despair and handing the job back to you. It is better to just let him do things *his* way, and if that results in combinations of pink and yellow or stripes and blossoms, so be it. All that is needed is that you summon up every bit of tact you possess and bring it into play. Maybe the wisest course is to withdraw a little and let father and baby learn to know each other in peace.

A Job for a Man

In the nuclear family today, it is, as a rule, the father who will have to provide the necessary support and encouragement if mother is to retain her self-confidence and breastfeeding is to run a smooth course. Once upon a time, extended families lived together. And at times of birthing, all the wise women of the neighborhood would come rustling in to surround the newly delivered mother in her bed, ready with all the necessary diversions, rituals, experience, and words of wisdom. In our time, the father very often finds himself alone and expected to fulfill all these roles simultaneously. Truly, this is quite a responsibility – and truly, a job for a man.

BREASTFEEDING IS A JOINT PROJECT

The Safety Net

Most people have some sort of a safety net that they can call upon when the situation demands it – a circle of friends, perhaps, or the new baby's grandparents. There are studies which show very clearly that it is not only father's support that is necessary, but at certain moments, the backing that friends and other family members can provide as well (Ekström, Widström, & Nissen, 2003a).

Not every person is capable of providing consolation and encouragement when things are difficult for you. Unfortunately, there may be too many people around who are very ready to talk about their own problems rather than yours. This is discussed in Chapter 6.

Lost Generations?

Grandparents, aunties, and other older members of the family may be a great help – or occasionally a hindrance. The generation of grandmothers who experienced breastfeeding problems in the 1970's and 80's are likely to have been exposed at the time to some of the most inappropriate ideas on the subject that ever held sway. You may find yourself hearing their stories once more before they fade into oblivion. Many, as a consequence, had to give up breastfeeding against their will and that may influence their view of breastfeeding now.

They may be eager to point to the virtues of and actual need for the feeding bottle, to which they themselves were once obliged to turn. But whatever their generation, the helper's own experience of breastfeeding is likely to determine their view of it, be it positive or negative, for the rest of their lives. Many people who have in the past had disappointing experience with breastfeeding feel a sense of relief at being able to talk about this, even after many years have gone by, if only to elicit an assurance that it was not *their* fault that they failed. Having obtained that assurance, such women can very well provide generous help and support – not necessarily with great enthusiasm, but at least in their role as dependable allies who have overcome their own reservations about breastfeeding.

The Information Deluge

Today's world is flooded with information. Many mothers are among those who look to the internet in their hunt for factual information and advice on breastfeeding. A hint, therefore, about using the internet sensibly – be critical about everything you find on the screen, and particularly cautious in accepting advice provided in chatter clubs and all sorts of forums. Are you sure it is impartial and well founded? The baby food industry is, for example, active on the internet, sometimes even creating breastfeeding websites of their own.

FEMININE AND MASCULINE SEXUALITY

Sexuality and breastfeeding are closely linked, although in our time this tends to be overlooked. Male and female sexuality naturally differ somewhat in their nature. For men, the issue of sexuality is very clearly focused on the act of insemination; the purpose of it is to deposit his sperm – this is a man's only opportunity to participate actively in the process of reproduction. A woman's sexuality can be considered to cover a broader spectrum for it is she who will be involved in all the events that follow insemination – pregnancy, birth, and breastfeeding. These processes have a lot in common with sexual activity and involve many of the same hormones. Oxytocin ("the love hormone") has a particularly important role to play (Uvnäs-Moberg, 2003). Some women experience the birthing process, especially its last phase, as an orgasm-like experience, despite the pain. Breastfeeding, similarly, has many sexual facets. The breast, and more especially the highly sensitive nipple, is an erogenous zone, in other words, one of the bodily parts nature has equipped as a means of stimulating sexual activity. Some women experience sensual, sexual, and even orgasmic sensations while breastfeeding. Others find that when they are experiencing a true orgasm, their milk is spraying from the nipple. And yet others experience none of this.

Rather than being concerned that sexuality and reproduction are closely associated, we can simply look on the linkage as another ingenious facet of nature's reproductive strategy.

THE BREAST AS A SOURCE OF PLEASURE – ALSO FOR THE BABY

Many words of disapproval and contempt, especially from women, have been devoted to the male fascination with a woman's breasts and the role of the breast as a sex symbol, sometimes portrayed as if it represents the very essence of femininity and sexuality. Is it not so that one could turn the tables and sense some delight in the fact that the preoccupation with the breasts experienced by men (and surely also by women) is a reflection of tender memories of early childhood? Or perhaps it is simply sufficient to note how men observe the pleasure that a woman experiences from erotic foreplay involving her breasts as an element in the whole sexual experience. Or can one validly look on the matter in both ways? For a woman, the breast can perfectly well perform a double duty – both as an erogenous zone and as a source of food for her baby. Men's obsession with breasts – and in particular with those that seem to be full of milk (even if it is only silicone) is surely perfectly innocent. Enough said!

FED UP WITH BREASTFEEDING PROPAGANDA?

The old debate about the status of women and mothers in society has flared up in a new direction in our own time. In spite of the fact that it is physically not possible to oblige a woman to breastfeed against her will, many women do find themselves exposed to strong moral pressure to breastfeed their children. Since in the western world, children reared on substitutes developed from cow's milk do not seem to suffer direct ill effects as a consequence, many mothers have taken the view that they should have a right to choose the bottle or the breast according to their own preference. They, therefore, tend to rebel against sometimes highly moralistic suggestions that a mother has a duty to breastfeed for the sake of her child. Anyone who has worked with breastfeeding for some years knows how strong and deeply rooted the feelings can be that are expressed on this subject. One also knows, however, how great the desire to breastfeed can be and how deep the sorrow when it fails. With such strong feelings in play, it is not surprising that a mother may object violently to any pressure exerted on her from the world around her when she has more than enough trouble dealing with her own emotions and frustrations. It may be hard to avoid awakening slumbering feelings of guilt in a woman who would gladly have breastfed, but for one reason or another didn't manage it, and who has not yet come to terms with the fact.

Remnants of Fictions and Fables Past

Moralizing, reproach, paternalism, and doubt as to a woman's abilities, both physical and intellectual – these run like a red thread though many of the curious notions and edicts handed down to past generations on the subject of breastfeeding (see Chapter 13 for examples). Nor have such things faded completely. As gardeners say, new weeds will spring up whenever they have the chance.

Why is it apparently so tempting for those charged with giving advice to young mothers during pregnancy and breastfeeding to devise rules that render life miserable, painful, and complicated? Recommendations to apply lemon juice to sore nipples, to shun a whole series of foods that may vaguely and theoretically disagree with the baby, to follow a balanced diet (whatever that is supposed to mean) spring up like mushrooms. Do they really reflect genuine sympathy and sound reason?

FEELINGS OF GUILT AND FAILURE

All of us tackle the challenges of life in our own way. When things go wrong, there are some who assume the whole burden of guilt: "I am not even able to breastfeed." Others will be ready to blame the hospital or the health workers around them: "If they hadn't forced the baby to drink from a bottle, he wouldn't have run into the problems he now has at the breast."

To feel guilty about certain things is only human. It's not always easy to shrug one's shoulders about a problem and cast it aside. When something goes wrong with breastfeeding, a number of things acting in concert may be to blame. Breastfeeding problems of one sort or another are unfortunately not uncommon. A study from Norway published in 2005 found that only 12% of mothers claimed to have experienced no breastfeeding difficulties at all during their babies' first year of life (Tufte, 2005). The same study found, however, that many women continue to breastfeed in spite of whatever difficulties they may experience. Häggkvist et al. (2010) found that during the first month, breastfeeding problems tended to lead to cessation of full breastfeeding. Fortunately, these early problems did not adversely affect breastfeeding performance in later months. Another study confirmed that having "too little milk" was the one reason why 42% of the women gave up during the first six months, while 15% cited worry, stress, and fatigue as the next most common reason (Norwegian Directorate of Health, 2009, p.38). Among the other causes of failure mentioned were having a baby who was sick from the start and separation of a baby from its parents. Less common reasons for failure are technical problems, for example, if the size or form of the nipples creates difficulties for a baby who is inherently a weak feeder. There may also have been inappropriate hospital routines and, in the worst cases, frankly incorrect treatment. Too little milk or a mother's concern about it is probably the most usual reason for a mother in any country to abandon breastfeeding (Camurdan et al., 2008; Taveras et al., 2003; Schluter, Carter, & Percival, 2006). It happens all too often that a mother shoulders a sensation of guilt for something that has nothing whatsoever to do with herself. Throughout the period of breastfeeding, it can be a good thing to get together now and again with a wise friend or with a health worker whom you trust, and talk these things through, trying to find out where problems arose and why they (perhaps) have persisted.

A "Good Mother" Is Not Necessarily a Breastfeeding Mother

If breastfeeding doesn't succeed for whatever reason, it is important to bear one thing in mind: *one can be a perfectly good mother without breastfeeding.* A good mother has a great many other qualities quite apart from producing milk. Providing a baby with the next most important things in life after food —warmth, responsiveness, confidence, and love, even a parent without milk producing glands (father) can play that role — and so can you!

If Those Around You Are Downright Nasty...

Particularly where there is a strong breastfeeding culture, neighbors, colleagues, relatives, and even perfect strangers may raise their eyebrows at the fact that a mother has resorted to the bottle and is not breastfeeding. Contacts with the healthcare team can also be upsetting if the questions raised are thoughtless or a tactless remark is dropped. To the question "Aren't you breastfeeding your baby?" there is no need to start explaining why, just have a standard answer ready to deliver to such a question. It is perfectly all right to say simply: "It's a personal matter, as I am sure you can understand."

Our underlying message in this book is that others have no right to come trampling in on your life and blurting out opinions of any sort as to what you or your husband should or should not have done where breastfeeding and breastmilk are concerned. Your situation, your preferences, your ultimate choices, and in particular, your feelings should be treated with respect. That is a principle you should maintain with all those around you, be they family, friends, or health workers.

SOME MYTHS AND PERSISTENT MISUNDERSTANDINGS ABOUT BREASTFEEDING

Breastfeeding does not require any special measures to succeed. Yet, it sometimes seems as if society takes a sadistic delight in imposing no end of commands, prohibitions, and rules on women who are pregnant or nursing. Examples of this abound down through the ages. The breastfeeding mother has been admonished variously to consume vast amounts of stout, milk, vegetable soup, or whatever other fluid the fashion of the day dictated. She has been warned to avoid cabbage, grapes, or strawberries. Sometimes, she was urged to take long walks; at other times, she was cautioned against bathing, dancing, walking, or any form of exertion. Needless to say, none of these rules, which were advanced with such conviction, had the slightest relevance to a woman's ability to produce milk. The only positive effect of imposing such rules was perhaps that adhering to them imbued the mother with a sense of duty done and greater self-confidence – now the milk would surely flow – and, of course, it often did.

Any woman entering motherhood for the first time is essentially a complete novice and is likely to listen attentively to everything she hears about the care and feeding of young children, irrespective of whether the source is a professional or an amateur. Some of what she hears will be well informed, the rest, unfortunately, may be pitiful nonsense, and it may be hard to know which is which. Even though sound knowledge of breastfeeding has grown encouragingly in many places, a lot of what is said and written is plainly incorrect. In the next few pages, we will take a look at some of the myths that still pop up on the most unexpected occasions. We will try to correct some of most common misunderstandings that they perpetuate.

Myth: Breastfeeding is complicated.

Reality: When breastfeeding functions normally, it is simple and easy.

Anyone who has experienced the whole rigmarole of washing, rinsing, and boiling feeding bottles, mixing the infant formula, getting it to the right temperature – and doing all this in the middle of the night – and who has had a chance to compare all this with successful feeding at the breast will readily acknowledge that breastfeeding is a great deal less labor intensive than bottle-feeding. It stands to reason, since breastmilk comes spontaneously, we have the ideal apparatus to deliver it, and there is nothing to be washed or boiled. Yes, the first few months may demand some effort to get things just right, but you have your reward in the months that follow, when you stop worrying about having enough milk, and simply know that you do.

Myth: Breastfeeding will tire you.

Reality: Breastfeeding won't make you tired at all.

Whatever may exhaust a mother, it will not be breastfeeding. The physical process of making and giving milk is so rational that it demands very little energy on the mother's part. The extra energy that a mother's body uses in transforming part of the food she consumes into breastmilk amounts to only a tiny percentage of the extra calories she needs while breastfeeding. If she feels weak and tired after having the baby, it is usually not due to breastfeeding. It is much more a reflection of the sudden move into a new and different phase of life, or perhaps a side effect of a lengthy and difficult delivery. The whole move into a new phase of life is bound to have both mental and physical repercussions. Some women sail into this new phase like battleships – strong and indefatigable. Others wake in the morning with an almost irresistible urge to sleep again for the rest of the day.

If breastfeeding is problematic, it can mean experiencing a tough and tiring period. All the same, the resilience of a human being is unbelievable. Even mothers who have struggled for weeks or months with breastfeeding will ultimately turn round and tell you that once they had conquered their problems and the milk was flowing, their energy came flowing back as well.

Myth: You must make sure to eat the right sort of food when you breastfeed.

Reality: Most people's everyday diet is perfectly all right.

Many mothers are concerned that they are not getting the right sort of food while they are breastfeeding. Firms advertising infant formula subtly exploit this concern when they put across to mothers the notion that a breastfeeding women needs to "nourish herself evenly throughout the day"– whatever that is supposed to mean. Any nutritionist will tell you that it is pure nonsense. Yes, a mother needs all the usual items in her food and she needs enough to drink, but none of this means that it is complicated to find the right diet. The truth is that the sort of food the average family eats every day is sufficiently balanced and complete for them all, including the breastfeeding mother. Take another look at Chapter 4.

Myth: Breastfeeding will ruin your figure.

Reality: Breastfeeding never ruined anyone's figure.

The breasts undergo some quite radical changes *during pregnancy*; the breast tissue itself is altered (see Chapter 1). This happens to every woman, irrespective of whether she breastfeeds or not. Apart from this, breastfeeding has only a very modest effect on the breast's composition and form. We have encountered various instances in which mothers have fed their babies over a long period from only one breast. And once the children were weaned, there was no visible difference between the two breasts at all. There are many women, especially those who tend to be flat-breasted at other times, who are only too happy with the full breasts with which they are endowed when they breastfeed. If there are any residual changes visible when pregnancy and breastfeeding are past, then they are surely trophies to look on with pride. A mother may point to her stripes (striae) that recall the birthing hours, and perhaps the varicose veins, all medals that honor the role she has played in carrying on the family line.

Myth: Not every breast is suitable for breastfeeding.

Reality: Almost any breast, whatever its size, can produce milk.

Breasts and nipples in very different sizes can produce and deliver milk. Most mothers, even those with barely visible breasts, can magically produce milk when it is needed (the same holds true for apes). When a baby is well latched on, both the nipple and the areola (the dark area surrounding it) are pulled out as far as necessary – anywhere from 2 cm to 4 cm, and perhaps further. Some mothers are afraid that their nipples are too flat or even inverted. That is rare, and in the period around delivery, such nipples often change their shape. Since a baby milks *the breast* and not the nipple, the shape of the latter is not of great importance. Occasionally, one does encounter such things as "difficult" breasts or nipples, but even here, some breastfeeding will usually be possible. Good positioning and latching on are what really matter. Babies are successful in taking milk from breasts of many different sizes, provided they get a little help to get started.

Myth: Your milk may be too weak.

Reality: There is no such thing as weak milk.

Even today, some mothers are exposed to the tale, handed around by mere chatterers, but on occasion also by health workers who ought to know better, that "Your milk may be too thin…" or "Your milk does not have enough nutrition." This sort of fable can only point to a lack of insight. Certainly, the fat content of breastmilk does vary quite considerably from one woman to another, but the concentration of other nutrients (sugar and protein) is relatively uniform in mothers. One has to realize that the exact composition of any mother's milk can vary considerably from the time she begins breastfeeding up to the point of weaning, and even between one feed and the next. The milk can never be "too thin" or "too weak" for its purpose, since the baby simply compensates for whatever variation there is by taking less or more of it. Even a mother suffering frank malnutrition can deliver perfectly adequate milk, though the quantity may be reduced and the standard may at such times only be kept up by drawing on her own physical reserves.

Even when a mother has continued to breastfeed for years, the quantities of nutrients in her milk will still be sufficient.

FULL BREASTFEEDING - FOR EVERYONE?

When we say that every woman's breasts can produce milk, we don't mean to claim that every mother can manage full exclusive breastfeeding for six months, let alone more. Even given the best advice and practical support, some mothers encounter the limit of what they can do very soon after delivery, while others never seem to encounter any limit at all. There is apparently no justice in the way Providence hands down capability in such matters, but when those who should be providing support flock in with confusing and even contradictory messages, a disappointing situation can only be rendered worse.

One such story is presented in the box below. It is the story of a mother's heroic struggle to attain the unattainable exclusive breastfeeding.

BREASTFEEDING FAILURE - ONE MOTHER'S CONFESSION

He arrived on the coldest and most beautiful day of the year. The delivery was just as smooth as the whole pregnancy had been. Lying there in the country hospital, I feel on top of the world, with a sunny view of the sea from my window and a perfect – no, an absolutely beautiful – baby at my breast. Now it's time for the next step in motherhood, isn't it? I have been taught that "Breast is best" and read the newspaper articles assuring me that breastfeeding is the way to rear healthy and intelligent children. So, of course, I shall breastfeed. Everyone can do that, they say, provided one makes a bit of an effort. Dire warnings from friends about sore nipples and sleepless nights are not going to dampen my ardor. I have bought a stock of nursing pads for a breastfeeding bra, and I'm all ready to gear up for the first session.

What follows, however, is something for which I'm not in the least prepared. I spend two days admiring my wonderful little boy, showing him off with immense pride to a constant stream of visitors, and putting him to the breast whenever he so much as murmurs. The experts in their white gowns have nothing but praise for the way he is positioned at the breast and takes a firm grip on it, and they hasten to assure me that however dry my breasts may be at the moment, they will soon be flowing with milk.

"But hasn't the milk come yet?" asks the older nurse, with a frown of concern all too evident on her face when I declare that I intend to go home, just as I had planned, two days after the delivery. "He's a bit on the slow side," she goes on as she sees the baby sleeping after a tiring night at the breast. "You need to wake him up and put him in place again," she tells me, "then we will see what happens." But the little one is not in the least prepared to take the nipple, he only wants to sleep. The nurse's serious face begins to register disapproval. "You will have to pump the milk and give him whatever you can produce, using the bottle," she suggests. Then she rolls in a milking machine and links me up to it, but only a few drops of milk appear. The tears, on the other hand, are now flowing in plenty. A quarter of an hour later, the nurse comes back to collect the pump. She takes it away without a word about the empty bottle – or about the tears.

"We don't think you should return home before your breastfeeding problem is solved," say the women in white. So there is my diagnosis. Just minutes ago I was an unbeatable and euphoric new mother, and now I am officially demoted to an unhappy postpartum case with breastfeeding problems.

Every eight hours, with a change of shift, a new helper comes striding in. All these people ask the same question, "Well, has the milk arrived yet?" But a new shift also brings with it some new views. Every midwife or nurse gazes at me with concern written on her face, yet each of them hastens to assure me that it is not at all unusual for the milk to turn up later than one would wish. Several times a day, my baby is laid on the scales, once before a period at the breast and again afterwards. "Ten grams more – splendid!" says the one. "Unfortunately, only 15 grams this time," says another later in the day. One truly wonders whether the two of them have read the same books. The one woman in white observes that the baby is getting a little restless and that it is time for a backup with some infant formula; yet another voice insists that for God's sake I should avoid resorting to the bottle. But then all of them, having argued the case for their own approach, end up giving me the most confusing advice of all, "It's your baby, so you have to decide." I? Me? Someone who can't even produce her own milk? Who says that I'm in the least qualified to decide what to do?"

On the morning of the fourth day, the most optimistic member of the team turns up to weigh my baby. This time, the results apparently move even her to despair. "He's now lost a bit more than 10 percent of his birth weight" she says. "We simply MUST give him some other food."

I find myself handed a bottle of milk and instructed to ask father to have a supply of infant formula ready at home.

Does this mean I shouldn't go on breastfeeding?" I ask. "Oh yes, you can carry on trying" the nurse consoles me, "but the main thing is that the little lad gets some food and puts on weight." She shows me how the milk has to be mixed and how I should wash the bottles. She makes an appointment for us with the out-patient department for the next day and sends us home to fatten the little one as best we can.

Convinced as I now am that he's on the verge of starving to death, I tackle things as if *my* very existence as well depended on it. "What happens if he doesn't put on weight?" I ask myself. "Will they come and take him away from me?" And so I redouble my efforts and my baby spends most of the next 24 hours with a teat in his mouth. He shall be fed, that's what matters now.

"How clever you have been, mother!" says the friendly lady at the out-patient clinic the next day. "He's gained 150 grams! Just carry on like that. Give the breast each time for starters, and then follow it up with the bottle."

All right, that sounds fair enough. I manage to follow the advice of the nurse at the well-baby clinic for just two days before I find myself facing a new helper at the clinic, once more with fresh ideas. "Do you really want to give the bottle each time?" She is a breastfeeding expert, and she frowns at the notion. "But surely you mean to put him on full breastfeeding." "Yes, of course, but can I?" "*Everyone* can breastfeed," says my new adviser briskly. "But you know you'll never get enough milk of your own if you come running with the bottle every time he's hungry." Now she is ready with her instructions. I am to breastfeed, 20 minutes at each breast, not more often than once every three hours. If he screams at other times, let father console him. Be firm, be calm.

Once again I do as I'm told. Except that I don't manage to be either firm or calm. Instead I feel a load of guilt pressing down on me, ever heavier as I endure the loud screams of my hungry baby upstairs, where father is valiantly rocking him, dancing, and singing to him. The load on my mind grows weightier with every drop of imitation breastmilk that he sucks from the bottle. Now, I tell myself, I have finally lost the battle. I'm not doing what I should do if I want a bright, healthy breastfed baby. I find myself crying when he's hungry and crying again when he's not. "But look how well he is!" says my partner by way of consolation. "That's just it," I sob, "such a splendid little boy and such a useless mother he has." In his handsome but serious little face, I am sure I see a sign of reproach.

Back to the well-baby clinic we go for a check-up and a turn on the scales. The little one has put on just enough weight, but no more than that. Weighing him after a breastfeed shows a gain of 36 grams. The nurse is not entirely satisfied. "Shouldn't we try the breast pump for a while?" I see a glimmer of hope – that way, I may be able to avoid depriving my baby of the good food he needs, and I jump at her offer to lend me an electric pump.

Motivated once more, I plunge into a new round of competition with the clock. Every three hours, they tell me, 20 minutes on each side, and I must warm up the milk from the last round of pumping, generally about 20 ml, and give as much milk substitute as is needed – pump each breast for 20 minutes each time, wash the bottle and the pump, and sterilize them…

The whole rigmarole is tiring, but perhaps that's a good thing. I can see that I'm doing my best and I'm not giving up. All the more disappointing when even now the milk barely amounts to 30 ml a time. The same story, over and over again. Now the nurse suggests that some medicines may help me, and writes a prescription for something that is supposed to get my milk flowing.

"Tell me now, do you find yourself thinking a lot about this milk business of feeding?" says the lady at the well-baby clinic when I confess to her that neither the medicine nor the pump have helped me to produce more milk than before. I gaze at her, dolefully I am sure. Is this the very same person who proposed a feeding routine that would take me eight hours a day (plus all the time I would need to clean up the equipment) and who now wonders if find myself thinking about the whole business? I see her shrug her shoulders as she remarks that I'm probably stressed and that *this* is the reason why I'm not producing enough milk. "If that's the case, I really can't help you," she concludes.

So it is that even the nurse finally labels me a hopeless case. I decide to do the same, with the full support of my family, who have long been concerned that I have been taking this breastfeeding business all too seriously. I go on for a few days before I surrender again. Surely something must be possible, if only I knew what? Everyone can breastfeed, they say! I call on an acupuncturist who is "nearly certain" she can help me. But she throws in the towel after four hours, and after using hundreds of needles and charging me a small fortune.

Everyone can breastfeed they say – yet I'm getting no further. Why not? None of the people around me can give an answer. Every spare moment I have I spent delving into the mystery, in books or on the Internet. Still I find no answer. My problem is just not supposed to exist, so it seems.

No one can do anything about it, either to ginger up these two miserable breasts of mine or dampen down the shame I feel every time anyone asks me why the little one is being bottle-fed. I can see the disbelief in their eyes when I try to make light of it and remark that I'm not all that talented at playing the role of a dairy cow. For everyone knows, don't they, that everyone can breastfeed? Am I stupid? Couldn't I be bothered? No one can shield me from the all too obvious skepticism I now meet at the clinic. "Still too little milk? What have you been up to? It seems very odd...."

What I'm experiencing just shouldn't be possible. What sort of person am I? A freak, perhaps? Am I imagining things? I get a glimpse of reality when I hear a rumor about an acquaintance of an acquaintance who had a problem like mine and who ended up with an undernourished baby. I dig up her telephone number and invite her for a cup of coffee. Fortunately, she's neither stupid nor evil. We spend a couple of hours exchanging thoughts and experiences, and both of us end up feeling less lonely than before.

All the same, I'm still obsessed with the miserably small amount of milk I have. I have black thoughts about the sort of life to which I may be condemning my baby – one tainted by allergy, middle ear infections, and a low IQ perhaps? Officially I have given up the idea of full breastfeeding, but my head is still full of it. I rebel at the idea of asking even more people for help and advice, but I know I won't solve my problem on my own. But I promise my partner that I'll try just once more. I call in a new helper.

She says, "We need a battle plan. The last attempt just has to be time-limited, maybe two weeks so you don't break your neck in the effort ... Let's chat on the phone every day..."

The way she says "we" brings tears to my eyes. She doesn't say "you" and certainly not, "You know best..." We're going to embark on this together, plan together, and perhaps ultimately admit defeat together.

She goes on, "This looks to me like a final all-or-nothing attempt. From what you've told me, I suspect that there's some physiological cause to your problems. You shouldn't expect that you'll be able to manage exclusive breastfeeding."

What she says disappoints me for a moment, but then I feel a surprising sense of relief. I realize that I'm already aware that I won't succeed. What I really want is to be acquitted; to hear a little voice saying to me, "You have done all you could. It is not your fault that you do not succeed fully breastfeeding. Not everybody can do it."

All the same I try again – another marathon by my standards. A breastfeed every hour, day and night, the nursing supplementer and the pump close at hand when I need them. I'm doing the best I can. It's not what you'd call exclusive breastfeeding, but it's good enough. When people ask about it, I feel I can hold my head high again. "The human body isn't perfect – now and again it lets you down" is the way I'm looking at it now. I have simply realized that there is *something* – and I have no idea what it might be, that makes it impossible for me to do something that should be in every woman's reach. Next time I may find out what it is, or perhaps I shall never know.

Bit by bit, the shame and misery have faded, though they are still in the back of my mind. But now I am busy discovering the young person who should have been in the middle of the stage from the start. When I wake in the morning, he's lying there beside me, smiling at me. I know he's thinking that his mummy and her breasts are the best things life has to offer. I've been acquitted.

"Mummy, I want to be cuddled" says the little one and throws himself into my arms. He will soon be two, and he's developing so fast that we joke with each other that if he had had more breastmilk, he would have become too smart for us. No allergies, no contact problems. Just a happy and lively young man with a zest for life and always coming up with new ideas. He's more perfect than I could ever have dreamed, even if he didn't get all that much breastmilk. I've long stopped feeling bad about my breastfeeding performance. But it seems absurd those two wretched breasts were capable of spoiling my first months as a mother; I can get furious when I think about it.

Breastmilk is what babies need. The health service people are absolutely right in following that line. But there is a risk of ever more preaching of the sort to which mothers are already exposed (and to which bright young ladies are so receptive) when the professionals who should be putting all this theory into practice being either not adequately trained, or simply not willing, to provide the help and support that mothers need.

I suppose it's true that you have to break eggs if you want to make an omelet. But it should be possible to support breastfeeding without breaking a mother in the process.

Chapter 12.
YOUR BABY GROWS – AND GROWS UP!

Finally, the time for supplementing the milk diet approaches. The term often used for this, weaning, can be confusing and might better be abandoned, since "weaning" has two different meanings. The first meaning refers to the process by which the baby ceases to be *exclusively* dependent on a diet of breastmilk and learns to accept some supplementary feeding; in other words, it moves from a pure breastmilk diet to mixed feeding. The second meaning refers to the later phases of breastfeeding in which the baby says goodbye to the breast altogether.

In this Chapter, we will take a look at both of these phases, in the order in which they arrive:

- Getting accustomed to solid foods along with breastmilk

- The phasing out of breastfeeding – when and how

LOOKING BACK

Supplementary Feeding – A New Phenomenon!

In the mid-1960s, Norwegian parents were strictly instructed by the health centers they attended to begin supplementary feeding when the baby was three and a half months old – 14 weeks – neither more nor less. A few years later, in the 1970s, the date for introducing supplementary feeding had shifted to four months, i.e., 16 weeks, no more and no less. In 2001, the World Health Organization informed the world that one of its expert groups had now concluded, after examining all the high quality studies on the matter that they could find relating to children's diet, weight, and well-being, that they could find *no* clear health advantage in giving a child any food other than breastmilk during the first six months of life. WHO's (2001) current message to health workers is that they should advise parents to begin solid food when their infants reach the age of six months. The

American Academy of Pediatrics also recommends exclusive breastfeeding for six months (American Academy of Pediatrics et al., 2005).

Development of Advice on Weaning

To give a broader picture of how the advice given to parents on this subject has evolved over time, we looked at some of the information that has been handed down both to parents and health workers in the course of a century. Much of what we read was from our own country – Norway – but we also turned to material from other parts of Scandinavia and Britain as well. Bearing in mind that this was a subject where women had traditionally followed their own judgment, we wanted to find out to what extent the "expert" advice being handed down was indeed based on scientific evidence and solid experience. How had these notions regarding breastmilk and the need for supplementation come into being, and how were they explained and justified? To understand this, we needed to start by going back in time. Norwegian and very likely European parents by that time, we may assume, belonged to a common medical culture. What was true for Norway was true for most European countries.

What Were Our Great- Grandmothers Told About Supplementary Feeding and Solid Food?

Very much to our astonishment it turned out that the answer to the question above was – "Nothing at all!" The printed advice being given to parents around 1900 makes it clear that if a baby under the age of three months was unable to feed at its mother's breast, it was deemed necessary to provide it with breastmilk from another woman. If that was not feasible, the baby would be given animal milk, although this often presented practical problems. Donkey's milk was considered preferable, but in Northern Europe, it was hardly obtainable. Mare's milk was another scarce item, rarely available in sufficient amounts. Goat's milk was a poor third choice, actually providing too little Vitamin B^{12} and folate (although they did not know this in 1900). If a somewhat older child needed a substitute for mother's milk, the parents would often turn to some form of thin gruel mixed with cow's milk and water. The many types of "baby cereals" that had come onto the market by about 1910 were not primarily intended as solid food. They were simply meant to complement breastmilk or its substitutes when these alone were insufficient. Doubt as to whether breastmilk alone could be sufficient to sustain a baby grew and blossomed in parallel with the increasing use of cow's milk and the feeding bottle. The people who were giving advice to mothers tended to base their views on their experience with artificial feeding and applied these to breastfeeding. The idea of "solid food" or supplementary feeding as an *essential* element in the young child's diet first seems to have made its appearance in the 1960s, at around the same time that small screw-top jars of mass produced "baby food" appeared on the market. They were marketed as necessities from then on, and were intended to supplement the purely milk diet from three to four months of age.

Many contradictory conclusions and incompatible points of view thus came to the fore, and they often proved to be based on variable and sometimes dubious arguments. Many of the advisors who insisted that infants should begin solid food at a fairly early age derived their inspiration from the infant food industry. Having mothers switch from breastfeeding to bottled and tinned infant food products was naturally very much in the interests of this industry which, during the period from 1900 to 1950, had developed into a big business.

WHAT FOODS DOES A BABY TOLERATE AND WHEN?

As pointed out above, it is now widely and authoritatively accepted that exclusive breastfeeding should be continued at least until the sixth month. If for any reason this is not feasible, breastfeeding may have to be supplemented, in which case, the first choice will be infant formula. In this situation, mothers often ask how early they can consider giving solid food. The answer appears to be that there is considerable variation from one baby to the next, and one should therefore be cautious. In some infants, for example, the digestive system seems to mature later than in others, and particularly in families where there is a history of allergy, the baby is more likely to react to food allergens if given solids before its immune system is fully operational.

WHAT IS "EXCLUSIVE BREASTFEEDING"?

By exclusive breastfeeding, we mean that a baby's diet consists of breastmilk alone, although it may be getting some vitamin and/or mineral support.

In recent years, the health authorities and experts of many countries have followed the view of the World Health Organization (2001) that most infants should receive breastmilk alone for the first six months of life, provided they are developing normally and their mothers have a reasonably problem-free milk supply. WHO makes it clear that most breastfed babies will not benefit in any way from supplementary feeding during the first six months of life.

Exclusive breastfeeding does not exclude the use of vitamins or other supplements, but breastmilk alone provides a baby with all its dietary needs until it is at least six months old. National health authorities usually provide advice on the exceptional situations where supplements are indicated. In northern areas, for example, with relatively little winter sunshine, it may be advisable for babies to receive Vitamin D (or cod liver oil).

Somewhere between the sixth and eighth months, many infants develop a need for supplementary iron, preferably provided from their food rather than separately. But there are many children who thrive on breastmilk alone for longer (see Chapter 3).

HOW DO YOU KNOW IT IS TIME FOR SUPPLEMENTARY FEEDING?

A baby usually manages to indicate when it needs more food quite simply by being very hungry and displaying a hungry interest in whatever food is within view, as well as wanting to get to the breast more often than usual. If by the age of six to eight months your baby does not seem to be interested in anything but mother's breast, you can try to encourage it to extend its culinary experience.

Supplementary Feeding: When?

It would be delightfully simple if there was a universal sign as to how one could recognize exactly the right moment to begin getting a baby used to eating food other than milk. Unfortunately, it is not so straightforward. The moment when teething begins, for example, is too variable to serve as a useful guide. Many have suggested that the infant itself provides signs that it is ready for solid food, by pulling objects towards its mouth and gnawing them enthusiastically. That, however, may simply reflect the fact that the mouth is a central part of the baby's "feeler" system that is used to explore and examine objects from its surroundings, rather than expressing a desire for food.

In parts of the world, parents put their faith in the stars and consult astrologers as to when their children should start taking solid food. All one can say is that one person's guess on the matter is probably as good as another's.

It has also been suggested that it is important to introduce new foods at an early stage so that an infant can become accustomed to new tastes and will not become too fastidious as it grows older. Others firmly reject that notion, maintaining that the process is one of maturation, not of acquired learning. In short, all you can do is to use the feelings and common sense with which nature has endowed you as parents, and assume that somewhere around the age of six months your child will be ready for a broadening of its menu. Always begin with one food item at a time, given in small amounts to start with. You simply use your fork to pulp some ordinary suitable family food on a plate and give it with a teaspoon.

Supplementary Feeding: What?

Once you have decided to start with supplementary feeding, you will find that no single individual can tell you with absolute certainty what that food should be. Many parents consider it wise to begin with porridge, gruel, or mashed rice. In Norway, a study of infant feeding around the beginning of the 21st century shows that two thirds of children were given home-made porridge as their first supplementary food, while a third were given a branded equivalent (Lande & Frost Andersen, 2005). Many types of cereals intended for preparing infant porridge are available to purchase, both with and without gluten.

Confusion in the 1980s

During the 1980s, the European Regional Office of the World Health Organization looked into the recommendations that were currently being made in three European countries regarding the time at which a baby should first receive solid food (WHO, 1987). It turned out that the advice being given in brochures issued to parents both as to *when* this type of food should be added to the diet and just *what sort of food* should be started were very different from one country to another. In Germany, parents were advised to give porridge from the first month of life onwards, in France only from the second month. Of 26 brochures for parents from England that were examined, only two discussed the introduction of supplementary feeding before the fourth month, while ten of 16 German brochures proclaimed that such supplementary foods as strained fruit or vegetables should be started in the first three months. In France, parents were receiving the same advice as in Germany, but by the third month of life meat, fish, and eggs were to be given as well. Comparing the 72 leaflets that were examined, some of which were issued by the health authorities and others by the baby food manufacturers, one was forced to conclude that parents were receiving contradictory, inconsistent, and highly confusing recommendations as to what food should be given to babies and at what time.

In the former Soviet Union, where the health authorities at that time provided standardized advice to all, mothers were instructed to start giving fruit juice as early as the second week, and strained apple in the sixth week, both intended to provide vitamin supplement.

Gluten Intolerance, Celiac Disease

Gluten is a protein to which some predisposed children react unfavorably if they are given large quantities too early in life. Relatively large amounts of gluten are found in wheat – it is the gluten protein that makes wheat flour ideal for baking. Gluten makes the dough firm, and it rises obediently when yeast is added, unlike the dough made from rye or barley flour, which contain little gluten and therefore end up as unleavened bread. It is clear that gluten intolerance, clinically manifested as "celiac disease," is relatively uncommon among children who have been breastfed. It is currently recommended that foods containing gluten should be introduced while one is still breastfeeding, with the mother continuing to breastfeed for a while, so the introduction of gluten is covered by a breastmilk "umbrella" (Ivarsson, 2005; Persson, Ivarsson, & Hernell, 2002; Agostoni et al., 2009).

Making Food for Baby

Whatever your baby is given in the way of solid food, it must be mashed or strained during the early weeks. Even then, one must realize that starting on solid food is quite a big change for a small individual. Until now, all the food the baby needed came flowing effortlessly in from a soft breast, so the baby might need to be quite hungry to accept porridge, gruel, or mash from a hard spoon pushed into its mouth.

Your Baby Can Smell and Taste

The fact that most babies soon take to strained and pureed food based on the varied items the family eats daily may well reflect the fact that the baby has already encountered many of these flavors. The taste of the adult food that mother had for dinner reached the unborn baby through the amniotic fluid, and a little later, it came to the breastfeeding baby in the milk. This is still a little speculative, but it is becoming an exciting topic for further research (see also Chapter 1). We do know for a fact that a baby is able to distinguish between a sweet taste (that it likes), bitter and sour tastes (that it does not like), and a salty taste (to which it is indifferent). It can also smell garlic, vanilla, mint, and alcohol. It recognizes the smell of its mother and prefers her smell to that of others. Just hours after it is born, this ability is apparent in the baby (Mennella, 2007).

THE BABY WHO SUDDENLY REFUSES THE BREAST

It can occasionally happen that a baby who has been happily breastfeeding suddenly refuses one day to take the breast at all; the problem may last for several days.

This can occur quite early, but sometimes the baby is three to four months old. Do not regard it as a sign that that your baby no longer needs to be breastfed. Various things can lead to such a sudden refusal – discomfort caused by teething, inflammation of the inner ear, a cold that makes it difficult to breathe through the nose, a change in the way your milk tastes during a menstrual period, your own diet (did you perhaps eat a lot of garlic yesterday?), hard physical exercise, or some other factor that may not be at all evident. If you don't want to begin weaning just yet, the main thing is to go on trying until things return to normal. Anne Lise Robak, an experienced mother-to-mother counselor, is familiar with these problems, and she has provided the story that follows, which also may give you some hints on what you can do:

What do you do with a breast refusenik? I have several times been contacted by mothers whose babies have quite suddenly refused to go on breastfeeding. They didn't know that anything like this could happen and were anxious to know what they could do about it. I ran into the same problem with my fourth child, who was three and a half months old when it happened. He was not ill; we hadn't been travelling;

I hadn't used a new perfume; I wasn't wearing scratchy or itchy clothing. No, there was no way I could explain what had happened, but however much or however little milk there was in the breast, he wasn't interested in it. He had quite simply gone on strike. I was reduced to despair, expecting the worst, and I began to think I had better give up the effort to breastfeed altogether. I remember how on that first day I was torn between the alternatives – should I give the little lad some other food? Just imagine him dying of hunger and thirst! Fortunately, common sense prevailed. I recalled the stories of infants who had managed without food and drink for up to a week, so surely my baby could carry on for a few hours more ...

I took care to offer him the breast every now and again, but he screamed his head off every time he was confronted with it. Finally, after I had tried many, many times and for a great many hours, he took a little nap, and in his half sleeping state he did take just a little. But when he awoke, he seemed to realize what he had been up to, and once more he forcefully pulled away from my breast and began to scream again, perhaps in some sort of protest.

It went on like that all day and most of the night (again he drank just a few drops while he was almost asleep). I had to use the breast pump to avoid overfilled breasts and to keep up my milk production. The next day started with the same misery, but I was obstinate enough to avoid reaching for the feeding bottle and giving him my expressed milk that way – I felt it might just prolong the problem. I was thoroughly upset to have been "rejected" like this by my own baby, and now and again I just broke down and cried. Things were made still worse by the irritation I felt that he "didn't seem to understand what was for his own good." All the same, I slowly began to realize that what was needed was more patience, more inventiveness, and a firm determination to do everything I could for him until things straightened themselves out. Among other things, I found that it seemed to help if I carried him around, calming him by letting him suck on my little finger as I did so...until the moment came when I stealthily brought to him to my breast, and a miracle *happened: he latched on, and so long as I went on walking around with him he continued to feed…If I tried to sit down, he would let go of the breast and start screaming again. Would I have to spend the coming months walking? Fortunately, I soon found that his protests at the breast were becoming less frequent, and I began to regain my confidence that the whole problem could be overcome. After about fourteen days, things were back to normal, and in the end, he was not weaned from the breast until he was two years old.*

It is precisely this experience – that it helps to carry the baby around with the breast temptingly exposed and just within reach, and that it is important to try to make the baby calm – that I have passed on to other mothers in the same situation. I know from their reactions how much it has helped them to solve their problems…

SOME GENERAL FACTS ABOUT DIETS

Broadly speaking, the rules that hold good for healthy feeding are the same for children and adults. Sweet treats, like honey and food with lots of sugar, unfortunately appeal to almost all children. Honey should not be given to a child less than a year old because it can contain traces of botulinum toxin that in the very young can be risky. And forget the salt habit – don't add salt to baby's foods, don't even sprinkle it on the meal.

The only important difference in the rules of healthy eating that applies to adults and infants concerns fat. A baby that is being fed on breastmilk alone is getting 50% of its energy in the form of fat - this is absolutely normal. In adults, the recommendation is that not more than 30-35% of the energy in the food should come from fat. As they begin to mature, between the sixth and 12th months of life, children still need more fatty food than adults. In early childhood, the stomach is still very small indeed and easily filled, bearing in mind the quantity of food that is needed. A teaspoonful of vegetable oil added to porridge, mashed potatoes, or rice provides a lot of additional energy from fat without occupying much space. A little goes a long way!

One Type of Food at a Time

A sound rule is to try introducing one new type of food at a time, always beginning with very small quantities (a teaspoonful or two) given as part of several successive meals. After beginning with a new food, wait for a few days before you introduce yet another one, so that you have a chance to see how your baby is reacting to the first.

It is not at all difficult to prepare food for a baby in your own kitchen, even though the glossy brochures advertising tinned or bottled foods would like you to believe the contrary. Your child's stomach is quite capable of digesting an ordinary warm meal, mashed finely with a fork if you don't have your own food processor. Potatoes, vegetables, and meat or fish can be included in the same proportions you would use in an adult meal. In a modern kitchen with a mixer and a deep freezer, you can easily prepare several portions at a time, freezing most of them for use later when the rest of the family is eating pizza. Ordinary, good, western-style food is varied and is just as good for babies as it is for older children and adults. It is also a good thing for the baby to become accustomed to eating the same food as the rest of the family whenever possible. However, so long as the child is still mainly dependent on milk, it is wise to let it take the breast *before* the warm meal, while it still has a healthy appetite. As the time for complete weaning from the breast gradually approaches, you can reverse the order.

Commercial Infant Foods

The main advantage of all the ready-made infant foods available in handy small containers in every supermarket is that they make things simpler. Now and again that is precisely what you need, for example, when the family is traveling, but it is hardly economical – you will have to pay the manufacturer for the work he has taken off your shoulders!

To Find Out More...

There is no shortage of good advice to be found on foods for infants – check with your local clinic on what they can provide or recommend. The internet and the bookstores are full of advice as well. But beware, some internet sites are designed primarily to sell you things, even if they do not admit it.

ALLERGY: IMMUNE PROTECTION GONE WRONG

Allergy is essentially a form of immune defense that has taken a wrong turn. Instead of the body protecting itself against dangerous intruders, it mistakenly calls up its immune defense mechanism to combat everyday newcomers which do not normally present a threat, such as foodstuffs, pollen, and housemites.

Allergists (physicians who specialize in allergy) point out that there are a great many people who *believe* they are allergic to a particular kind of food or react badly to it, but they are not in reality suffering from allergy at all. Quite commonly, they go on to restrict their diet, avoiding certain foods, for no good reason.

Adverse reactions to food and to certain components of breastmilk may occur, not only as true allergies, but also as other forms of intolerance. True allergies can give rise to serious reactions (including "anaphylactic" states) that demand acute medical help. It is vital that parents of allergic children are aware of the condition and know what to do in case of an emergency.

Allergy is fortunately rare: two to five percent of children are believed to suffer from true food allergies, and only a small percentage of them have severe reactions (Høst, 1994). The fear of possible allergic reactions and the belief that a child or infant has adverse reactions to a food or a component of the breastmilk, unfortunately, too often leads a mother to restrict her own diet or that of the child. These restrictions can be quite limiting, and often serve no good purpose. There is actually no strong evidence to support the idea of restricting the diet (Brandtzæg, 2010; Agostoni et al., 2009; Thygarajan & Burks, 2008). It can be quite confusing to diagnose reactions to food, and any modifications to the allergic mother's or child's diet should be made only in consultation with healthcare personnel.

Scientists have devoted a lot of attention to young children whose siblings or parents are allergic, since such children may be more prone than others to develop allergies. It is difficult to carry out such studies perfectly, since one never knows in advance how and where an allergy may appear or which child is likely to be sensitive to which substance. It can also be extraordinarily difficult to determine what foods a given child has been exposed to and when. As all sufferers from allergy know only too well, it may only take a minute amount of allergen to fire off a reaction. This sort of information is vital for any proper study of individual allergy. Despite such problems, the results obtained to date show that exclusive breastfeeding for at least four months can confer a measure of protection against developing allergy, particularly the sort that manifests itself as an atopic eczema (dermatitis), cow milk allergy, asthma, and wheezing in childhood. The protective effect is stronger in high risk infants (Friedman & Zeiger, 2005; Agostoni et al. 2009; Thygarajan & Burks, 2008; Høst et al., 2008). Any breastfeeding also reduces the risk for recurrent wheezing and development of atopic dermatitis, and the effect is more marked if breastfeeding is continued for a longer period, e.g., up to four months (Odijk van et al., 2003).

Essentially, it seems that breastmilk helps the baby's immunological defenses to mature appropriately, so the overall tendency to allergy is lessened. Conversely, if you give a baby cow's milk during the first weeks of life, this process of immune maturation is likely to be deranged. This is particularly unfortunate in the case of a child with allergic tendencies, who has a particular need of breastmilk to get through the early weeks of life without undue risk.

Also relevant is the fact that during the first few weeks of life (one does not really know how many), the baby's intestinal wall is much more inclined than later to allow large molecules (for example, proteins) to pass from the intestine into the bloodstream. For most newborn infants, this doesn't pose a problem, but if a baby is predisposed to allergy, the arrival of a foreign protein (e.g., as a component of cow's milk) in the bloodstream can cause the baby to become oversensitive to it. The next time the same protein arrives, the baby may experience an allergic reaction to it. Most infant formulas are largely composed of cows' milk unless otherwise marked. It is therefore particularly necessary that this special group of babies be fed on breastmilk – and if possible *only* breastmilk for the first six months of life. Finally, *if you have a familial predisposition for allergy* and you want to try giving any new and unfamiliar foods for the first time, if possible, wait until the baby is six months old, and then proceed cautiously, adding only one new food at a time and keeping a careful lookout for any sort of unwanted reaction. Make a note of precisely what you have given and when!

WEANING FROM THE BREAST

Voices Around You - Is It Time to Stop?

One irritating aspect of continuing to breastfeed an older child can be experienced if those around you, no doubt with the best intentions, try to persuade you that it is time to stop. "It puts too much of a strain on you" says one voice. Of course it's not true – you are producing less milk, now that your child's needs are increasingly met by solid food. If you are only giving the breast once or twice a day, as is likely at this time, the child will be taking only a few deciliters (ounces) of milk a day. It may be only a little, but it remains just as important and valuable in that second year as it was in the first.

Some people seem surprised that it's possible to go on breastfeeding as long as you wish. But as we have seen, whenever milk is taken from the breast, it provides a signal for production to continue.

Some mothers who go on breastfeeding for a long time are actually confronted with moralistic objections from those around them, "Go on, admit that you're only doing it for your own enjoyment"! There's only one answer to that, "For *our* enjoyment!"

Weaning From the Breast– Some Statements from Modern Norwegian History

Our old friend, Leopold Meyer, recommended in **1899** that exclusive breastfeeding should continue for ten to 11 months, followed by a transition period of four to six weeks, during which the child would progressively become adapted to solid food (Meyer, 1899). He pointed out, however, that from the seventh month onwards, it could be desirable to "provide a little solid food," as a back-up to the breast. In his firm view "…continuing to feed a child at the breast when it is more than a year old is entirely improper. At that time, the quality of the milk is no longer sufficient. The child needs other forms of food, and the mother's constitution will be weakened by such an unnatural prolongation of breastfeeding."

When Axel Johannessen wrote in **1902** that the child should receive breastmilk for some nine to ten months, he clearly intended this to mean that it should be given nothing else – in other words, exclusive breastfeeding would continue for the first nine to ten months of life (Johannessen, 1902).

Kristiane Skjerve recommended in **1916** that an infant should be fed at the breast for the first nine to ten months of life, after which she suggested that weaning should take no more than four to six weeks (Skjerve, 1916).

Alex Brinchmann considered in **1929** that "feeding with breastmilk can be continued for nine months without risk to the child" and the context makes it clear that he had exclusive breastfeeding in mind. Like Meyer, however, he believed that in case of need, a mother might begin the weaning process when her child was only six months old (Brinchmann, 1929).

All the authoritative statements one finds from the above period (1899-1930) point to the fact that if a mother's milk supply is sufficient, her baby can be reared on breastmilk alone for as long as a year. None of the books known to us, however, suggest that breastfeeding should ever continue for longer than a year.

On the contrary, some writers in later years tend to adopt the view that breastfeeding should last substantially *less* than twelve months. Alfred Sundal, writing in **1939** (and other authorities in the late 1940s), cited nine months as the proper duration of breastfeeding (including two weeks for weaning, meaning that progressive withdrawal from the breast began when the child was only eight and a half months old; Sundal, 1944). And finally we might quote Smedberg and Ødegaard, writing in **1964**, who declared quite simply that "the baby may be weaned at the age of four to five months..." The 1960s were truly the darkest days for breastfeeding. But the revolution was nigh!

It is not really possible to judge from the appearance of an infant – or for that matter any young mammal – when it is ready to say farewell to its mother's breast. In some species of animals, the moment for change is determined simply by the fact that the mother is ready for another pregnancy to assure the continuance of the race. At that time, she will become more interested in the males in the flock than in her brood. In some instances, one can actually see how the mother animal is becoming irritated by the way her ever bigger and stronger young tug at her teats and struggle to get to her udder. But according to the books, these things differ considerably from one species to another, as regards the behavior both of the mother and her litter. So can one say just when the moment has indisputably come to finish with breastfeeding? Once more, we may well look back to the literature provided for parents a hundred and more years ago. Two of the authors of the old books that we quote below refer to "an old and well-established belief" when they seek to justify their views on the duration of breastfeeding. That old belief states "...the child shall breastfeed for the same length of time that it developed in its mother's body" (Meyer, 1899) or in similar terms that "the baby shall spend nine months in its mother's body and nine months at its mother's breast..." (Brinchmann, 1929).

These quotations from one small country about the supposedly proper duration of breastfeeding all dated from the first six decades of the 20th century. They probably reflect contemporary Western pediatric practice and clearly show how the writers of the day insisted on an ever shorter period of breastfeeding. One wonders whether the advice given reflected the inability of mothers to continue any longer, or whether the recommendations in themselves led to an ever shorter duration of breastfeeding. We are very inclined to put our money on the second explanation.

The Duration of Breastfeeding - What Is Our Conclusion?

To be quite honest about it: no one really knows how long breastfeeding should continue, and there is probably no universal rule. It is up to every mother and baby couple to find out for themselves how long they want to continue. Whether they want to persist with breastfeeding after the first year and on into the second, third, or even the fourth year of life is a private matter for them and them alone, dependent on their wants and feelings. In the old days, when breastfeeding for many women was the only reasonably dependable means of family planning, that alone was sufficient reason for some women to continue with it for very long periods (see Chapter 13). Thomas Ljungberg has suggested that the "natural" duration of breastfeeding in humans is some three to four years, arguing that the much shorter period of breastfeeding that has become widely accepted is precisely the reason why young children have such a need for soft toys and other things to cuddle in the cradle... (Ljungberg, 1991).

Breastfeeding the More Mature Baby

The recommendation now provided by WHO, confirmed January 2011 (Baby Friendly Canada, 2011), is that infants should be exclusively breastfed for the first six months of life to achieve optimal growth, development, and health. Thereafter, infants should be given nutritious complementary foods and continue breastfeeding "up to the age of two years or beyond."

This is realistic advice. As we have seen, virtually all mothers are able to go on producing at least some milk for this period, provided they continue to put their babies to the breast.

As the baby approaches its first birthday, by which time you will be introducing it to solid foods and the occasional cup of water, milk or juice, breastmilk will no longer be playing such a central role in nutrition. It is, however, worth bearing in mind that even half a liter a day of breastmilk will still be enough to cover a third of the child's needs for energy and protein and half of its Vitamin A requirement, as well as providing almost all the Vitamin C it needs. To say nothing of the fact that breastmilk continues to provide a child with a higher level of immunity and protection against infection, right through the second year of life and beyond if breastfeeding continues for a longer period. That can be a real blessing if the child begins nursery school.

For many mothers and their babies, however, it is the coziness of breastfeeding that is appealing, whether it be in the waking hours of the early morning, providing a welcome break during the working day, or calming a little child who has woken in the night and finds everything frightfully dark and spooky.

Many look back on the later phases of breastfeeding as the most rewarding. Now the child is old enough to experience everything more intensely and to show the real joy he or she finds in breastfeeding. Now the child knows very well what the breast is for, and will soon be setting out to feed itself! I (Elisabet) remember the hungry look on my one-year-old's face when he was sitting in the changing room of the public bath and saw all those juicy breasts parading past him!

The End of Breastfeeding

Deciding when breastfeeding should end, as we have said above, is a matter for you, your baby, or both of you. However it happens, you don't need to take leave of breastfeeding with a heavy heart. It may be a part of what is sometimes elegantly called a baby's process of socialization – coming to realize progressively that there is a big world out there, that it cannot expect to remain forever everyone's center of attention.

The Right Way to End Breastfeeding

At some point, of course, you will feel the time has come to round off the whole process. When that time comes, it will be both in the child's best interest and your own to plan the process, making the change over a long period, preferably a number of months. There are, however, children who wean themselves willingly within a very short time.

To start with, try giving the breast after a solid meal, when the child is no longer so hungry. After a while, you can replace one of the daily breastfeeds with another fluid, offered in a cup.

The best thing is to replace the midday breastfeed first, and later the morning and evening sessions. Your child will find it easiest if the lunchtime feed is the first to go. Nature has wisely arranged matters in such a way that when you are breastfeeding less frequently, for example, only once a day or every other day, the let-down reflex is relatively slow to respond. Most children will, bit by bit, lose interest in a breast that seems so unwilling to react.

Some children are more persistent (perhaps stronger willed?) than others, and it may be a problem if the mother feels that she has had enough of breastfeeding, whereas the child does not, or vice versa. The child may have taken it into its head that it has no intention of abandoning the breast, whatever mother may say. We have encountered many such stories and heard of all the ways in which desperate mothers try to make the breast less seductive. Some try applying unattractive potions to the nipple, ranging from mustard to the bitter juice of the gentian root, others deck the nipple with a plaster as a sign that it is now out of bounds. The most drastic step of all is simply to withdraw – no longer offering the breast at all – in the hope that the child will soon forget the whole business.

If the baby does go through a phase of needing more contact, for example, if it falls ill and you go back to more frequent breastfeeds, your milk production will soon increase to cope with the renewed demand.

Such interruptions apart, you will find that with this process of gradual weaning from the breast, the number of feeds declines as the weeks go by. Ultimately, you find that only the cuddly session in the morning or a goodnight feed in the evening remain. And then, one day, you will realize that you have omitted even those, and that a week has already gone by since the last breastfeed. So it is that the two of you have taken a big step towards independence, but carrying with you the happiest memories of how it all was and knowing that it has provided you with a firm foundation for a good and lasting relationship as mother and child.

It Still Isn't Quite Finished!

As weaning from the breast progresses, your milk production will gradually decline so that your breasts again become smaller, regaining more or less the volume they had before you became pregnant. For quite a while after you have stopped breastfeeding, however, there will still be some milk in your breasts – indeed, it may continue to be present until you become pregnant once more. This doesn't mean, however, that you need another pregnancy in order to breastfeed once more! There are many accounts of mothers who have taken a child to the breast successfully, in some cases even after the menopause (Hormann, 2006). For those of us who have grown a little older and will no longer bear children (or perhaps have never borne them), it is comforting to realize that breastfeeding is such a simple process that everyone who wishes can produce some milk in her breast.

Part 3

Glimpses into the History of Breastfeeding: What Happened and Why?

Chapter 13.
A GLIMPSE INTO THE HISTORY OF BREASTFEEDING

Where breastfeeding is concerned, a very sound reason to take a brief glimpse at the past is that one can learn so much from the dramatic events that led to its decline and the way in which it rebounded. It is hardly ancient history; some of the most astonishing events were played out within the lifetime of people who are still around to tell the tale – and who were intimately involved in them.

IN THE BEGINNING THERE WAS BREASTFEEDING

Breastfeeding is as old as humanity. The process by which women bear children and nurture them to maturity has been basic to the survival of our species. From the ancient past, small stone figures portraying wonderfully fat women, generally with massive hips and buttocks, and large breasts obviously well filled with milk, have been found in an area that stretches from western Europe to Siberia (Figure 13.1).

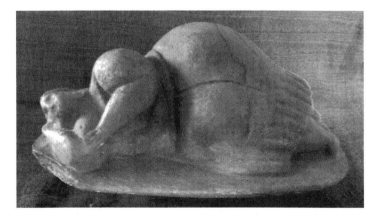

Figure 13.1. *A fertility symbol dating from the Stone Age: Venus from Malta.*

Source: Photo by Michael Dukes. Used with permission.

Some even date back to an era of nomadic hunter-gatherers some 20,000 years ago. We do not know why these small figures were made, but it is reasonable to suppose that they played a role in fertility rites. This is suggested by the distribution of bodily fat stores in these images, reflecting the typically female pattern of fat storage the system builds up as a reserve of energy for pregnancy and breastfeeding. A second and much later harvest of stone figures, again generously proportioned, dates from the time when agriculture developed and permanent settlements appeared, a few thousand years before Christ. Many of these have been recovered in the "fertile crescent" – the area of Mesopotamia, Babylonia, and Assyria, where western culture was born.[7] From that same era and area, massive numbers of smaller elegant female figures have been recovered, often made of baked clay.

In those times when a mother did experience problems of one sort or another in breastfeeding her baby, the solution nearest at hand was to summon help from another woman who was lactating successfully, and we know that this was a commonly recognized practice. The Code of Hammurabia Babylonian book of laws dating from 1800 B.C., contains explicit provisions on the duties and uses of a wet-nurse to breastfeed a child other than her own.

MORE THAN FOOD ALONE

While breastfeeding is, and has been through history, a normal part of human life, it has also been surrounded by an aura of solemnity and symbolism. Various statues from Ancient Egypt portray the goddess Isis breastfeeding a pharaoh at one or another of the cardinal moments in his imperial life – birth, coronation, or death. The feeding of the pharaoh at the breast of Isis perhaps reflected the divine blessing that rested upon him.

An echo of more everyday concerns with breastfeeding in Ancient Egypt is to be found in the health regulations set out in the Ebers papyrus, dating from 1550 B.C. "In order that a woman shall have sufficient milk in her breasts, take the bone of a swordfish, heat it in oil, and use it to massage her back." Or, alternatively, "Let the woman sit cross-legged and eat hot steaming durra bread dipped in sauce, while you massage her body with the juice of the poppy." This is perhaps a piece of advice worth trying?

---

7   This is the area that today comprises Syria, Jordan, Anatolia (in Turkey), Iraq, and
    Iran.

The Greek-Turkish statue of the goddess Artemis, two versions of which were excavated in Ephesus on Turkey's Mediterranean coast, is also instructive. She is endowed with some twenty breasts, embellishing her body from her neck to her midriff. Bearing in mind that both copies of the statue date from 200 A.D., this is quite a creditable achievement for an 1800-year-old. It is small wonder that this version of Artemis has long been seen as a symbol of a copious flow of milk.

Many spokesmen for the various religions have, down through the ages, made pronouncements on breastfeeding. The best known is the edict of the Prophet Mohammed, laid down in the Qur'an about 600 A.D., to the effect that a baby should be breastfed for two years - a rule well compatible with modern teaching. But there is some room for adaptation with the added provision that "…should the parents, after due consultation, agree that weaning shall take place earlier, this will not be held against them…" (Pickthall, 1948, V 233).

BREASTFEEDING, JUSTICE, AND THE LAW

In the Far North, one finds some ancient edicts on breastfeeding, perhaps less flexible than those laid down by the Prophet. The Ancient Christian Civil Law which was in force in Norway by 1387 (Weiser-Aall, 1973, p. 17) rules that "…it shall be the duty of the husband to ensure that breastfeeding does not continue longer than through two seasons of Lent and up until the third Lent…" (i.e., up to the third year of life). The fines to be imposed on any unfortunate husband who failed to observe the rule were not inconsiderable – for permitting his wife to breastfeed longer, his penalty would amount to three marks in silver – at the time the value of two or three head of cattle. Should it turn out that the husband had actually conspired with his wife to flaunt the regulation, the penalty would be doubled and taken from his personal estate. It has been suggested that rules such as these were not merely a means of levying taxes, but that they reflected serious concern on the part of society that couples might be tempted to engage in a form of family planning; knowledge of the fact that breastfeeding inhibits fertility proves to have been very widespread. At the time, both lawmakers and governments were very occupied with the need for population increase, especially since by 1400 the recurrent plague known as the Black Death had wiped out half the population. Not that this is the only explanation that has been offered; the rule may simply have been intended to promote adherence to the Church's rules on fasting during the forty days of Lent. Breastfeeding women were namely exempt from the fasting rule, and that alone might have induced a woman with a healthy appetite to nurse her baby just that little while longer…

This very same Ancient Christian Civil Law also imposed on neighbors the duty to provide assistance at the time of delivery, and to remain with the new mother until the baby had been put to the breast. Perhaps romanticizing a little, it is easy to suppose that people in those times understood that the process of birthing was not truly complete until the baby had ceased to take its nutrition from the umbilical cord and commenced to feed at the breast. Yet the explanation for this particular rule may also have been more prosaic; it could have represented an attempt to counter the practice of infanticide, all too common at the time among unwilling and unhappy mothers, as we saw in Chapter 6. The Christian Church was vigorously opposed to this practice – often seen popularly as a late form of abortion. Once a baby had been fed at the breast, however, it acquired the right to the protection afforded every individual by the law. To deprive it of life from that moment onwards, thus constituted a criminal offence. And perhaps this first skin-to-skin contact with the mother, stimulating the release of oxytocin – "the love hormone," would banish any lingering thoughts of infanticide.

NORTHERN WOMEN AND THEIR WORK

High infant mortality was not always directly linked to difficult economic conditions (Lithell, 1999). However, there was a clear relationship between deprival of breastfeeding and high infant mortality; the former might in turn be linked to the mother's employment, which was not always compatible with frequent breastfeeding sessions. A mother who found herself forced to perform heavy physical work far away from home in order to maintain herself might well find that she had no opportunity to breastfeed. However, there were even situations in which working women under relatively comfortable conditions encountered this problem. For example, the linen workers in Sweden's Hälsingland province were unable to breastfeed because it was not compatible with the nature of their day-to-day employment. Linen making was an important source of welfare in such an area, and employment in the linen trade demanded skill and carried with it a high status. It could not be entrusted to mere unskilled workers, but it also required intense concentration and skill throughout the day. If a woman so employed sought to breastfeed during her working hours, it was feared that this could adversely affect the quality of the product – and the risk of losing her job might be too great for a mother to take.

ICELAND: THE ISLAND OF THE SAGAS WHERE ONLY THE STRONG SURVIVED

A Danish physician, Biarne Povelsen, has put on record a remarkable account of the situation of breastfeeding that he encountered in Iceland when he spent time working there in or around 1772. He describes how the Icelandic mothers of the day made no attempt to breastfeed their offspring for more than the first week of life (Ólafsson, 1772). After that, they were handed over to one of the neighbors or an elderly relative, who set about feeding them with fresh cow's milk, together with minced fish or meat. Among the more moneyed classes, there was also provision for them to receive cream and butter. The result, not surprisingly, was an appallingly high incidence of infant deaths. A mother had to deliver as many as 10 to 15 children in order to hope for three survivors. Not that there was anything wrong with an Icelandic mother's ability to breastfeed; we know that among the poorest families, where there was no money to pay for anything other than feeding at the breast, most of the children survived. No written evidence has come down to us that might explain how this massive mistrust of a mother's own milk had come about in 18th century Iceland; we can only speculate on the reason for it. Iceland was at the time a country where natural resources were very scarce, and it was necessary to limit the size of the population to a level the nation could support. One means of ensuring this was to limit the period during which women would deliver children. A massive bridal dowry was therefore required, and that could only be built up through many years of savings. As a result, most women were well advanced in adulthood before they were able to marry and begin their reproductive career. Since infant mortality was so high, it was necessary to have many pregnancies in rapid succession in order to ensure the family's continuation. By strictly limiting the period of breastfeeding, fertility was maintained, and one pregnancy followed another. The notion seems to have taken root that the few children who survived the brutal regime to which they were subjected would be the most likely to develop into strong and sturdy adults. The price paid, however, was a high one in terms of women's health, required as they were to bear so many children in vain.

That it was possible for such rigid attitudes to change, even at that time, emerges from another report from Iceland, penned 70 years after the first, in 1842, again by a physician, Dr. A. Schleisner, who had similarly spent a period working in Iceland. He writes that it was still the general custom to entrust the care of babies to others, who would feed them on cow's milk and suchlike, but he added that in the capital of Reykjavik and other trading centers, a midwife trained in Copenhagen had succeeded in persuading mothers to breastfeed, with the gratifying results that one would expect as regards the health and survival of their children.

WHO WAS CONSIDERED TO UNDERSTAND BREASTFEEDING?

Throughout the ages, breastfeeding counseling has been traditionally viewed as a matter that would be entrusted to "wise women," traditional birth attendants and midwives. The field was very much dominated by women, a fact that may perhaps help explain why, for a long time, breastfeeding was not taken seriously in male-dominated academic circles as a matter warranting scientific scrutiny, especially not by the medical profession.

When, however, in the course of the 19th century, it became customary for women to enter a hospital for their deliveries, it became necessary for medical men to form a view on how newly born infants, as their patients, should be nourished. The actual process of breastfeeding seemed to merit little in the way of academic interest and was regarded with something approaching indifference or contempt. And when, the clinicians concerned began to develop their views and pet theories on the matter, they unfortunately did so with scant regard for the available evidence or for scientific logic. Perhaps that was to some extent understandable; it was, after all, a field from which men had traditionally been almost entirely excluded.

Breastfeeding Research - Of a Sort

As early as the late 17th century, a number of books had appeared on the health and illnesses of infants and children, and some of these devoted some attention to the question of feeding. By 1789 a British doctor by the name of Michael Underwood had produced a three-volume work on diseases of children, in which he presented some of the earliest known work on the composition of human breastmilk. Insight into such matters at the time was naturally restricted by the analytical methods available, such as, for example, knowledge of the acidification and fermentation process as compared with animal milk, particularly that of the cow. Underwood was struck by the fact that fresh breastmilk remained usable for several days, even at room temperature, though the reason for this could not be found with the methods available to him, which relied primarily on observation. It is interesting to note that several of these early researchers advanced the hypothesis that the milk might contain certain important substances that would be destroyed by boiling. Since the scientists of the day had no means of determining whether that was in fact the case, such suggestions remained untested almost down to our own time.

For that matter, Dr. Underwood very properly asked himself and his readers how it could be that animals had so few problems with breastfeeding as compared with humans; alas, he could find no clear answer to his own question.

DISCIPLINE RAISES ITS UGLY HEAD

The first authority to suggest that there was a need for more discipline and order in the feeding of infants seems to have been the English pediatrician Hugh Smith, who as early as 1792 published his "Letters to married women." In his letters, he urged mothers to feed their babies at fixed times of day, namely 7 and 10 a.m. and 1, 6, and 11 p.m. Just that – without any argument to support it. Later authors took up this idea with a degree of enthusiasm, which at the present day we find difficult to understand. Today we have a clearer picture of the physiological processes underlying a human being's natural breastfeeding pattern, regular or otherwise. And in retrospect, we can document, using firm historical data, the catastrophic consequences the notion of feeding by the clock ultimately had for breastfeeding.

A Double Message to Mothers

Society has at times held curiously conflicting views about the new mother and her correct behavior. According to the traditional lore both of Islam and Christianity, she was unclean and had to be considered as a heathen, literally standing outside the religious community and deprived of its protection during the first 40 days after giving birth. In Islam, this period has traditionally been doubled to 80 days if the baby is a girl. During this time, a woman was forbidden to enter the holy place, be it a mosque or a church, and in the Christian community, she had to pass through a cleansing ceremony ("the churching of women") before she could again be admitted alongside respectable people. Yet at the same time, the new mother was assured that she was blessed, and told that she had fulfilled her feminine duty by bearing a child – a matter for celebration.

All this meant that a woman received a double message regarding her role as a mother, positive and negative at the same time; she was blessed for having performed her duty, yet at the same time, looked down upon as an unclean heathen. The psychologist Berit Ås has developed an interesting theory that this seeming inconsistency was in fact one of a series of techniques developed by society to keep women in their appointed place (Ås, 1999). This "double punishment" as she calls it, served to confuse the individual by providing mutually incompatible messages ("Damned if you do and damned if you don't"). So the new mother, vulnerable as she was because of the acute changes she was undergoing both physically and mentally following delivery, would be a particularly easy victim of the general process by which women were repressed and their rights contained by society.

Another Double Message - About Milk

Even though a mother's own milk has always been regarded as ideal for her baby, and though mothers have so often been urged and expected to breastfeed, one sees that there has often been another double message as regards the quality of her milk. It has, on the one hand, been extolled as a veritable elixir of life, while on the other, it has been dismissed as mere hogwash. Colostrum in particular, with its golden-yellow hue, has raised suspicions and seeded fantasies. The Greek physician Soranus, who practiced in Rome around 100 A.D., emphatically counseled women to refrain from putting their infants to their breast during the first three weeks of life, since the milk at that time was in his view too "strong" for them to tolerate. The fashionable Parisian physician Jacques des Pars, who was active around 1450 A.D., similarly considered that a mother should not breastfeed during the month that she was supposed to remain in bed following delivery, since in his view the milk had been stored too long in her body and must therefore be deemed unclean. Given such views, it is hardly surprising that the women of Paris in his day experienced problems with breastfeeding.

To take one last example of these curious professional opinions: the English pediatrician Thomas Bull in England wrote in his "Hints to Mothers" published in 1848 that women who had born a child for the first time were particularly unlikely to provide a sufficient amount of breastmilk during the first four days; those who could afford an alternative were advised to feed their infants with diluted asses' milk or to use cow's milk with added sugar during these early days. Dr. Bull did ordain that the infant should be allowed to determine the feeding time during the first ten days, but that was the limit of freedom – thereafter, a four hour routine must be imposed.

The Positive Side of Injustice

Like the proverbial donkey, however, the new mother was cajoled with the carrot as well as the stick. Even apparently illogical advice could have its compensations. So long as a young mother was regarded as "unclean," she was not permitted to engage in any form of housework whatsoever. She had to be provided with all her meals, lest she be tempted to prepare food herself. Should she ignore such prohibitions, which were to be found in both Christian and Islamic tradition (Eberhard-Gran, Nordhagen, Heiberg, Bergsjø, & Eskild, 2003), any food that she prepared would be deemed to be unwholesome and the household would be regarded as doomed to a series of misfortunes. The new mother, therefore, had no reason to challenge the rules banning her from involvement in housework. She could relax with a clear conscience, something that might otherwise have been difficult for a conscientious homemaker.

So it was that throughout the greater part of Europe and Asia, new mothers down through the ages spent the first few weeks after delivery in bed with their babies, while other women cared for the home and, where necessary, the animals. Visitors naturally brought food with them, knowing full well that they should not expect the nursing mother to wait on them. It was an ancient and sound tradition.

THE WET-NURSE

Some mothers have always been concerned about the real or supposed failure of their milk supply. Whenever the problem seemed to exist, relatives, friends, acquaintances, and professional wet-nurses moved in to provide support. Sometimes any woman who had a breast to offer – grandmother included – was considered eligible. The best qualified, however, was very often the professional wet-nurse. Many a poor woman has, down through the ages, found herself obliged to sell her milk to those of better means, often being forced to leave her own child to be looked after by her family, deprived of her milk. She was, however, in a strong negotiating position with those who needed her services and had the resources to pay for them. They, in turn, would require that she provide sound and reliable support (Figure 13.2). Books on infant care dating from before 1900 all sought to formulate the standards that a wet-nurse should meet.

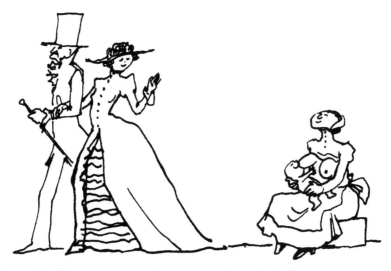

Figure 13.2. *The wet-nurse assumed an important place in the family.*

Source: Cartoon by Ellen Wilhelmsen. Used with permission.

The most fundamental demand was that the wet-nurse should have milk in her breasts. The other requirements vary greatly with the writer, but most medical texts from the 17th and 18th centuries provided advice on the demands that the family should make regarding the wet-nurse's health, the freshness of her breath, her skin color, and the color of her hair (red hair was often considered dubious). In earlier times, there was a belief that the wet-nurse's personality would be imparted to the child through the milk. This latter issue was the subject of a learned debate held at the University of Oxford as early as 1605, but the outcome of that debate is not known since only the invitation has come down to us.

Since it was often considered that the wet nurse should have born her own child at approximately the same time that the foster-child was delivered, she often had very little opportunity to feed her own baby before leaving it in order to exercise her profession. The employer was, however, advised to determine how the wet-nurse's own child looked, since this might provide some indication as to whether or not she was a good breastfeeder. Other writers suggested that the wet-nurse's own confinement should have been three, four, or as many as seven months beforehand.

Breastfeeding - A Matter of Free Will

As we pointed out above, a wet-nurse was in a strong negotiating position with her potential employer, for it is a fundamental fact that a mother cannot be forced to breastfeed, something which has always been known intuitively or at least recognized of necessity. Her employer was dependent upon her coming to work willingly and without reservations; otherwise, her let-down reflex would not work and the foster-baby would look in vain for its milk supply. The source of milk had to be tempted and beckoned, not commanded.

Leopold Meyer, who was the source of many of the ideas about infant care in Denmark and Norway in his day, deplored the fact that in Denmark almost all the women seeking employment as wet-nurses were unmarried mothers and that it was virtually impossible to obtain information from any reliable source on their state of health or their morals. Syphilis and tuberculosis were real problems among these women and presented a danger to the foster child. These problems were particularly likely to arise when a poor wet-nurse had been obliged to earn a meager living by engaging in prostitution.

Problems with the Wet-Nurse

Such were not the only problems that could arise if one took a wet-nurse into the home. Since her presence was so important to the family and to the survival of its youngest member, she was in a position to be quite demanding if she had the wit and inclination to do so. Should she have engaged in prostitution, she could well become a source of much tension and suspicion in the family. At the same time, there would be a need to ensure that she cared properly for the baby – a matter in which she might well fail, being entirely untrained, for as a rule, it was only fate and misfortune that had driven her to seek work as a wet-nurse and child-carer. According to a baby-book of the day, the lady of the house should, therefore, ensure that the wet-nurse tucked the baby properly into its cradle after a night feed, that she kept the nursing room at a proper temperature, and that she allowed sufficient air into the stove to avoid the risk of carbon monoxide poisoning. There was plenty of opportunity for error and one must wonder why mothers let it happen. Sometimes the mother and the wet-nurse would find themselves competing for the baby's favors, with the mother not uncommonly losing out.

The practice of wet-nursing survived longest in pre-revolutionary Russia and in France. In both countries, there was an established tradition that country women took city children belonging to the nobility and the upper middle classes into their homes and cared for them there (Drake, 1940). It seems astonishing today that such an unnatural approach to infant feeding was so long-lived, surviving as it did from early times down to the early years of the 20th century. It must have been painful for the mother, and at the same time disingenuous, for the women who offered their services as wet-nurses often were not among God's chosen. Most large towns in France had their wet-nursing markets where such services were bought and sold. At one stage, the French authorities found themselves obliged to threaten them with economic sanctions, as it was reported that foster babies had repeatedly been "lost" from the carriages conveying them to the wet-nurse's home from the market place where the bargain had been struck, and no doubt an advance on the agreed salary had been paid.

Record Breaking Wet-Nurses!

Around 1900, a well-known French pediatrician, Pierre Budin, responsible for child nutrition in a foundling hospital (to which children abandoned by their mothers were admitted), published a remarkable account of his experiences. Various physicians had been struck by the fact that women often proved capable of breastfeeding several children alongside their own. For that reason, Budin recruited 14 wet-nurses whose duty it was to breastfeed as many foundlings as possible. How many they could provide for depended on circumstances. At a given moment, the 14 nurses were caring for 50 infants, and each wet-nurse was deemed to provide some 40 feeding sessions a day. Even for a professional, this proved too ambitious. Budin estimated that 34 breastfeeding sessions daily was the most that a woman could manage without risk to the health of the foundlings, her own baby, or herself. When the milk production of each of seven wet-nurses was meticulously recorded over a four month period, it was found to average 1.5 liters daily, but when the demand on the staff was greatest, an average of no less than 2.5 liters was attained. Budin remarked that the total milk production by the group he monitored was closely related to the current demand, even in the case of women who had been breastfeeding for more than a year. Budin sought to assess the quality of the milk to the extent possible with the methods available in 1907 and noted no significant change where women had been breastfeeding for as much as a year. Such findings are not surprising in light of today's knowledge, but they must have been greeted with some astonishment at the time. Budin was French, and Englishmen have always held remarkable and sometimes critical views on the French diet, which might explain why his important findings, published as they were in an exemplary manner, were ignored in the Anglo-Saxon world (Wickes, 1953).

The institution of the wet-nurse faded gradually as bottle-feeding became more dependable and more convenient. Meyer, as noted, discusses wet-nursing in his small book on child care published in 1898 for Danish and Norwegian parents. But in later books published in that part of the world, it faded away. From 1920 onwards, it had virtually disappeared into the realms of historical curiosities, along with the dinosaur and much else from the world's past. Fortunately for those infants in the western world most in need of human milk, which their own mothers were unable to provide, milk banks arrived. The very first was established in Vienna in 1900, and the first in North America (in Boston, Massachusetts) started in 1910.

LACTARIUMS WITH DROPS OF MILK

All the same, with the disappearance of the wet-nurse, a degree of confusion did arise. How were needy babies now to be fed? One answer was provided in the form of distribution systems for specially produced and treated dairy milk of the highest quality, often from specially selected herds of cows, serving those babies who were considered to need more supplementation than the breast could provide. In Sweden and some other European countries, publicly funded milk kitchens were set up. The Swedish and the French project, both named "drops of milk" ("Mjölkdroppen" and "Gouttes du lait," respectively) had both a practical and an educational purpose. In Sweden, bottled cows' milk was distributed to the homes where it was needed. To counter criticism that this could discourage breastfeeding, as undoubtedly it did, mothers who were still breastfeeding received a modest payment. What is more, the project staff not only delivered milk to the front door, they inspected the home to check for the possible presence of bottles of breastmilk substitute from other sources. If a mother was found to be in possession of a feeding bottle for which she could not account, she forfeited her regular breastfeeding premiums. The staff soon learned to suspect certain mothers – and certain grandmothers, as well – of improper feeding practices: "…they ignore the rules and feed the babies according to their own outdated and dangerous notions" (Stenhammar, Ohrlander, Stark, & Söderlind, 2001, p. 60).

In 1905, when the project was introduced, the children were being fed eight times in 24 hours. By 1940, the scheme of things had become more mainstream, with an average of five feeds daily at fixed feeding times – 6:00 and 10:00 a.m. and 2:00, 6:00, and 10:00 p.m. If nothing else, this provides a reminder of the extent to which breastfeeding is subject to the whims of history.

In France, as the practice of wet-nursing progressively disappeared, the authorities established lactariums or dairy milk agencies, some 18 of which were still functioning as late as 1994 (Merlin, 1994). In a country where the infant formula industry had grown in strength and influence and the State had long seemed indifferent to the breastfeeding issue, the lactariums had a role both in public education and policy support.

In Russia, too, milk kitchens were common as late as the early 1990s, operating on very similar lines to the systems established in France and Sweden. The dairy milk supplied was from specially certified herds, and it was sterilized before it was distributed to make assurance double sure. A mother would be referred by her health center to such a milk kitchen if it was considered that she was unable to breastfeed, for example, because she was suffering from an infectious condition.

THE INDUSTRIAL REVOLUTION CHANGES THE WORLD

Between 1850 and 1930, the industrialization of society led to fundamental changes in the style and nature of daily life, especially in the western world. There were a whole series of revolutionary changes in many areas of life. During this period, urbanization proceeded apace: farming families moved into the towns since it was there that the men (and to an increasing extent women and children) could sell their labor, labor for which there was now less demand in the agricultural sector. Mothers, too, were caught up in this process, slowly but surely being drawn away from the home and into the factory.

BREASTFEEDING MOVES INTO THE HOSPITAL

The eclipse that breastfeeding was to experience in relatively modern times clearly began when it moved away from the circle of the extended family, in which it was a visible and prominent part of life and where there was no lack of experienced mentors and positive examples. From there it moved first to the mean and over-filled quarters in which urban workers were obliged to live; then the hospitals opened their doors to women going into labor. An ever greater proportion of working class town mothers chose to deliver in the hospital, rather than in the confines of their overcrowded homes. And as these women moved into the hospital, so did breastfeeding, thus becoming a matter for which the institution assumed responsibility.

This transition was bound to have consequences. For thousands of years, both the birthing process and its natural sequel in breastfeeding had been the joint responsibility of society's women. Now for the first time, breastfeeding had become a matter governed by the rules and views of the hospital staff, despite the fact that the latter had no experience or tradition in guiding or assisting mothers to pursue it successfully. Some doctors simply assumed that breastfeeding was a process natural to every mother, in which she could engage without any need for tuition. When that assumption proved to be at fault, those who had responsibility for the well-being of the new mother and her baby all too often demonstrated a lack of the practical insight that was called for when problems with breastfeeding arose (Liddiard, 1946).

Since mother and child fell into different administrative classes in the hospital, it was considered natural to keep them apart. A baby would be placed under the care of pediatricians or nurses in the infants' ward, while its mother would remain in the delivery or post-delivery ward, where the necessary obstetric and gynecological care could be ensured.

It was obvious that when it was time for feeding at the breast, mother and child would have to be brought together; five half-hourly sessions daily were arranged for this purpose. During the night, it was deemed better that both mother and baby should rest undisturbed. Should a baby become inconveniently hungry in the course of the night, the nurses considered it most appropriate to administer a feeding bottle, and usually saw this as a rather enjoyable part of their task in the infants' ward.

But Who Knew Anything About Breastfeeding?

The physicians of the day in the newly created speciality of pediatrics, the general nurses working alongside them, and the hospital's midwives received no scientifically based and practically oriented training in the task of supporting a new mother who had difficulty in making milk in a reluctant breast or coaxing it out when the baby needed it. Breastfeeding was a non-subject in the medical curriculum; one only needs to glance at the medical textbooks in use at the time to see that the subject was barely mentioned, if at all. Only in our own day have the medical textbooks begun to provide information of practical use on the subject, and even now, most of them provide very little in the way of advice in dealing with breastfeeding problems.

GENERATIONS OF ADVICE ON BREASTFEEDING–PART I

The Duty to Breastfeed

Books on infant care or written to provide advice to new mothers have long stressed the virtues of breastmilk and the fact that it was a mother's duty to provide it (Meyer, 1899). They were often backed by highly derogatory remarks as to the character and personality of women who failed to do so:

> ...She should be thoroughly ashamed of herself, unworthy of being a mother... (Meyer, 1899, p.8).

> As Nature has placed in the bosom of the mother the natural food of her offspring, it must be self-evident to every reflecting woman, that it becomes her duty to study, as far as lies in her power, to keep that reservoir of nourishment in as pure and invigorating a condition as possible (Beeton, 1859, p.1034).

> ...Every mother is capable of breastfeeding and every mother must indeed do so, for her child's sake (Sundal, 1939, p.70).

> ... For such reasons, it is the absolute duty incumbent on every mother to rear her baby on breastmilk... (Monrad, 1952, p. 62).

Such moralization has in our experience only tended to defeat its own purpose, perhaps because the recipient felt an urge to defend herself against these demands which were being made upon her, interfering as they did in a matter that was an intimate one involving only herself and her baby.

When Things Go Wrong, Just Blame the Victim!

Quotations in boxes throughout this chapter paint a sad picture of the abysmal level of breastfeeding knowledge over a century now past. Even pediatric nurses had no resources to fall back on other than their own experience and common sense – which were sometimes sufficient, but which on other occasions left them standing helplessly by as a baby remained hungry and inconsolable, despite the fact that its mother seemed to be in perfectly good health. When that happened, the simplest course was to explain away the cause of the misery by blaming the victim – it was all too easy to assert that the mother was guilty of her failure to breastfeed. Had she not been told how important breastfeeding was? Had she not been commanded in no uncertain terms to do her duty? Had she not been told, quite simply, that she *must* breastfeed her baby?

As for the doctors, they consoled themselves with the belief that many a woman was simply not equipped by nature to nurse her baby. The reasons advanced for such a belief were numerous and fanciful. It could be that the woman in question was too refined – or perhaps not refined enough. Perhaps she had lived unhealthily, or maybe she was just not strong enough to breastfeed? Others pointed to the fact that levels of breastfeeding had fallen drastically in the period between 1920 and 1950, suggesting that genetic selection was involved. Since, so ran the argument, the babies of mothers with an inability to breastfeed now survived to maturity thanks to bottle-feeding, the next generation of women would inevitably comprise a higher proportion of individuals genetically endowed with similar breastfeeding difficulties. In the course of a few generations, therefore, the majority of women might be expected to be incapable of breastfeeding. But like many of the other explanations for breastfeeding failure offered at one time or another, this is scientifically just not true.

YET MORE REASONS WHY THINGS WENT WRONG

It is not difficult to trace yet other factors that over a hundred years led to the decline in breastfeeding. Just a few of the most prominent causes are mentioned in the paragraphs below.

The Dictatorship of the Clock

The industrial revolution altered popular notions of *time*. Until then, it was the waxing and waning of daylight that determined the pattern of the day. However, with the arrival of gas and electric lighting, which extended the day, and of factories with their fixed working hours, the clock became an essential element in daily life. Factory employees worked and were paid according to a scheme of things dictated by the clock; it was perhaps not unnatural that the notion soon arose that the pattern of infant feeding, too, should be determined by the fingers on the dial (Milliard, 1990). So it was that the new arrival must be taught to respect the need for regularity and learn that it was pointless to scream in the hope of attracting food merely because it was wanted. The unfortunate infant, coming into the world as it did with a need and expectation for feeding on demand (see Chapter 2), was not in a position to argue the matter. Protest as it might, loudly or softly, it had to learn discipline and respect for a timetable. Such was the theory of the day, resulting as it did in much fruitless protest by small voices and many hungry little stomachs. The theory also meant that many a breast well filled with milk was deprived of the chance to play its role, and all this because of unfounded beliefs as to the manner in which a mother should care for and feed her child.

GENERATIONS OF ADVICE ON BREASTFEEDING –PART II

Good – And Less Good – Advice

From 1870 to 1970, the litanies of praise lavished on breastmilk and on mothers who dutifully were to provide it were complemented by attempts to provide advice on the matter. Much of that advice, viewed in the light of today's knowledge, would necessarily render breastfeeding difficult for many women and entirely impossible for some.

Regularity and Discipline Were the Catchwords of the Day

The baby was to be permitted only short periods at the breast, preferably not more than 10-20 minutes. After that time, so ran the conventional wisdom of the day, the baby would "merely be swallowing air." It was also deemed advisable to provide as few feeding sessions as possible, with intervals as long as possible between them, so the infant's digestive system could "rest and relax." After all, so it was argued, the digestive system should not be expected to labor continuously; work and rest must alternate. Such rules, unsupported by science though they are, were at the time proclaimed with immense conviction. Mothers received dire warnings that failure to observe these principles would result in a new portion of milk reaching the baby's gut before the previous portion had been fully digested, a situation that could have catastrophic consequences. Quite apart from this, insistence on order and regularity was a means of instilling discipline into the child:

> … In many instances the consequences are considerably more serious; the digestive process will be entirely deranged and serious disorders of the digestive system may well ensue…. (Meyer, 1899).

...Obedience in infancy is the foundation of all later powers of self-control; yet it is the one thing the young mother nowadays is most inclined to neglect... (Truby King, 1908).

The careless, shiftless and ignorant mother, whose child is....given the breast whenever he cries for it, is injuring both the health and character of her child....he is acquiring the slipshod ways of his parents, and without discipline in self-control, he grows up self-willed and unable to adapt himself to our customs, and is neither physically nor morally a credit to the race... (Fairbairn, 1914, as quoted by Liddiard, 1923).

In particular, traditional breastfeeding practices and beliefs were condemned as outdated:

...if one sought to know how often a small infant should be put to the breast, the true answer would all too often be "as often as you can manage" or "whenever it cries" or "when it is restless." Such practices are antiquated and thoroughly reprehensible... (Meyer, 1899).

During that century of misunderstanding, one piece of disastrous advice was followed by another in the North as well as in the South. The advice was conveyed through the books for parents and are thus available to us today, as frightening examples. Our examples are naturally mainly from the North:

... there are limits to the quantities of milk a baby can drink, and one must not be tempted to provide a feed merely because it is restless or demanding; the immature child is unable to discern the difference between a real need for food and a mere liking for taking the breast... (Monrad, 1952).

... The infant shall have its meals at fixed intervals, which must not be excessively short.... (Meyer, 1899).

...The more strictly one adheres to the feeding timetable, the more tranquil and healthy the child will be... (Brinchmann, 1929, 1943).

... As soon as the flow of milk has been established, one must accustom the child to fixed and regular feeding hours. Most infants born at term and healthy breast-fed babies can be satisfied from the time of birth onwards by five feeds daily... (Monrad, 1952).

... Once the doctor has explained the timetable for feeding, set the times for feeds, and determined how much the infant needs, you must adhere strictly to these rules, neither providing intermediate feeds nor deviating from the set hours. It is particularly necessary to ensure a complete pause in the feeding program at night. Although babies may during the first few days of life protest this regularity by crying, they very soon adjust to it.... (Dahl, 1964).

If these, then, were to be the rules and the clock was to determine the pattern of feeding, how was a mother to persuade her baby to fall into line? Dr. Meyer was firm on the matter– she would need to tackle it with strictness and determination: "One must realize and respect from the first moment the need to follow the clock when deciding the moments at which the infant shall be put to the breast."

Should the fact that the infant was crying be occasioned by an irritating nappy or a troublesome flea, the mother had the right to attend to the matter, "but she must resist firmly any urge merely to take the baby up in her arms and walk around with it. ..."

As Meyer sees it, the cunning little infant would otherwise "soon learn that it could achieve this merely by screaming, and from then onwards, it will no longer be content to lie still." The mother is urged to steel herself against such things, turning a deaf ear to the baby's signals. He realized full well that many a mother would find it painful to suppress her natural instincts to this extent: "... no one likes to hear a small child cry and for the mother it may almost be heartbreaking. For that very reason she should be firmly convinced that, even though it may seem that she is depriving her child, she is in fact enriching it; she needs to know that she is making here a small sacrifice for the sake of achieving a greater good...."

In Meyer's view, this is the way to teach a baby to wake and take food during the day according to the clock and to sleep at night. Today we might interpret it differently; the unfortunate infant simply surrenders, abandoning any attempt to make known its needs and ensure that they are met. But Meyer knows no mercy.

Distrust of Breastmilk - And the Search for a More Dependable Alternative

Towards the end of the 1800's, researchers at Harvard University in the USA came to the conclusion, based on their studies, that there could be considerable variations in the composition of breastmilk. They attributed these variations to the fact that human milk production could supposedly be influenced by many factors, though they admitted that the nature of these factors was unknown. This could mean, as they put it, that many women would prove incapable of producing milk of sufficient quality to meet their children's needs. This supposedly scientific conclusion came to seed a widespread lack of trust in the ability of modern women to breastfeed their children adequately.

It is remarkable how widely and rapidly this distrust took hold. It represented, after all, a drastic change of view on a matter in which women had functioned, almost always successfully, for millions of years. No one, it seemed, stopped to consider the fact that it was the child which was regulating the breast's milk production, with its appetite and its enthusiasm for the nipple.

Pediatricians - And Producers - Reap the Benefit

By the time that distrust of breastmilk arose, pediatrics had come to the fore as a new medical speciality. In the United States, these developments were virtually simultaneous and the new profession had a need to announce its arrival and attract clients. In that connection, it was not inconvenient that new problems with breastfeeding appeared to have been identified and might call for a specialized approach.

At that time, too, marketing was developing as a major influence on society, and the producers both of tonics and of infant foods based on cereals and on dairy milk were quick to promote them to mothers. Dependent as the latter were on the information and advice provided on the label of these new products, they were likely to follow it in good faith. The results commonly fell short of the producer's promises, and the widespread use of these products was reflected in faulty nutrition and in health problems among the children for which they were destined.

THE PERCENTAGE METHOD: AN ACADEMIC APPROACH

In the hope of countering the problems arising with commercially inspired products, a group of researchers at Harvard University towards the end of the 19th century sought to develop a systematic approach to breastmilk substitution. In all seriousness, they developed a wide range of "formulas" for infant feeding, all based essentially on cow's milk, but each differing somewhat in its percentage composition from the others (Figure 13.3). The "percentage method" that they employed was based on the belief that even fractional variations in the composition of milk could have consequences for a child's growth and well-being. Having determined an individual baby's nutritional needs (using a method that was claimed to be scientific, but was in fact highly obscure) the pediatrician would prescribe the most appropriate formula, with ingredients precisely chosen to meet those needs. Such an individualized product might, for example, be a mixture of cream, cow's milk, calcium salts, barley water, malt soup, whey (from dairy milk), condensed milk, olive oil, boiled water, and lactose. It was hardly possible to prepare such a mixture in an ordinary domestic kitchen. To keep the control, special milk laboratories were established in the principal American cities from which all the many formulas could be supplied. They were to be made available, however, only with a prescription written by a pediatrician – a provision negotiated by the American Medical Association, ever watchful of its members' interests (Apple, 1987).

Many parties had reason to be content with this arrangement: the pediatricians developed a wider circle of patients, the laboratories earned well on their products, the dairy industry watched its sales expand, and mothers believed that they were acting in the best interests of their offspring. The only individuals who were perhaps less content were the infants for whom the formula was intended. They often became sick and failed to thrive, but no one, after all, was asking their opinion on the matter.

SCIENTIFIC THINKING AND THE SPIRIT OF THE AGE

A Time for Mutual Congratulation

The medical profession as a whole was happy to welcome what was perceived to be a new and modern approach to infant feeding, backed by the percentage method and the establishment of a chain of milk laboratories. Its arrival was as an American physician of the day put it:

...not only a great scientific achievement in itself, but also the means of changing the whole trend of professional thought upon the subject and of establishing this science of infant feeding upon an exact and rational basis (Westcott, 1900).

It was a time when anything smacking of exact natural science was greeted with unbounded enthusiasm. In many areas, applied research had indeed resulted in miraculous advances, benefiting many and enhancing daily life in a manner that few would have believed possible. Pasteur had discovered how pathological bacteria could be identified and combated. Semmelweis had shown how a simple measure, such as hand washing, could prevent life-threatening infections among women giving birth. In the course of only a few decades, the incandescent lamp, the steam locomotive,

A New Method of Calculating Milk Percentages. L. Emmett Holt, New York.

Formula obtained from milk containing different percentages of fat.

		A 7 % Milk	B 6 %	C 5 %	D 4 %	E 3 %	F 2 %	G 1 %	Per cent.	Per cent.
I	1 ounce in 20 has Fat.	0.35	0.30	0.25	0.20	0.15	0.10	0.05	with Protein 0.175	Sugar 0.225
II	2 ounces in 20 has Fat.	0.70	0.60	0.50	0.40	0.30	0.20	0.10	with Protein 0.35	Sugar 0.45
III	3 ounces in 20 has Fat.	1.05	0.90	0.75	0.60	0.45	0.30	0.15	with Protein 0.50	Sugar 0.65
IV	4 ounces in 20 has Fat.	1.40	1.20	1.00	0.80	0.60	0.40	0.20	with Protein 0.70	Sugar 0.90
V	5 ounces in 20 has Fat.	1.75	1.50	1.25	1.00	0.75	0.50	0.25	with Protein 0.85	Sugar 1.30
VI	6 ounces in 20 has Fat.	2.10	1.80	1.50	1.20	0.90	0.60	0.30	with Protein 1.05	Sugar 1.35
VII	7 ounces in 20 has Fat.	2.45	2.10	1.75	1.40	1.05	0.70	0.35	with Protein 1.20	Sugar 1.55
VIII	8 ounces in 20 has Fat.	2.80	2.40	2.00	1.60	1.20	0.80	0.40	with Protein 1.40	Sugar 1.80
IX	9 ounces in 20 has Fat.	3.05	2.70	2.25	1.80	1.35	0.90	0.45	with Protein 1.60	Sugar 2.00
X	10 ounces in 20 has Fat.	3.50	3.00	2.50	2.00	1.50	1.00	0.50	with Protein 1.75	Sugar 2.25
XI	11 ounces in 20 has Fat.	3.80	3.30	2.75	2.20	1.65	1.10	0.55	with Protein 1.90	Sugar 2.45
XII	12 ounces in 20 has Fat.		3.60	3.00	2.40	1.80	1.20	0.60	with Protein 2.10	Sugar 2.70
XIII	13 ounces in 20 has Fat.		3.90	3.25	2.60	1.95	1.30	0.65	with Protein 2.25	Sugar 2.90
XIV	14 ounces in 20 has Fat.			3.50	2.80	2.10	1.40	0.70	with Protein 2.40	Sugar 3.15
XV	15 ounces in 20 has Fat.				3.00	2.25	1.50	0.75	with Protein 2.60	Sugar 3.35

From 4 per cent. milk..............From 5 per cent. milk

To obtain 7 per cent. milk use upper 16 oz..............upper 20 oz.
To obtain 6 per cent. milk use upper 20 oz..............upper 24 oz.
To obtain 5 per cent. milk use upper 24 oz..............all
To obtain 4 per cent. milk use all..............................remainder after skimming off 2 oz.
To obtain 3 per cent. milk use remainder after skimming off 2 oz..remainder after skimming off 3 oz.
To obtain 2 per cent. milk use remainder after skimming off 4 oz..remainder after skimming off 5 oz.
To obtain 1 per cent. milk use remainder after skimming off 8 oz..remainder after skimming off 8 oz.

With Formulas I to V, enough sugar should be added to raise the amount to 5 per cent.
With Formulas VI to XV, enough sugar should be added to raise the amount to 6 per cent.

One ounce milk sugar by weight in 20-oz. mixture adds 5 per cent.
One ounce milk sugar by volume in 20-oz. mixture adds about 3 per cent.
One even tablespoonful in 20 oz. mixture adds 1.75 per cent.

1 oz. 7 per cent. milk...	27.5
1 oz. 6 per cent. milk...	25.0
1 oz. 5 per cent. milk...	22.5
1 oz. 4 per cent. milk...	20.0
1 oz. 3 per cent. milk...	17.5
1 oz. 2 per cent. milk...	15.0
1 oz. 1 per cent. milk...	12.5
1 oz. fat-free...	10.0
1 oz. whey..	10.0
1 oz. milk sugar by weight......................................	116.0
1 oz. milk sugar by volume......................................	72.0
1 even tablespoonful of milk sugar..............................	44.0
1 oz. barley flour by weight....................................	100.0
1 oz. barley water (1 tablespoonful to a pint)..................	2.0
1 oz. malt soup extract...	80.0
1 oz. condensed milk..	132.0
1 oz. olive oil by volume.......................................	245.0

Figure 13.3. *Ingredients of various infant formulas designed according to the percentage method.*

Source: Holt, L.E. (1911). A new method of calculating milk percentages. American Journal Of Obstetrics and Diseases of Women and Children, 64, 556.

and the sewing machine had appeared. Horses were giving way to the new automobiles, which with their rubber tires were immeasurably more comfortable than the wooden-wheeled wagons of the past. . .

Surely, the percentage method represented just another such step forward on the road to a better world (Rotch, 1890). Or perhaps not?

BOTTLE-FEEDING AND ITS PROBLEMS - EVEN IN AMERICA

A View from the Clinic

Meanwhile, an American investigator, Dr. H.J. Gerstenberger, was struggling to create a suitable mixture of fats to incorporate in something he proposed to call Synthetic Milk Adapted, S.M.A., a brand which indeed subsequently reached the market and still exists today. Gerstenberger was a pediatrician with long and broad experience in his profession. In one of his scientific papers, he mentioned, almost in passing, the fact that the use of S.M.A. proved much less satisfactory when his product was used "in institutions and among the poor or middle classes, especially in instances where the child is less than a month old."

He continued:

One can usually pick out from a group of dispensary patients the breast- fed from the bottle-fed, and in an institution, this can be done practically without an exception. There are, however, some infants who do well under the worst conditions and on most any kind of food; but they are exceptionally resistant little human beings and by no means speak for the innocuousness of the food that they have received or the environment in which they live (Gerstenberger & Ruh, 1919).

Innovations for Infants

The arrival of *rubber*, and of the means of processing it into usable forms, was to have important consequences in the field of infant feeding as elsewhere. It provided a solution to the problem of bringing milk directly into the baby's mouth. An infant is very capable, with the help of its reflexes, of mastering the complex process of taking the milk as it spouts forth from the mother's nipple and sending it on its way, but that same infant is not ideally designed to drink from the necks of bottles. Many attempts had been made to solve the problem, even including the use of the animal nipples, taken from slaughtered cows or goats and mounted onto the neck of a bottle. Some tried inserting a rag into the neck of a bottle, so the milk could be sucked out slowly. In institutions where there were many children to feed, it was not unknown to bring a goat, donkey, or other lactating donor animal into the house and lay one baby at a time up against the udder to feed as if it were just another kid or calf.

Teats (Rubber Nipples) - Popular from the Start

The first rubber teats came onto the market in 1856 and went a long way towards solving the problem of bringing milk to the baby. The original teats were stiff, evil smelling, and equally evil tasting. Once flexible latex rubber teats became available, which was only the case after 1900, they became immensely popular since babies, who delight in sucking, immediately applied their sucking reflex to the task of drinking milk. It is unfortunately true that this process of feeding by suction is entirely different from that of milking the mother's breast, which involves quite a different mode of use of the mouth's musculature. Many babies never become accustomed to feeding in these two different ways, and are likely to abandon the complexities of breastfeeding in favor of the simple process of sucking on a rubber teat.

WOMEN'S HEALTH: GOOD AND NOW BETTER THAN EVER

With the exception of overworked mothers in factories, the health of most mothers during the period from 1870 to 1950 was, as a rule, no worse than it had been in previous generations. In that respect, there was no reason to believe that they would be less physically capable of breastfeeding than their predecessors. On the contrary, in various respects, women now had opportunities to attain better health than ever before. The arrival of effective contraception rendered it possible for the average woman to avoid unwanted pregnancy, and as the 20th century progressed, the methods available became increasingly acceptable and within reach of all. In the western world, women bore fewer children than had earlier been the case; the burden of an excessively large family was essentially a thing of the past. In many countries, women were living longer than their male contemporaries. In areas where nutrition had been poor, good food became accessible to all. And as the professional and health services increasingly succeeded in identifying the causes of disease and countering them with improved hygiene, better living conditions, new vaccines, and antibiotics, infectious illness was, to an important extent, deprived of its potential to harm and kill.

There was no rational reason, in terms of physical health or social conditions, for the sudden demand for artificial replacements for breastmilk, a demand that nevertheless arose as society passed from the 19th century into the 20th century. Those women whose daily duties in the factory prevented them from full breastfeeding did have a need for substitutes, but they were often unable to afford those that were marketed; and the substitutes were often of dubious quality.

Unscientific Science

In that period of change, extending as it did over two generations from the 1870's to the 1930's, scientists still groped largely in the dark when they sought to understand the similarities or differences between breastmilk that was the natural diet of human babies and dairy milk that was natural only for calves.

The percentage method soon proved to be both impractical and ineffective. It had from the start been based on highly dubious science and guesswork as to a baby's nutritional needs, and the results of its introduction did not meet the expectations that had been voiced. The system created around it was cumbersome to operate and maintain, falling well short of the quality control standards that one would apply today. Some of the milk laboratories failed to provide milk formulas that conformed to the physician's instructions.

In 1932, physicians came to agree that where there was a need to provide supplementation, a simple mixture of dairy milk, water, and sugar, which had often been used successfully (but which perhaps appeared too simple to meet the desire for sophisticated solutions), was as acceptable as anything else. For the next 40 years, such simple mixtures as these played a growing role in infant feeding. There was apparently no need for anything more complicated.

Chapter 14.
THE WORLD'S LARGEST HUMAN EXPERIMENT

In the 1930s, by which time artificial infant feeding was firmly taking root, at least in industrialized countries, it was deemed necessary to develop exact (and if possible standardized) nutrition plans for babies. By now, the overall composition of cow's milk was reasonably well known since it was everywhere on the market and the customer wanted information about it. The farmers and the dairies were also supposed to supply a standardized product.

HANDY RULES?

Given these facts, physicians considered themselves sufficiently well qualified to estimate, at least approximately, how much cow's milk a baby would require daily, taking into account their own experience and what was known about the amount of breastmilk that should normally be ingested daily. The estimated total volume of milk to be given each day was then divided into portions to be administered at fixed intervals, generally allowing three or four hours between feeds during the day and a longer break during the night.

The arguments advanced for avoiding nighttime feeding sessions were not particularly well founded. They comprised little more than a belief that consuming food at night was immoral and unnecessary. An adult eating at night would merely put on weight, and since adults did not need a meal during the night, so ran the argument, neither did infants. Night is the time for sleeping!

It was further decreed that each feed should normally be allowed to last twenty minutes. And once the physicians had proceeded this far in drawing up rules and schedules for artificial feeding, they unhesitatingly set about applying them to breastfeeding as well. As we have seen earlier, this was hardly a new notion; the idea that babies needed to be fed at regular intervals had been advanced as early as 1792.

It would seem that the staff of obstetric units and health centers accepted these ordinances unquestioningly as being both logical and convenient. It obviously simplified things if one could tell mothers that they should follow a standard feeding timetable, irrespective of whether they were giving the breast or the bottle, human milk or cow's milk. The inevitable result was that mothers, who were by nature continuous breastfeeders, found themselves and their offspring subjected to a feeding plan that allowed a baby to breastfeed only four to six times a day, instead of feeding continuously, hence departing from the procedure for which the breasts had been designed. The four to six times a day feeding pattern soon proved too little for many a breast. Given the long intervals, the breast received too little stimulation; the pituitary gland, therefore, produced too little oxytocin and prolactin for the mother to maintain her milk production at a sufficient level to meet her baby's needs. Ever more mothers were experiencing difficulties in producing sufficient milk for their offspring. But when they presented themselves to their health workers with this problem, the latter could only advise them to turn to the bottle and provide supplementary feeding that way. They might also contrive to suggest saving milk by skipping a breastfeed now and then, so the baby would, at least during the next session at the breast, be able to have a really good and adequate feed. The consequences can all too easily be imagined.

Science Was Still in the Dark

Around 1900, knowledge regarding cow's milk and what one could and could not do with it was still emerging. Scientists and the producers of breastmilk substitutes were still groping in the dark as to how dairy milk might need to be modified to render it safe and suitable for the feeding of tiny humans rather than hungry calves. Existing knowledge at the time was deficient regarding the composition of both human and cow's milk and the manner in which the composition of breastmilk might (and indeed did) change during the course of a feeding session.

In 1902, Professor Axel Johannessen, a well-known pediatrician, wrote in his book for parents, called *Parents and Children…A Book on Domestic Duties,* that "…Science has not yet contrived to determine the relationship between the nutritive properties of milk and the mother's general state of health, and one is not uncommonly astonished to observe how a child

HERE IS ONE EXAMPLE OF THE SORT OF ADVICE WITH WHICH A BREASTFEEDING MOTHER IN THE 1940S MIGHT FIND HERSELF FACED:

Amount of Breast Milk: Some Simple Rules for Mother to Follow (Sundal, 1939, p 73)

First quarter (months 1-3): one sixth of the child's net body weight

Second quarter (months 3-6): one seventh of the child's net body weight

Third quarter (months 6-9): one eighth of the child's net bodyweight

What is one to make of such advice? One is tempted to say that rules like this were not likely to be comprehensible, except perhaps to a mother well versed in mathematics, who recalled which were the numerator and denominator, respectively, of a fraction, and who understood how to use them, as well as being intuitively aware of when months 3-6 began and ended. Quite apart from this, the rules only made sense in practice if one knew the baby's net body weight. We recall very well the scales, white enameled contraptions, which one could see in many a home in the 1940s and 1950s, a sure sign that there was a baby in the vicinity. The rules quoted above were to be found in the manual of infant feeding that her father bought for her mother when Elisabet came into the world in 1940 and was duly weighed (Figure 14.1).

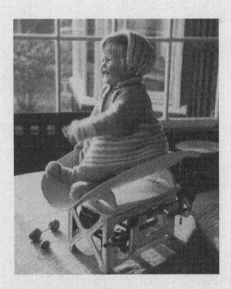

Figure 14.1. *Elisabet on the scales*

Source: Photo provided by author. Used with permission.

may thrive despite the fact that its mother is weak and apparently in poor condition…" (Johannessen, 1902, p. 36)

There was no easy means of determining how a baby might best be reared on dairy milk. The composition of human milk was destined to remain largely obscure for researchers until 1954 (Hytten, 1954). Not surprisingly, the normal variations in the composition of breastmilk that occurred, not merely over time, but also in the course of a single feeding session, led to discrepancies in the analytical findings obtained with different samples. Nor was it realized that babies, as a matter of course, adapt to such variations by taking more or less milk, as dictated by their stomach and their appetite (Mitoulas et al., 2002).

Two Faulty Conclusions with Fatal Consequences

The fact was that, at the time, the baby was regarded as no more than the passive recipient of its mother's milk, and when the results of analyses differed from one study to another, it was concluded this must be due to differences in the composition of the milk produced by individual mothers. That, in turn, could be due, it was argued, *either* to the fact that their children had very different needs *or* to the fact that the milk of one mother differed from that of another, because some women were simply not able to produce sufficiently high quality milk.

Both conclusions were, in fact, wrong. The latter notion indeed reduced some mothers to despair and hardly cheered the health workers caring for them. People began to doubt seriously whether modern women were really capable of sound breastfeeding, or whether human milk was adequate to satisfy a baby's needs. These unfounded fears prepared the ground for the disastrous swing to artificial feeding that was due to follow.

Cause and Effect - But Which Was Which?

So it was that things began to go wrong and no one understood why. Mothers found that, despite a deep desire on their part to breastfeed, the milk trickled only reluctantly from their breasts. The advice obtained from the professionals hardly helped matters. The baby that found a rubber dummy (pacifier) thrust into its mouth at regular intervals – so very different from mother's nipple – became confused. Taking milk from the bottle rather than the breast required that the muscles around the mouth had to be used in a different way (Chapter 1). It was a small wonder that many a baby soon chose the path of least resistance and abandoned the breast in favor of the bottle, which merely needed to be sucked to extract the milk it contained.

This, in turn, meant that in many cases the generous flow of milk that a mother had experienced in the maternity ward progressively dried up, until no more than a trickle remained. Those who were called upon to provide an explanation shook their heads in puzzlement and expressed the view that the causes were unknown, but probably complex.

1967: WHY DO "MODERN" MOTHERS NO LONGER BREASTFEED?

In 1967, a writer in a WHO Monograph devoted to Infant Nutrition in the Tropics and Subtropics valiantly set out to "explain" what had gone so drastically wrong with breastfeeding in industrialized countries.

His thoughts on the matter were typical of those expressed by others who found themselves puzzled by the mystery of the disappearing milk. He made five points:

1. One must realize that many more mothers were now employed outside the home than had been the case in earlier times.

2. In modern society, women were embarrassed to breastfeed their babies in full view of others; breastfeeding had, therefore, become an obstacle to social contact.

3. Many effective, relatively cheap, and heavily promoted breastmilk substitutes were now available, designed specifically for babies.

4. With emancipation, women had gained access to the many other activities and entertainments which they could enjoy in modern society.

5. Failure of breastfeeding had quite simply become a general trend…

Even with such reasoning, the basic cause of the decline in successful breastfeeding remained entirely unexplained. It was striking that an English investigator who had examined 1100 cases of breastfeeding failure in Liverpool found that in 40% of cases there was simply no explanation as to why a mother had not managed to breastfeed her baby. All the same, he managed to define three categories of possible "causes" which in his view were at least credible:

1. *Psychological causes,* such as lack of enthusiasm on the part of the mother, her fear of failure, or other "emotional tensions sufficient to derange the vital let-down reflex."

2. *Insufficient emptying of the breast.*

3. *Insufficient stimulation of the nipple by the infant's feeding motions,* leading to reduced production of the milk stimulating hormone prolactin.

With the hindsight of 60 years, we can at least give the third of his arguments a nod of approbation; here he was indeed on the right track (Figure 14.2).

Others remained confused, misinformed, or simply uninterested in the fact that across the world something had gone wrong with breastfeeding. There were those who blamed the mothers who supposedly had lost interest in the practice, while others simply shrugged their shoulders and turned their attention to making supposedly better breastmilk substitutes. Surely, if one tried hard enough, it would be possible to find out precisely what made breastmilk so special, and then make a perfect copy of it? Hospitals, for their part, were very interested in developing correct routines for infant feeding–and having done that for bottle-feeding with cow's milk, they unthinkingly applied the same procedures to breastfeeding mothers. Babies and mothers were separated, and the number of breastfeeding sessions was reduced. They did what they believed was best – and the results were appalling. And, all the time, the use of the feeding bottle filled with cow's milk went on growing…

THE WORLD'S LARGEST HUMAN EXPERIMENT …ON BABIES

The fact that bottle-feeding was perhaps not in reality as simple as it was put up to be emerges from various papers published in the pediatric journals of the time, which report one attempt after another to modify dairy milk for the purpose (Gerstenberger & Ruh, 1919). Somewhere in the shadowy background to such reports one discerns the unfortunate mother who can do so little to help her sick infant since her own milk has been analyzed and found wanting.

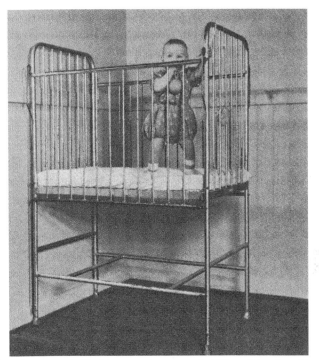

Figure 14.2. *Some remarkable things were done to small children. Taken from Monrad, S., Moderens bog" (The book of the mother) Gyldendal 1952, page 57.*

In the meantime, it had become more than obvious that in industrialized countries, a remarkably large market for infant formula had come into being. The growth of that market brought with it what soon amounted to, and later was described as "the largest nutrition experiment ever carried out on human beings"(Hendrickse, 1976). It was an experiment without a starting hypothesis, uncontrolled, and without any well defined goals or justification. Its only starting point was the theory that when feeding human babies, one could perfectly well get away with the use of bottles, filled with the milk that was species-specific for four-legged ruminants.

To put it simply, there were several reasons why this vast experiment came about. Breastfeeding seemed to have run into problems. No one understood why, but it was tempting to look around for an alternative. In an increasingly technologically oriented society, such an alternative seemed to be available in the form of infant formula. What is more, there was money to be earned by selling these substitutes for mothers' milk, sufficient reason for the commercially minded to engage in it.

So it was that the experiment began: nobody, it seems, had the slightest notion as to what the results of this experiment might be – and nobody seemed particularly interested in even considering the point.

AND THE TIME SEEMED RIPE FOR IT...

Various parallel developments at about the same time almost seemed designed to foster the spread of bottle-feeding. One of the first may have been the development of the rubber teat, while another was perhaps the work of Pasteur who discovered how any infective organisms that might be present in cow's milk could be eliminated by pasteurizing it at a sufficiently high temperature. Yet another factor seems to have been the invention in 1895 of the milking machine, adapted to the cow's particular anatomy, which virtually eliminated the role of the milkmaid, and rendered it possible and profitable to operate large-scale dairies. Cow's milk found its place on the menu, not merely as a food or an ingredient in cooking, but as an essential element in maintaining public health. It soon became marketed not so much as a mere commodity, but as a health food.

AMERICA LEADS THE WAY

In the United States, the proportion of babies fed at their mother's breast fell more rapidly than anywhere else. As late as 1911, 58% of American women had breastfed their babies for at least 12 months, i.e., more than half of all children were breastfed for at least a year. Fifty years later, in 1961, a mere 28% of women were found to be breastfeeding their babies at the end of the first week of life, which is to say that two thirds of mothers made no attempt even at the outset to feed their offspring at the breast (Woodbury, 1925; Meyer, 1968). America was, of course, the country which had adopted industrial development most eagerly, which had gone on to modernize its industries with unequalled success, and which prided itself on providing its people with everything they could wish for in terms of material benefits, including good health. That was very much the case with women of the middle classes, who were the first to abandon breastfeeding.

Perhaps the Bottle Was Better?

Why was it that in the USA the womanly art of breastfeeding dried up first and in the course of only a few decades? For that is what happened. In the ecstatic rush to the bottle, there were even some individuals to be found proclaiming that cow's milk actually presented advantages over mankind's own breastmilk. In addition, feeding from a bottle seemed to offer practical advantages: the mother was less tied to her baby, and the health workers around her with responsibility for infant feeding could, with their very own eyes and measuring appliances, determine precisely how much milk a baby had ingested.

The combined influence of sales pressure by the burgeoning baby food industry and the enthusiasm expressed by doctors for what was perceived as a scientific approach to infant feeding was to prove catastrophic for breastfeeding – a trend that emerged first in the United States, but was soon disseminated across much of the world. In the course of the 1920s, the frequency of breastfeeding was found to be falling to a worrying degree in much of Europe as well.

The Race to Develop Unnecessary Products

Meanwhile, the industry had begun to search assiduously for ways in which it might create temptingly saleable variants on the theme of infant formula. The very first product specifically designed for infant feeding was patented as early as 1867 by the German chemist Herr Prof. Justus von Liebig. In all modesty, he called his product "The perfect infant food." Whether such a description would have been acceptable to the food control authorities of the 21st century seems at least doubtful, for this so-called perfect food was, in fact, a mixture of white flour, cow's milk, malt extract, and baking powder. Whatever its merits or lack of them, the perfect food was an instant success in the market. Ambitious researchers and businessmen like Liebig and Nestlé smelled the sweet smell of a commercial breakthrough, and they lost no time in pressing ahead. The merchant and pharmacist Henri Nestlé was based in Switzerland, one of the many European countries where there was a long tradition of dairy farming. He had succeeded in 1863 in producing the first tinned condensed milk, an innovation that essentially solved the problem of storing milk in edible condition over long periods and laid the basis for industrial involvement in the processing and sale of dairy products. Soon thereafter, Nestlé developed his own variant on the original baby food theme in the form of "Nestlé's Milk Food," and from the 1870's to our own time, the approach has meant good business for Nestle and his successors. The first products to reach the market were not, when judged by later standards, particularly suited to the feeding of young infants, but thousands of eager parents flocked to the shops, impatient to pay whatever was demanded, so they might provide their offspring with the best and most scientific food that money could provide (Anderson, Chinn, & Fisher, 1982). Other industrialists followed in the wake of Liebig and Nestlé. As early as 1883, there were no less than 27 patented baby food products on the British market alone. What was the basis of such products? Many were based on various types of flour; in England, for example, we find among the most typical products on sale:

- Boaden's (rye and wheat flour)

- Prince of Wales Food (potato flour)

- Plumbe's (pea, bean, and potato flour)

In later years, malted products, such as Mellin's Food and Horlicks, gained in popularity.

According to the book by Leopold Meyer, Nestlé's farine lactée (lactified meal) and various unspecified brands of "Special Baby Meal" were popular in Denmark. Around 1900, gruel was being widely used throughout Scandinavia. It was based on sago, semolina, or other coarse flours that had been boiled in a mixture of milk and water for 45 minutes, and then pressed through a sieve.

What was not always made clear, either to parents or to doctors, was that products such as these were primarily intended for use in children older than six months. Nor was it realized at the time that these products were deficient in various vitamins and minerals; the concept of "vitamins" was not advanced until 1924.

Neither the baby foods based primarily on milk nor those in which milk was mixed with cereals were free of problems. Often they were wrongly used, either given too early in life or used in illnesses that had been neither thought through nor properly diagnosed. It is hardly surprising that they were responsible for ill health, and even death, among young children (Wickes, 1953).

All in all, the situation that had been created in the baby food market by the time the First World War ended was one of sheer anarchy, with many initiatives reflecting ignorance, thoughtlessness, or mere guesswork. Another 20 years were to pass before researchers began to gain some insight into the problem of adapting cow's milk for feeding human babies. It was not until the late 1920s that physicians succeeded in formulating products based on cow's milk (modified dairy milk mixtures) which were reasonably well tolerated by infants. Even though various individual workers had found that it was sufficient for the purpose of feeding babies to add water and sugar to dairy milk, their ideas were generally brushed aside by others who had devised more exotic (and therefore more saleable) solutions. In the end, however, the simpler approach won the day. When there was a genuine reason to provide artificial feeding in early life, all that was needed was to dilute dairy milk with water to reduce the protein content, and then to add sugar to provide sufficient energy.

The Target Group

The mothers most in need of breastmilk substitutes were unfortunately those who could least afford them. Many of the mothers working in the shadow of the industrial revolution ended up by improvising their babies' meals as best they could; turning to rusks (dry biscuits) and pre-chewed food, and perhaps even administering a drop of brandy when the screams from the cot became too insistent.

Oddly, economic disasters sometimes led to a return to more natural practices. In a footnote in his book "Das Kapital," Karl Marx wrote that when the American Civil War led to the closure of the spinning mills in England because of the collapse of raw cotton supplies, one positive consequence was that the unemployed spinning workers at last found time to breastfeed their children, even though they themselves had precious little to eat (Marx, 1954, p. 372).

Dr. Julius Sedgwick was a breastfeeding enthusiast who provided inspiration to many, and numerous others flocked to work with him for little or no monetary reward. But in general, there were too few individuals like him, seeking to learn about successful breastfeeding instead of improving on the food originally intended for calves. Today we realize how thankful we can be that people like Dr. Sedgwick ensured the maintenance of the tradition through a difficult period.

THE HEALTH SERVICES - A THREAT TO BREASTFEEDING?

Unhappily, many professional health workers had become the most convinced advocates of what was seen as the new and progressive means of feeding infants with the help of the bottle. With unbridled enthusiasm, they proclaimed the message. Many of them remained convinced that

FIGHTING THE GOOD FIGHT - IN THE USA

In 1920, an American medical journal published a paper on the "principles of hand milking." It is of interest for several reasons. The author was a pediatrician, Dr. Julius Sedgwick (1921), and it was based on a lecture he had delivered to the American Pediatrics Association. In his own clinic for newborns in the city of Minneapolis, he led an active breastfeeding support program, and he opened his lecture with the remark that over the years, many in his audience must have heard him expressing his views on the subject. At that time, breastfeeding was still relatively common in the USA, though the decline had clearly set in. Dr. Sedgwick had built up a research program in his clinic with the intention of determining whether the decline was due to the fact that mothers were no longer capable of breastfeeding. He had a suspicion that the fault might lie in a lack of knowledge and failure to understand the technique needed to establish and maintain milk production. The further his work proceeded, the more unlikely it seemed to him that there were mothers who were truly incapable of producing milk. Sedgwick realized that the infant's desire for milk – and its insistence that the breast provide it – was by far the most important factor in maintaining the milk supply. He had what we would today regard as a thoroughly modern understanding of the physiology of breastfeeding, and he had a staff of well-trained consultants advising mothers. Over a period of a year, he followed the course of breastfeeding in every one of the 1000 new mothers passing through the clinic during that time. At the moment of their discharge from his clinic, every single one of these 1000 women had milk in her breasts. Sedgwick's program extended to every child born in the city of Minneapolis, including premature infants, which he believed had a very clear need for breastmilk, a view warmly shared by today's pediatricians. Since electric breast pumps were not available at that time, hand milking was needed. He described how the mothers of premature babies continued with hand milking over a period of several months. After that, as soon as each baby had become stronger and better able to use the muscles around the mouth, it would be put to the breast. Inverted nipples did not appear to stand in the way. Nearly 3000 infants studied by the clinic were followed up until the age of nine months. Three months after delivery, 93% of the children were still being breastfed, after six months 84%, and at the age of nine months, no less than 72%.

modern mothers were, whatever they were told to do, incapable of breastfeeding or obstinately unwilling to try it. Many physicians regarded with contempt the primitive, apparently arbitrary, and irregular practice of feeding babies at the breast. The bottle, ever ready to provide its premeasured and accurate contents at dependable intervals, was in their minds clearly preferable. According to their theories, it rendered better control possible and enabled one to apply pure scientific principles to infant feeding, very different from the situation in which a mother, with unbuttoned dress and exposed breast, sat messing around, unmethodically and imprecisely feeding the old-fashioned way.

GLOBAL CAMPAIGNS: DOWN WITH THE BREAST, UP WITH THE BOTTLE

An English-language report issued in 1917 by the authorities of the then British colonial administration of the Caribbean Islands complained that "most of the children suffer from over-nursing, their mothers keep them at it for 16 to 18 months; during the last seven or eight months, the children draw an abundant supply of a highly un-nutritious fluid from the breast" (Colonial Medical Report, 1917). During the 1920's, British health workers geared up for a determined effort to teach mothers in colonies across the world to adopt correct artificial feeding. In 1925, the Colonial Administration in Malaysia was able to recall, with evident satisfaction, that as recently as 1922 "some mothers had not even seen a clock and those who had could not understand what it had to do with the feeding of an infant ... Now, the majority of mothers understand the clock and feed their children regularly by it, and the boat-shaped bottle is accepted in most homes" (King & Ashworth, 1987, p. 1315).

THE WHO STUDY THAT WOULD HAVE SHOCKED MANY... HAD IT ONLY BECOME KNOWN

Between 1975 and 1978, the World Health Organization carried out a thorough large-scale study of the situation of breastfeeding in nine countries. A finding common to all of them was that the more often mothers had been in contact with the health system the less likely they were to breastfeed (Figure 14.3). Unfortunately, WHO did not see fit to publicize this unwelcome finding, and the final report on the study only referred to it in the vaguest possible terms (WHO, 1981 p.149).

Ten years later (1984-1988), other investigators found precisely the same thing when, in a similar study, they looked at breastfeeding practices in nine Latin American countries (Pérez-Escamilla, 1993). The higher the percentage of deliveries conducted under the supervision of health workers, the shorter the period of breastfeeding.

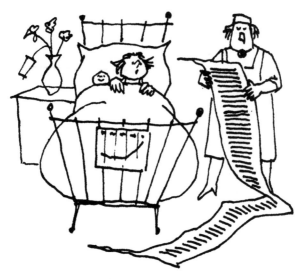

Figure 14.3. *The more contact with the health system, the less breastfeeding.*

Source: Cartoon by Ellen Wilhelmsen. Used with permission.

Most people have a healthy respect for health professionals and tend to listen to their advice. Not only do they follow their instructions, they also follow their example. Health workers, for their part, are not always aware of the influence they have on the public's behavior and the extent to which they are emulated. On occasion, they may even advise their patients on matters on which they themselves are not necessarily well trained, for example, good practice in breastfeeding.

It is not at all unusual to see a relatively well-paid health worker in a developing country, having spent her working day with young mothers (and in contact with a climate favoring breastfeeding), returning home to her own bottle-fed middle class baby. There have also been times when certain manufacturers of breastmilk substitutes have competed with one another to provide doctors with young children a year's free supply of breastmilk substitutes – if they were willing to take up the offer.

SUPPORTIVE INFLUENCES – AND THE OPPOSITE

Commerciogenic Malnutrition

The notion that malnutrition might be directly due to commercial influence was one of the colorful and, at the same time, very precise concepts introduced by Derrick and Patrice Jelliffe (1978), a married couple whose research on breastfeeding peaked during the 1960s and 1970s. Working primarily in tropical countries, they had perceived that something very alarming was happening to breastfeeding. The feeding bottle occupied an ever more prominent place, and in its wake, one observed increasing problems with ill health, diarrhea, and poor growth among young children. In many cultures, there was a long tradition of giving supplementary feeding from the time a baby was very small, sometimes merely as a symbolic or ritual practice after birth, and often with adverse effects on the baby's well-being.

Practice in developing countries tended to follow hard on the heels of that in the industrialized west where infant feeding was concerned. In the cities, where the market economy first developed, the population soon found itself with money to spend, and it was not very long before multinational corporations, some of which had become the major producers of breastmilk substitutes, began to cast their eyes on the new and rapidly growing opportunities for profit offered by the market in developing countries. Systematic campaigns to promote the sale of their products were created and carried through. The marketing program was from the start aimed directly at mothers. In some hospitals, the manufacturers employed uniformed nurses who distributed free samples and corresponding advice to mothers in the maternity wards. Glossy books and posters, replete with illustrations of glamorous, well dressed, and distinctly modern mothers, together with their strikingly healthy babies, and in the middle of the scene, the inevitable feeding bottle, strove to present the notion that this was the sort of world into which every baby might wish to enter. At the same time, more subtle methods were – and still are – employed to sow doubt as to the qualities of breastmilk and a mother's ability to provide it. Such material is cunningly contrived, suggesting without precisely saying as much, that a woman should be in real doubt as to her ability to feed her baby herself. Perhaps that was only to be expected – the manufacturers do not, after all, produce breastmilk substitutes in order to help women breastfeed.

HEALTH WORKERS SOUND THE ALARM

Earlier in this Chapter, we touched on the way in which the former European colonial powers sought to convert mothers in their far-flung empires to "civilized" infant feeding. Not all traveling Europeans, however, believed that to be the right approach. One of the first to recognize and describe the problems that followed in the wake of bottle-feeding was the British doctor Cecily Williams, who delivered a lecture in Singapore in 1939 under the title "Milk and murder" in which among other things she argued that "...misleading propaganda for artificial infant feeding should be regarded as a "murderous activity." Dr Williams put into words the conclusion to which many health workers were now coming to, with many more to follow, deeply concerned as they were to observe how parents were being seduced to use breastmilk substitutes. Many of them could not afford the branded products, and some were using instead ordinary powdered milk or sweetened condensed milk. To save on the costs of milk powder, some would often use less than the quantity recommended on the package – many, for that matter, were illiterate. And the water was often contaminated. Even today, in many city slums, clean water is nowhere to be found.

Lack of Self Confidence - A Recurrent Problem Among Women

It is not easy to understand why women so readily lose their self-confidence and faith in their own physical ability to produce good milk. True, the very first drops of mature milk that find their way out of the nipple may seem a little watery, certainly when set alongside full cream dairy milk. But the breastfed baby thrives on breastmilk, and grows and matures splendidly on it.

WATERY MILK?

It was in Niger that Elisabet met a young Tuareg mother, 18 year-old Mariamma, who had borne a child by a Frenchman, and now lived together with him. The baby lay in her lap as we talked; he was two months old, fat and happy, and fully breastfed.

"But I'm not sure..." said Mariamma, "Perhaps I ought to start bottle-feeding."

"But why?" I asked her, "He certainly doesn't look as if he's being deprived of anything."

"No, but I'm just not sure that my milk is good enough."

"What makes you think that?"

"Well, I don't eat all that well," murmured Mariamma a little sadly. "I only eat French food. It's a long time since I tasted camel's milk. That's why I'm not sure that my milk is good enough. Frenchwomen all use bottle-feeding – probably because with their diet their milk isn't as good as it should be..."

IS THE INDUSTRY QUITE DEAF?

It soon became increasingly clear that in places where hygienic conditions left a lot to be desired, the use of powdered milk could and did lead to significant health problems, the risk being most marked in the tropics. For this reason, the United Nations' special working group on nutrition problems, the Protein Advisory Group (PAG), convened a series of meetings in the early 1970s with leading personalities from the infant food industry to make entirely clear to them the serious consequences of the way in which their products were being marketed. The perhaps naive view of the well-thinking doctors who sat in the PAG was that the onward march of marketing in this area, extending into ever more countries, must be due to the fact that the planners and managers had not realized the health risks to which their activities were giving rise. Surely, they asked themselves, people in industry were not ill intentioned?

OR PERHAPS THEY SIMPLY DON'T LISTEN...

In their role as WHO experts, Derrick and Patrice Jelliffe attended some of these meetings, and Patrice recalled how on one occasion a field trip was arranged to the slums of Bogota, Colombia, to give the participants from the baby food firms an opportunity to observe firsthand the problems for which they were responsible. None of the industry representatives, however, had time to visit the slums that day; only the WHO experts turned up–and they had been there before (P. Jelliffe, personal communication, 1998).

HOW MARKETING MANIPULATES THE HEALTH SERVICES

The marketing campaigns in developing countries, which became ever more intensive in the late 1960s, were modern and aggressive, and were conducted through all imaginable channels. One of the major routes used, and one which industry had found to be profitable on earlier occasions, was through hospitals and health workers. On every continent, the message was designed to spread emphatically the news of the excellent qualities of their infant formula. Many physicians had long been accustomed to visits from the drug industry's detail men, and they now saw no reason to spurn the advances of the baby food manufacturers.

The effect was precisely as might have been expected. The food manufacturers had rightly anticipated that the high road to a mother's purse strings was through the health services. Such services are well organized and staffed with highly qualified professionals, and those professionals are accessible and commonly susceptible to persuasion, except perhaps when their political or social views render them unusually critical…

THE WHO CODE OF MARKETING OF BREASTMILK SUBSTITUTES

In the course of the 1970s, a whole series of larger and smaller organizations across the world confronted the issue of the unethical marketing of breastmilk substitutes. The English group War on Want published a pamphlet that vigorously attacked the industry. Its title "The Babykiller" pointed to the feeding bottle as the murder weapon. A small Swiss group known as "The Third World Working Party" (Arbeitsgruppe Dritte Welt) produced a German version of the pamphlet under the heading "Nestlé tötet Babies" (Nestlé kills babies). The firm in question took the working group to court and sued them for damages. When the verdict was handed down in 1976, Nestlé was awarded a miniscule sum in symbolic damages, while the judge strongly recommended the firm to move away from the sort of marketing practices around which the case had revolved. It was a classic example of a pyrrhic victory – the sort of victory that is, in fact, no more than a defeat.

WHO Marketing Code Comes Into Being

In 1979, WHO and UNICEF held a joint meeting in Geneva on the subject of infant feeding. Once again, it was clear that the uninhibited marketing of artificial foods was leading mothers to abandon breastfeeding. What was happening presented both a moral problem and a health challenge. It also became increasingly clear that for the industry it was the profitable market that really mattered. The firms struggled desperately against the drawing up of a code of marketing behavior, i.e., a set of rules, on which the two United Nations bodies were known to be working. The companies concerned, usually battling among themselves for the market, now found themselves united against a common enemy, namely the consumer organizations. For the industry, the situation was both absurd and unprecedented. In a move savoring of desperation, the industry created its own advisory council on nutrition, the ICIFI (International Council of Infant Food Industries). When at a given moment it became clear that the World Health Organization would indeed draw up a code, one that would limit the industry's ability to market these products as freely as it wished, the firms sought to take a leap ahead by launching a marketing code of its own. In May 1981, the whole issue was brought up before WHO's highest consultative body, the World Health Assembly. The Assembly, in which all the member states of WHO are represented, decided to recommend that each member state should take steps to implement the WHO Code in the manner best suited to its own national system. The Baby-Friendly Hospital Initiative introduced in later years is fully compatible with the provisions of the Code. The principal elements of the Code are provided in the Annex to this book.

What Does the WHO Code Say?

The WHO code proved to be an eye opener for many people who up to that moment had scarcely realized how unconscionably the baby food industry had exploited the market with a cynical disregard for whatever consequences this might have for the small consumer. In the form in which it was adopted, the WHO Code declares that the industry shall not offer or distribute free samples of breastmilk substitutes to mothers, nor shall they provide them with feeding bottles or teats. The health services, for their part, shall not allow its premises or its staff to play any role in marketing. The Code specifies very clearly what shall and shall not be said in industry-sponsored printed matter on infant feeding, and rules that any free supplies to hospitals shall be provided only at the specific request of the latter, and shall be used only for mothers who are unable to breastfeed. This latter principle has unfortunately proved to be capable of flexible interpretation, effectively providing an escape clause for firms eager to exploit it as an excuse for distributing free supplies for so-called emergency use. The Code has 39 clauses, and it lays responsibility for its implementation and maintenance jointly in the hands of health workers, health services, the public health authorities of member states, the manufacturers, and WHO itself.

Have Health Workers Forgotten the WHO Code?

Today very few health workers - or their institutions or organizations – seem to be aware of the fact that they bear a joint responsibility for upholding the principles laid down in the WHO Marketing Code. A shortened version of the Code's provisions is in the Appendix to this book.

The Hidden Battle Against Breastfeeding

With the adoption of the WHO Code in 1981, the marketing process went largely underground since direct and uninhibited marketing to the consumer was now frowned upon. Such indirect marketing still continues, but it can be quite difficult to recognize it for what it is.

Information or Marketing?

Marketing is often decked out in the guise of "information." The producers of breastmilk substitutes do not hesitate to assert that they have a moral right to inform the public. The term "information" can, however, mean various things (Dukes, 2005). Where marketing is concerned, true information is only one element in the total process. Marketing can be looked upon as a three-headed ogre, one of the heads comprising factual information, another education, and the third persuasion. Information in the strict sense of the word means the provision of facts, while education involves the provision of a point of view, and persuasion involves a deliberate effort to convince the potential customer of a particular matter. All three are important elements in the marketing process, but none of them stands alone. Certain particularly subtle forms of marketing can go a long way to educate and convince the customer – while misleading him or her, as is evident from many past and present examples in the field of breastmilk substitutes.

Companies marketing breastmilk substitutes cling assiduously to their right to "inform" the public, but all too often the information is carefully and subtly selected in order to destroy the breastfeeding tradition. That may, for example, be achieved by undermining a mother's faith in her ability to produce milk or by stressing the fact that the quality of breastmilk can be variable. Now and again, the information that is put across is quite simply false, but much more commonly it is merely confusing and sometimes contradictory within itself.

Only a few years back, the leaders of the new Russia believed that they were doing mothers a service by permitting foreign producers of baby food to establish themselves in the country. On one occasion, I (Elisabet) was asked across the table by former President Yeltsin what I thought of the policy. When I expressed much doubt as to whether this was a useful solution for Russian children, he hurriedly changed the subject, enthusing instead about the sow's ability to feed so many piglets!

Powerful Friends with Loads of Money

For many European countries, the production and export of breastmilk substitutes is now a thriving sector of business. One might add that since the ingredients of these products are hardly expensive, the producers can certainly be assured of a high profit margin. Thrive it does, but as a rule, it represents only a small part of the total turnover of the vast pharmaceutical or food producing companies who own the business, and the latter are, as a rule, multinationals enjoying close political contacts. Small wonder, then, that where breastmilk substitutes are concerned, the marketing practices of these firms have scarcely been tampered with by the authorities – whatever the WHO Code says. How enormous some of these multinationals are is very evident if one compares their turnover with the national budget of some medium-sized countries (see Table 14.1), and the influence they are capable of exerting on the authorities (and do not hesitate to use to their own advantage) can readily be imagined.

Table 14.1. Financial Strength of Companies and Countries (U.S. $ billions)

COUNTRY OF COMPANY	Source	Gross domestic product or company revenue
USA	2	14657
UK	2	2247
Poland	2	468
Wal-Mart *(supermarkets)*	1	421
Norway	2	414
Royal Dutch/Shell *(fuel)*	3	368
Exxon *(fuel)*	1	354
Nigeria	2	216

Toyota *(cars)*	3	203
Nestlé *(foods)*	3	104
Procter & Gamble *(household)*	1	79
Pfizer *(drugs)*	1	67
Unilever *(foods)*	3	59
Glaxo Smith Kline *(drugs, babyfood)*	3	46
Merck *(drugs)*	1	46
Uganda	2	17
Laos	2	6
Central African Republic	2	2
Gambia	2	1

Sources: 1. Fortune 500, 2011; 2. International Monetary Fund, 2010; 3. Wikipedia, 2011.

These comparisons of wealth and power have to be set against the fact that in many countries the authorities still do not appear to take breastfeeding too seriously. All the same, when visiting China in 2003, I (Elisabet) was a little taken aback when visiting that national shrine "The Forbidden City" to discover that the reverse side of the admission ticket sold to me was embellished with the name and emblem of a well-known multinational producer of baby foods, together with a photograph of Young Pioneers, complete with red scarves and happy smiles, each holding aloft a product of the firm in question. Influence at the very highest levels indeed....

Will They Manage to Break the Code?

In 1996, an informal group of voluntary organizations, the Interagency Group on Breastfeeding Monitoring (IGBM), carried out a well-planned study of the current marketing of breastmilk substitutes in four countries. A total of 29 bodies were involved, most of them attached to churches, including the World Council of Churches (Interagency Group of Breastfeeding Monitoring, 1997). Four countries – Poland, Bangladesh, South Africa, and Thailand – were examined. The investigation extended to marketing directed at mothers while they were still in the maternity ward, as well as campaigns seeking to influence the health system.

In all four countries, it was found that products were being marketed in a manner that breached the WHO Code, both in advertising and through the distribution of free samples to mothers and to health workers. According to the Code, samples may only be provided and accepted where they are to be used in an investigation or in research. Sample distribution as recorded in the study did not meet this requirement.

The WHO Code goes on to say that industry employees shall not pose as health workers in maternity wards, nor shall they seek to contact mothers in any other way. Alas, in all four countries, mothers who were interviewed declared that they had been approached directly by salespersons from the industry.

The study, which was published in the British Medical Journal (Taylor, 1998), concluded that in all four countries there had been systematic contravention of WHO's ethical standards for the marketing of breastmilk substitutes. This commonly involves the provision of false information, as a result of which mothers who wish to breastfeed are much less likely to do so. The reactions to this investigation, which had met the rigid standard that applies to all publications in the British Medical Journal, tell us something of the political pressure that the manufacturers concerned can bring to bear when it suits them. The Anglican Church's highest organ, the Church of England Synod, had essentially promoted the study in order to determine whether there was reason to maintain a boycott of the Nestlé Company's products, which the church had imposed during the years 1991–1994. The boycott had then been allowed to lapse, pending new and clear evidence that Nestlé was indeed acting in breach of the Code. Now such evidence was at hand in a study that met the highest scientific standards. Great was the disillusionment of the various consumer organizations, especially IBFAN (see below), when in July 1997, meeting at York, the Synod accepted the findings of the report – but voted against resumption of the boycott. Just a few months later, according to Allain (2002), the Synod accepted a donation of £100,000 from Nestlé. Ah, well.

The Sooner, The Better

The most effective form of sales promotion for any individual firm is when hospitals are seen or believed to be using its products, more especially when such a hospital proves willing to distribute samples of them to its patients. To induce hospitals to do so, firms are willing to provide gifts and donations, large and small. Particularly popular are benefits that can only with difficulty be funded from an ordinary hospital budget, such as funds to participate in conferences, special equipment for a department, or simply invitations to lunch and to dinner. Some hospitals have been so besieged by insistent sales representatives that they have ultimately imposed a timetable, with each producer in turn allocated a week during which it can distribute its products. A Russian proverb says that the only free cheese is to be found in the mousetrap – much the same as the American saying that there is no such thing as a free lunch. Both phrases reflect, very precisely, wisdom won through painful experience. For a producer, it means a great deal if mothers observe that it is his products that are in use in the hospital – "recommendation by association" as it is called. Not knowing that those products have been supplied free of charge, any mother is likely to conclude that the hospital has selected them because they are the best available. And beyond that, market analysts have found how strong brand name loyalty among mothers tends to be. If a mother has started to use a particular brand at the outset, she will hardly be likely to later switch to another, provided her baby is doing reasonably well...

Chapter 15.
SO WHAT CAN ONE DO?

The marketing of breastmilk substitutes needs to be regulated to protect mother and child against the ill effects of misleading arguments and improper use of information, both of which can lead a mother to abandon breastfeeding without having any valid reason for doing so. Such regulation can take as its starting point the WHO Code, which for several decades has demonstrated its relevance and its moral force. It has indeed been brought up afresh on numerous occasions in the World Health Assembly. Member states have frequently underlined their need for it. It remains the standard on which national law and regulations on the matter are based.

On the other hand, where member states have sought to implement the Code within their borders, one weakness has emerged in the sense that it is often unclear where, within a country, the responsibility is supposed to lie for the enforcement of its principles. The health system is unlikely to have the power to impose sanctions on any commercial party for breaches of the Code, and the firms themselves deliberately sabotage its provisions. If marketing is to be regulated according to the principles laid down in the Code, it is necessary to provide the rules with a firm basis in national law, enjoying sufficient political priority and with provisions for the imposition of sanctions. The Code can be regarded as an important instrument in the implementation of the various global and regional Conventions on Human Rights, and more particular, the Convention on the Rights of the Child.

If these things are to be achieved, all interested parties and individuals will need to exploit, patiently but persistently, the relevant mechanisms, for example, with respect to human rights, which are at hand. Politics, it has been said, is the art of the possible, even if the consumers whose interests are at stake are the smallest members of society, without a voice and without a vote. So far!

BREASTFEEDING IN THE NORTH

The history of our own times is the story of events that we as authors have ourselves experienced and to which we have been able to contribute. Both of the present writers were very much involved in the interaction between Norway's mothers and the health professions that developed from 1967 onwards. For Elisabet, it all began when she gave birth to Ingerid in 1965 and to Jon two years later. Anna-Pia became the mother of Malin in 1986 and Ada in 1996. Both became active in Ammehjelpen, the organization that grew up to support breastfeeding mothers, Elisabet from 1967 when she founded it, and Anna-Pia from 1987 to the present day.

It was purely by chance that Elisabet encountered the fact that breastfeeding could ever be a problem. Visiting the health center with her breastfed baby in 1965, she was handed a brochure on the subject. It hardly made for inspiring reading: "Relatively few mothers," it solemnly declared "indeed only some 30 percent of the total, produce sufficient milk to carry their babies through the entire period of breastfeeding. Only one mother in two manages to supply her baby with all the milk it needs for as much as three to four months. Many find much earlier than this that their milk supply is failing" (Njå, 1965, p. 4). Very encouraging words for a new and uncertain young mother! The pediatrician who had written them probably meant no harm—at the time, these things were either true or thought to be true. But how many mothers had enough self-confidence to believe that they belonged to the happy 30% who had sufficient milk? Elisabet turned to a good friend, Eira, who had a baby of the same age. Looking around, both of them had the feeling that many mothers were struggling to provide sufficient milk. Then Eira remarked, "It once happened to me, too, I lost my milk, but after a little while, the milk was there again." Elisabet's face must have betrayed her astonishment, but then Eira went on to tell how she had experienced a bout of flu when her baby son was about six months old and her milk supply seemed to dry up. However, she recovered from the flu in a matter of days, and she was obstinate enough not to give up on her breastfeeding. So every time the baby cried for food, she put it to the breast, empty though it might seem, and sure enough, within days the milk was flowing again as plentiful as ever. Elisabet was fascinated by the tale. Could it really be true that the milk could vanish and then return without more ado? That was when she began to delve into the how and why of breastfeeding. And she has being doing it ever since, throughout a reasonably long existence, and she is still finding more questions and answers.

1967: THE YEAR WHEN BREASTFEEDING IN NORWAY STRUCK ROCK BOTTOM –AND THEN BEGAN TO FIND ITS WAY BACK

The modern history of breastfeeding was played out to a large extent as the swinging '60s gave way to the progressive '70s. It was one of those periods in which, on all sides, people began to question old dogmas and turn accepted rules on their head. Everything that we had learned from our parents was called into question. Like unruly four-year olds, we began to ask all sorts of questions – subjecting our parents (and other authorities) to an inquisition they must have found irritating. And all the time, we were asking, "Why?"

THE MYSTERY OF THE VANISHING BREASTMILK

Up to this point, we have naturally concentrated our attention on why, across the world, something went wrong with breastfeeding. For that is indeed what happened, more or less everywhere during the first half of the 20th century. Mothers found that their milk supply failed, and no one knew why. There were those who blamed the mothers themselves, while others simply shrugged their shoulders, considering that it was not a matter of great concern. Much energy was expended on improving infant formula. But very few asked the essential question: what had gone wrong with breastfeeding? Hospitals were occupied with developing correct routines for infant feeding, and having done that for bottle-feeding with cow's milk, they unthinkingly applied the same procedures to breastfeeding mothers. They did what they believed was best – and the results were appalling. As we now know, separating mother and baby was not a sound idea, nor was it sensible to limit the number of breastfeeding sessions, but that is what happened.

While many believed that mothers had simply lost interest in breastfeeding, we were confronted with a very different reality: a host of unhappy mothers were constantly writing and ringing us, anything but content with (or indifferent to) the fact that their breastmilk was drying up.

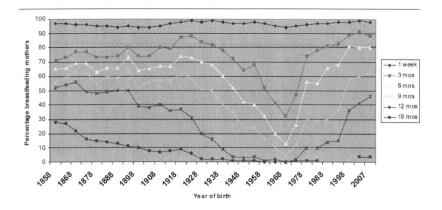

Figure 15.1. *Frequency of Breastfeeding in Norway over a Period of 149 Years*

Sources: Øverby, Kristiansen, Frost Andersen, & Lande, 2008; Kristiansen, Lande, Øverby, & Andersen, 2010; Lande et al., 2004.

Figure 15.1 is based primarily on data from the three largest hospitals in Norway's three principal cities. Women giving birth in these three hospitals during the period 1858-1988 were more or less routinely asked by the hospital how long they had breastfed their previous child, and their answers are reflected in the graph. Data for this analysis relates to 9150 participating mothers (Liestøl, Rosenberg, & Walløe, 1988). Although the information is based on what mothers claim to recall (i.e., it is retrospective), we have good reason to believe that it provides a reliable picture of trends. It is, in any case, the only available information on the matter. For the period 1988-1998, Elisabet worked with Rosenberg, adding data from a study undertaken by the Nutrition Council in 1998 and 2006-2007. For each individual year during the period 1858-1998, the analysis shows the percentage of mothers who were breastfeeding at the time they were discharged home from the clinic (i.e., when the baby was about a week old) and the numbers still breastfeeding at three, six, nine, 12, and 18 months. The breastfeeding data from 1998 onwards were retrieved from the Norwegian infant nutrition surveys (Øverby, Kristiansen, Frost Andersen, & Lande, 2008).

Over the entire period, Norwegian mothers had been doing their best to breastfeed during their stay in the maternity clinic or birthing center, and virtually all of them were producing milk at the time of their discharge.

What had changed, however, was the pattern of feeding once they were back at home. From about 1928 on, breastfeeding at home had gone into steep decline, reaching rock bottom some 30 years later. The proportion of babies being breastfed at three months fell from 70% to under 30%. The proportion still being breastfed at 12 months had dropped from 30% to almost zero.

And then, from 1968 on, it was as if a miracle occurred: the frequency of breastfeeding began to rise once more. At the very least, it was time to abandon the theory once advanced by some parties that that the initial decline in breastfeeding had been due to some genetic change in the female population. Within a decade, breastfeeding had returned to the level seen before the Second World War. For a time thereafter, the curve flattened out, but it began to rise once more at the beginning of the '90s. At first the phenomenon was dismissed by some as a mere quirk of fashion that would soon pass; others viewed the recovery of breastfeeding as part of a transient "green" trend – whatever that was supposed to mean in this connection. The rise of breastfeeding continued, sometimes in fits and starts, but inexorably and confidently. From today's perspective, the rebirth of breastfeeding certainly does not appear to be a mere quirk of fashion; it seems to be more of a lengthy and often difficult process in which mothers and their faithful allies succeeded in overcoming the unhappy consequences of earlier ignorance and poorly founded ideas about infant nutrition. Quite simply, mothers learned anew the art of breastfeeding, and they often did so in the face of practical obstacles. Why? That is the question we shall try to answer in this Chapter.

THE BREASTFEEDING REVOLUTION IN NORWAY: THE EARLY YEARS (1968-1975)

If there was one spark from elsewhere that ignited the dramatic recovery of breastfeeding in Norway, then it was certainly an example from the USA. In October 1956, a group of seven American mothers, among them some persons of great determination and blessed with organizational talent, came together and established an association known as La Leche League International (LLLI). The new body was designed to make available to a wide audience the considerable experience and knowledge regarding breastfeeding that the seven pioneers had acquired, having realized that there was a tremendous call for practical information on the matter. American mothers proved to be a great deal more motivated to breastfeed their children than many people had imagined. The seven also committed their experience to print in a book entitled *The Womanly Art of Breastfeeding*. In Norway, Elisabet tracked down a copy of this book when she was expecting her second baby, and she found the explanation of Eira's "miracle." The American ladies had been working on the matter for ten years, and they knew what they were talking about. Here clearly, was an example to follow, full of wisdom and sound advice.

What followed was a series of five complementary developments:

1. A Folder for Mothers

In June 1967, Elisabet embarked with social anthropologist Eli Heiberg on the writing of a compact little folder designed to be distributed to mothers during their stay in the maternity ward. The original title "Why a Mother Should Breastfeed Her Baby" may have been a little solemn and slightly moralistic, but the reception that it received, both from the mothers and from most of the health workers who read it, was entirely positive; what is more, the message worked. The more milk mothers provided for their babies, the more they produced. Intent on following the path further, the authors of the folder turned to the country's prestigious Board of Health. There they met Dr Gro Harlem Brundtland, later destined to become Director General of the World Health Organization. At the time, she had just received her Master's degree in the United States, her thesis centering on the problem that modern mothers were no longer breastfeeding. What was more, she herself was pregnant. As Dr Brundtland's subsequent autobiography recalls (Brundtland 1997, p. 131), her next step after meeting the authors of the folder was to present it to her male colleagues on the Board of Health and persuade them that breastfeeding was indeed a subject with which the health authorities should be concerned. The text of their folder was submitted for comment to all who might be regarded as competent in the field, and by early 1968, it was officially in print, though now under the less pompous title: "How to Breastfeed Your Baby – Some Advice at the Start." Distributed to all mothers entering maternity clinics or visiting health centers, it was well received. To date it has been revised and updated eight times, and has been translated into 10 languages. During the 40 years of its existence, more than a million copies of the Norwegian edition have been printed. In a country with a population of less than 5 million, this was sufficient to provide one copy to every woman becoming a mother for the first time during this period. This was a rather more than the authors originally expected.

2. Ammehjelpen Arrives

In 1968, a journalist with a woman's weekly read the brochure and became fascinated by the topic. Her subsequent article traced the history back to America's La Leche League and led to a flood of letters and telephone calls to Elisabet and Eli from mothers who, having unsuccessfully tried to breastfeed their babies, had now found someone who could tell them why they had failed and how they could succeed. Among the writers of letters were some by women who were positively interested in helping others and who saw a need for Norwegian mother-to-mother support groups inspired by the example of La Leche League. Very soon afterwards, ten women met to consider emulating the American model. As a result of this meeting, a national Norwegian movement came into being under the rather pompous name of "The Breastfeeding Mothers' Mutual Aid Association." A more compact title was soon found – Ammehjelpen – literally meaning "Breastfeeding Support." The women taking that initiative were mothers of small children. None of them had organizational experience, but they learned to improvise. They wrote to housewives' associations and to organizations promoting health. They descended on the National Broadcasting Corporation and found that their message resonated with the producers of programs for housewives. Shortage of cash was a recurrent problem, but they induced a pharmaceutical company to print both headed notepaper and a small prospectus for them, and they collected the considerable sum of 50 dollars for an envelope-addressing machine that somehow delivered pale blue labels, while filling the flat where it was housed with the pervasive smell of methylated spirits.

Naturally, there was an occasional setback on the way. For example, in 1971, when the group began ward rounds in a hospital in Oslo, it turned out that the daughter-in-law of the hospital's obstetrician was seeking breastfeeding advice, both from Ammehjelpen and from her father-in-law. Alas, the advice given by the worthy doctor was diametrically opposed to that which Ammehjelpen was providing. The daughter-in-law followed Ammehjelpen's advice and breastfed successfully, but Ammehjelpen's views were clearly now less welcome in the hospital, and its ward rounds were abruptly terminated.

Although the coming of Ammehjelpen had been welcomed by the health authorities, the health sector as a whole was at first suspicious of what was happening. Could an army of mere mothers, storming the professional barricades, properly question the teaching on infant feeding that leading physicians had been declaiming for generations? Was there a good reason to abandon familiar routines? Some of those concerned felt that Ammehjelpen's insistence that a baby must decide for itself when it was to be fed was little short of an invitation to anarchy. Such a feeding would surely play havoc with the baby's digestive system that would have no resting time! On the other hand, there were health workers who had felt for years that there must be a different and better way of tackling the feeding issue, and who were easily convinced when they saw the results of the new approach. But time, as they say, heals most wounds, and over the years, the opposition faded. By the time Ammehjelpen celebrated its first 25 years of work in 1993, there was nothing but praise from health workers who had over the years seen how this form of mother-to-mother support enriched the whole process of care. During those years, many of Ammehjelpen's voluntary breastfeeding consultants obtained professional qualifications, again a development that helped the health sector move away from old prejudices and controversies. And, last but not least, Ammehjelpen received the state's official blessing in the form of a prestigious prize that is awarded annually to persons or institutions that have made a significant contribution to health education – another form of acknowledgement of what has been achieved.

3. A Whole Book About Breastfeeding

In the 1970's, there was an evident need for more printed material. An attempt to translate the American *The Womanly Art of Breastfeeding* into Norwegian stranded on the fact that, however valuable the original book was, an attempt to transpose it for use in a different environment could hardly succeed; the translated text would tend to appear stiff and pretentious. Some felt that there did not seem to be a potential market for a book about breastfeeding, "Is it really possible to write a whole book just about that?" Finally, however, Elisabet encountered a sympathetic soul who provided the vital spark that was needed, "Why not write a book yourself on the subject?" Well, after all, why not? Many nights later, towards the end of 1969, the manuscript was delivered to a publishing house that was at least willing to help this eager young lady. The book was allocated a place in one of the publisher's series of cheap paperbacks, meaning that it could be printed on light, low-cost paper in a small format. Very practical, however, for one could read the book and breastfeed at the same time! Soon the publishers discovered that there were a great many more mothers than they had imagined who were anxious to read a book on this curious subject, and from then onwards, a reprint was found to be necessary almost every year. By the time the last edition reached the bookshops in 1995, the book had sold more than 74,000 copies, many of which were being handed down among friends and families from one generation to the next. It was translated into Swedish and Danish, reaching sizeable new audiences and contributing to the fact that a Swedish breastfeeding association – Amningshjälpen – saw the light of day.

4. A Ministerial Working Group on Breastfeeding

In the meantime, Norway's health authorities extended their involvement. When the Ministry of Social Affairs created a Working Group in 1974 charged with "examining the social and practical conditions conducive to breastfeeding and developing proposals for measures to encourage breastfeeding," Ammehjelpen was prominently represented, providing three of the Working Group's six members. The measures recommended in its widely distributed report issued in 1978 were a decade ahead of any similar initiatives at an international level. In particular, its "Ten Steps to Successful Breastfeeding" were destined to be adopted in the WHO/UNICEF Baby-Friendly Hospital Initiative ten years later. Though it may have appeared to be brief and bureaucratic in style, it was read thoroughly.

The Breastfeeding Working Group went on to develop further initiatives. They sent a questionnaire to all Norwegian maternity centers regarding the procedures they had in place regarding breastfeeding and the feeding of the newborn. The investigation was first performed on data from 1973, and was later repeated using data collected in 1982, 1991, and 2000. The study was performed once more in 2009. Astonishingly, there was on every occasion a 100% response. The findings document the massive changes that have taken place in maternity wards during this period (Heiberg Endresen & Helsing, 1995; Eide, Heiberg, Helsing, & Paalgard, 2003). In 1973, for example, 58 % of the centers had permitted the mother and her baby to be together for less than five hours daily, the time being divided over some four to six feeding sessions at fixed hours. What this meant in practice was that more than half the babies spent the greater part of the day alone in a cot in the nursery, watched over by a pediatric nurse who fed them with cow's milk mixtures, infant formula, or sugar water when they cried or appeared hungry between the prescribed breastfeeding sessions. Meanwhile, their mothers lay apart in another ward, often with painful, milk-filled breasts, waiting for the moment when they would be permitted to breastfeed according to the timetable. By 1998, 25 years later, not a single hospital in Norway was practicing this artificial separation of mother and baby, and today it is entirely normal for the institutions to encourage mothers in their care to be together with their infants 24 hours a day. The mother has also regained free access to her baby. The strict regime of disciplinary rules, regularity, and controls, which by the beginning of the last century had taken hold of the process of baby care and the practice of maternity units, is a thing of the past. It has made way for a new tradition involving treating mother and baby as an inseparable unit, and having a receptive and respectful attitude towards both of them.

5. The New Feminism

Alongside all these specific developments restoring breastfeeding to its proper place, one must recall a more general trend in society that clearly played a role. This was the growth of the new feminist movement, which endowed women with a greater sense of confidence in this, as in so many other fields. Towards the end of the 1960s, numerous rebellious ideas were busy germinating and growing just below the surface of society. In 1970, the first new feminist groups came into being and found themselves at first regarded as dangerous insurgents. "Bra burning" – were we to expect that in Norway as well? Yes indeed, and more than a few of the rebels were recruited directly from the ranks of Ammehjelpen. In that circle, we had already learned how rewarding it was when women banded together, how much common ground we found to talk about, and last but by no means least, how important mutual support and the building of each other's self confidence could be. "Sister solidarity" was the name we gave to it at the time. Those of us who were active in both the feminist and the breastfeeding movements sometimes found ourselves developing something of a split personality, since not all the breastfeeding supporters around us were equally sympathetic to the new and radical feminist point of view. Feminists on the other hand, at least in Norway, had little difficulty in approving of breastfeeding. They simply maintained that there is no alternative to pregnancy for making babies, and there is no truly worthy alternative to breastfeeding for making them grow. The feminist approach must be to make breastfeeding accessible to every woman, both in practical and in physiological terms. What any individual of her own free will then chooses to do in her own life is naturally her own business.

Once again, the Jelliffes had put into words a fundamental principle underlying breastfeeding. As they put it, "Breastfeeding is a confidence trick." Self-confidence is the real key.

UPS AND DOWNS ACROSS THE WORLD

The Norwegian experience was remarkable, but one must also look at what was happening to breastfeeding elsewhere. As the century ended, there was a modest swing back to breastfeeding in a number of industrialized western countries, such as England and Wales (see Table 15.1), and it took many by surprise, including those who were actively working to spread knowledge of the subject. Meanwhile, the positive trend initiated earlier in the United States by La Leche League continued.

Table 15.1. Frequency of breastfeeding at the time of discharge from maternity units in England and Wales (Bolling, Grant, Hamlyn, & Thornton, 2007.)

Year:	1980	1985	1990	1995	2000	2005
Percentage of mothers breastfeeding	67	65	64	68	71	77

The fact that the renaissance of breastfeeding was less dramatic in some countries than in others can be explained in various ways. Women determined to breastfeed could find themselves faced with a number of practical obstacles. One such obstacle was the brevity of the maternity leave commonly permitted for working women. In the 1960's in Norway, maternity leave was commonly little more than six weeks prior to delivery and six weeks after birth, with no possibility of negotiating anything better. Yet it was as if the renaissance of breastfeeding was unstoppable. Figure 15.2 shows how, at a time when ever more women in Norway were seeking employment outside the home, the proportion who were breastfeeding nevertheless continued to rise. How is one to explain it all?

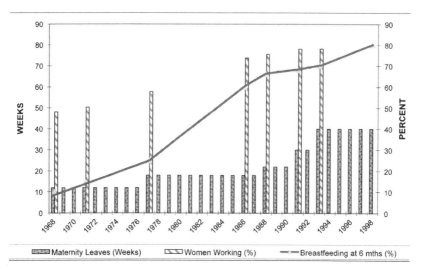

WEEKS / PERCENT

Maternity Leaves (Weeks)   Women Working (%)   Breastfeeding at 6 mths (%)

Figure 15.2. *Maternity leave and proportion of working women in Norway, 1968-1998*

As we have seen, the breastfeeding trend was already rising when maternity leave was very brief, and it continued to do so when the period of leave was only modestly lengthened. During the period 1977-1988, maternity leave in Norway was still limited to a total of 18 weeks, and the proportion of women in paid employment rose from 60% to as much as 75%, yet breastfeeding went from strength to strength. It was, quite simply, what women wanted, however problematical it might be. It was only secondarily attributable to any initiative from the authorities or the health sector. That said, however, it was a fact that in Norway provisions on maternity leave have developed more generously than in some other countries, and the authorities have taken breastfeeding and women as a whole seriously. The Ministry of Social Affairs provided a little financial support, but more importantly, sought the advice of mothers, and listened to their replies; the role of the Breastfeeding Working Group has been touched on above. The National Board of Health developed and has maintained a critically positive view of these developments. Over the years, Ammehjelpen has come to enjoy much support from the Norwegian health authorities, both in the form of financial assistance and in the way in which the organization has been consulted on matters relevant to breastfeeding. All these various forms of support and encouragement have continued to the present day. Table 15.2 shows how extensive breastfeeding has now become in the five Nordic countries.

Table 15.2. Breastfeeding during the first year of life in the Nordic countries.

	Full breastfeeding			Any breastfeeding			
	1st week	4 months	6 months	1st week	4 months	6 months	12 months
Denmark							
1995	86[1]	60	17	93	75	61	18
1996	98	51	-	-	-	-	-
Finland							
1995	-	10	0	-	61	40	-
2000	-	15	1	-	66	51	26[2]
Iceland							
1995	88	46	5	97	83	77	13
2001	93	48	14	98	81	68	13
2003	92	48	12	98	79	67	15
Norway							
1998/99	96	44	7	99	85	80	36
Sweden							
1997	94	69	42	98	84	74	-
2000	93	68	33	98	83	72	-
2002	91	68	32	98	83	73	-

Sources: Health Statistics in the Nordic Countries 2003. (2005) NOMESCO (Nordic Medico- Statistical Committee, 73, Copenhagen. (NOMESCO (Nordic Medico-Statistical Committee) 73, (2005), Health Statistics in the Nordic Countries 2003.)

[1]   *1 month*
[2]   *11 months*

THE NORDIC SITUATION

There are several lessons to be learned here, especially from Norway and Sweden. The first and most important is that the breastfeeding movement was initiated from the mothers and by the mothers. It was *not* someone acting on behalf of the mothers, wishing to convince them to breastfeed. Ammehjelpen, for example, has always underlined that they are there for those who want support and practical help. In the case of Ammehjelpen, therefore, it was the problem-owners themselves who took action. Ammehjelpen continues to exist and assist fellow mothers, as it has done for half a century.

The second lesson from the Nordic countries is that once breastfeeding has again become universally accepted as a normal part of motherhood, the only essential decision for a woman to make is whether she wants to become a mother at all. If she does, then she will quite simply expect to breastfeed. There is no need for a separate decision on the latter issue. When a woman has decided that she wants to have a baby, she should be ready to feed it in the species specific way of humans and with species specific milk. If she is among the few percent who do not want to or do not feel that maternity is right for her, she should be left in peace with her decision and not be scorned because of her choice.

Breastfeeding - A Human Right?

In spite of all the ups and downs, advances and repulses, to say nothing of the ingenious inventions of the producers of breastmilk substitutes, breastmilk and breastfeeding remain the only sound and normal basis for rearing in early childhood. That, we can be sure, will remain so in the future. The advantages of human milk, attuned as it is to the needs of the human child, have been documented to the hilt. It could hardly be otherwise for it involves the transfer of a specifically designed liquid food from one human body to another that is intimately allied to it. The infant has, in this way, access to all the resources of its mother's body to supply it with exactly what it needs. Understandably, the demands that the process makes on a mother's mental and physical system may occasionally become too great for her to handle. When that happens, one can be content with the fact that the dairy industry has devoted some of its research to adaptation of cow's milk. One can be content, too, that the human being is an omnivore, strikingly tolerant to the milk of other species.

The Mother's Rights to Breastfeed

What can we draw from the relevant international, legal human rights instruments regarding mothers' rights to breastfeed their children? Especially viewed from the standpoint of human rights law, it is undeniable that if a country has ratified the Conventions on Human Rights, and in particular, the UN Convention on the Rights of the Child (ratified by 190 out of the world's 192 states by 2011) in its article 24.1 on the right of the child to the enjoyment of the highest attainable standard of health, mothers in that country have a legal right to breastfeed their children and to be assisted in making it possible for them to do so. It follows that the State, as the number one duty-bearer for the realization of the agent of human rights that it has ratified, has an obligation to ensure that the mother's rights in this matter are respected, protected, and realized by appropriate policies and by ensuring the implementation of specific duties of relevant institutions and services. Such things do not happen by themselves. One only needs to look back to earlier chapters to see how little respect was paid to these matters in the past. The essential point here is that a mother should never be prevented from breastfeeding because of obstacles which society is capable of removing. It is clearly an obligation of the States to ensure that no barrier is laid across the path to breastfeeding.

The Rights of the Child to be Breastfed

Since the baby cannot talk, it cannot express its claims as a right-holder in legal language, but in many other ways, the human baby does contrive to make known its wants and preferences. The child's rights in these and other matters flow directly from the provisions of the UN Convention on the Rights of the Child. Perhaps the most relevant of the Conventions' provisions is that, to quote it literally: "States parties recognize the right of the child to the enjoyment of the highest attainable standard of health…" (Article 24.1). It is incontestable that the milk of its own species represents a golden standard in this connection, an essential instrument for the attainment of the highest possible level of health. Viewed in the light of the Conventions on Human Rights, it is abundantly clear that a baby has an inalienable right to mother's milk and to the breastfeeding process. And, one must emphasize once more, it is the State which is charged with ensuring, within its own borders, that these rights are respected in daily practice.

Enthusiasm - And Tolerance

In today's world, it is easy to become confused. Things are not as they once were. In the past, breastfeeding often seemed out of reach because of the false rules and ideas that abounded. Today, in many countries, breastfeeding has become the norm. Some false teachings persist, but true knowledge and understanding are now abundant. Unfortunately, it can happen that truly knowledgeable individuals are not always readily at hand when a mother has need of them, and as a consequence, some women will – sometimes for good reasons and sometimes for bad reasons – seek the solution offered by a breastmilk substitute in a bottle. Many a woman in that situation knows how much she misses the breastfeeding experience, but her frustration in that regard is only made more painful if she finds herself stigmatized and criticized for what she is doing, as if she is not doing her best for her baby. We have said it before and we must say it again: it is (very fortunately) not possible to force any woman to breastfeed against her will. One still encounters women who, for one reason or another, do not succeed in breastfeeding. The one may have started incorrectly, another may have had no access to the help and support that she needed, and a third may actually have been misled by incorrect information. There are, too, those who have to forfeit the experience of breastfeeding because of some problem in the area of mental or physical health. It is unfair and bitter for such women if, in addition, they feel criticized. Many of the pleasures and rewards of breastfeeding that we have discussed here can, when the need arises, be experienced by concerned parents, even when bottle-feeding is necessary. When we declare that breastfeeding is a true human right both for mother and child, that view should be adopted with the necessary provisions and reservations. On occasion, the proponents of breastfeeding have been condemned as preoccupied with policing young mothers or imposing their views, perhaps even terrorizing women into putting their babies to the breast. It is almost impossible to talk or write about breastfeeding without displaying one's own enthusiasm, but that enthusiasm must not lead to contempt for those women who, for one reason or another, turn to artificial feeding as an alternative.

BREASTFEEDING AND ITS ALLIES

A fortunate characteristic of our own time is the ease with which global contacts can be established and maintained between people with similar needs and interests, a fact that has been fully exploited by a range of voluntary organizations. Since a breast is a breast everywhere in the world and greedy multinational corporations are also very much the same all over the globe, the movement offering resistance to artificial baby feeding has necessarily chosen to organize itself on a worldwide basis. Two organizations have become particularly prominent in this area of the consumer movement. One is the International Baby Food Action Network, better known as IBFAN, and the other is the World Alliance for Breastfeeding Action, better known as WABA.

IBFAN (International Baby Food Action Network)

IBFAN is a network with a flat structure. It was created more than a quarter of a century ago, when WHO's International Code of Marketing of Breastmilk Substitutes was formulated in 1981. IBFAN concentrates the bulk of its efforts on inspecting the manner in which the multinational corporations selling these products exploit – often unconscionably – all possible means of attack in the intense and ongoing battle for customers. The intention of the Code was to ensure that only those few women who were truly not able to breastfeed would buy these products. Attainment of that ideal would, however, limit the market to a size that would be commercially unattractive. Firms, therefore, continued to engage in vigorous efforts to convince women that breastfeeding was difficult, scarcely justified the effort involved, and industrial products based on cow's milk were equally acceptable.

Within IBFAN, there is a specialized office known as the International Code Documentation Center (ICDC), which every third year publishes a valuable overview entitled "Breaking the Rules." In its pages, one finds detailed reports from every part of the world on the manner in which the provisions of the Code are being breached by a range of named companies, in a sense *shaming* the companies by *naming* them as Code violators. ICDC also provides courses to train lawyers in the drafting of national laws and regulations in this field. IBFAN's work extends beyond the Code, involving issues of maternity protection, legislation on contaminants, and collaboration with the Pesticides Action Network to name but a few examples. IBFAN's work is based on the premise that protection is necessary if the promotion of breastfeeding is to have the slightest chance of success. Most IBFAN groups work at the grassroots level in protecting, promoting, and supporting breastfeeding in nearly all the countries of the world. Viewed locally, it may be difficult to distinguish between the initiatives taken by IBFAN and other global or national bodies, but the movement as a whole benefits greatly from the work undertaken by IBFAN.

WABA (World Alliance for Breastfeeding Action)

WABA is younger than IBFAN, having been founded in 1990 at the time of the Declaration, which provided the basis for the Baby Friendly Hospital Initiative (BFHI). WABA was specifically created to follow that initiative, which became known as The Innocenti Declaration. We personally joined WABA perhaps because it had in practice a somewhat broader base and program than IBFAN. Elisabet was both a representative of IBFAN Europe at its establishment in 1981 and a member of WABA's governing body for many years. She remains active in the organization, to the extent of donating all income earned on the present book to WABA, which has its headquarters and secretariat in Penang, Malaysia. With its small office, WABA can point to an impressive list of achievements. Every year it supports World Breastfeeding Week, which on each occasion devotes in-depth attention to a particular theme, and in this way has assembled a great deal of valuable information material. In addition, the organization has been actively involved in such issues as legislation governing maternity leave, the possible presence of contaminants in breastmilk, and dialogue with the feminist and women's movements, to cite only a few examples. WABA also collaborates with other organizations and is, for example, a member of the Pesticides Action Network. It has also been very much involved in the problems arising in countries where AIDS is widespread, and it seeks to disseminate up-to-date material on this and other matters affecting breastfeeding. The organization was at an early stage involved in human rights issues. One might well summarize things by saying that, while IBFAN undertakes a great deal of work within in a relatively focused field, WABA works less in depth, but over a broader field. In fact, the two organizations complement one another perfectly.

BREASTFEEDING IN TODAY'S WORLD

Both IBFAN and WABA are examples of the global consumer movement that has grown up in recent decades. They bring together the accumulated wisdom of the wise women of yesterday and today, and the energy and idealism of young men and women. Today's wise woman can ensure that her voice is heard, thanks to the Internet.

International comparisons of breastfeeding rates, such as that attempted in a project for the European Union (Istituto di Ricovero, 2003), are somewhat precarious since the methods of data collection vary, but certain impressions can be obtained. Data from some English-speaking countries are summarized in Table 15.3. Figures from other parts of the world seem to show that, while initial breastfeeding is today common, the extent to which it is continued during subsequent months varies widely. The considerable differences in the maintenance of breastfeeding after a number of months point very clearly to the fact that breastfeeding is, in part, dependent on political factors. The influence of rules governing maternity leave has already been mentioned, but health policy in general, commercial policies, and policies on women all play a role in determining how straightforward or how difficult it is for mothers to breastfeed. Within countries, too, there are some marked variations, for example, as between various provinces in Canada.

Table 15.3. Prevalence and Duration of Breastfeeding in Four Countries

Country	Date	Percentage of infants being breastfeed			
		Ever breastfed	At 6 months	At 12 months	Source
USA	2001	65.1	27.0	12.3	1
Canada	2005-9	87.5	47.2	14.0	2
Australia	1995	84.0	49.0	(data unavailable)	3
New Zealand	2001	68.0	61.0	(data unavailable)	4

Sources:
1. National Immunization Survey 2001, as cited by Li, Zhao, Mokdad, Barker, & Grummer-Strawn, 2003.
2. Scott, J.A., Binns, C.W., Aroni, R.A. (1995). Infant Feeding practices in Perth and Melbourne - Report 1 (p. 72), as cited by Australian Breastfeeding Association: ABA's Five Year Plan for Australia, ABA, East Malvern, Va., (undated). Retrieved on August 3, 2011, from http://www.breastfeeding.asn.au/advocacy/plan.html.
3. New Zealand Ministry of Health, 2002.

Variations in the pattern of breastfeeding also reflect the knowledge and attitudes about breastfeeding that a mother encounters in her immediate environment. These, in turn, are influenced by society's attitude toward women and by a woman's attitude about herself and her femininity. Where attitudes in a community are not particularly sympathetic and knowledge is scarce, it can be difficult for an individual mother, even if she wishes to breastfeed, to maintain confidence in her ability to manage it. Even if she is constantly being assured that "breast is best," those whom she approaches for support will often, in their gestures and choice of words, convey a belief that she has precious little hope of succeeding. It may be hard to find anyone who can genuinely advise her in solving whatever problems she may encounter. Instead of helpful guidance, she may be offered breastmilk replacement products. This is unhappily still the day-to-day experience of women in many of the world's countries, even though there are many fortunate exceptions. Perhaps one could put it like this: Mothers have been exposed to a gigantic conspiracy, designed to cast doubt upon their ability and their will to breastfeed. It takes a great deal of courage to face up to such an intense degree of mistrust, to defy health workers who provide confusing and unhelpful advice, and to challenge the messages handed down by an industry bent on doing its best to impose milk from ruminant animals on as many human infants as possible, seeking to persuade us that it is as good as our own milk – and to those friends and prophets of gloom who assure us that our milk will very soon dry up, and that it is entirely healthy for a baby to cry. In this book, we have discussed factors that in the past led to a catastrophic fall in breastfeeding in Scandinavia and elsewhere. But in Scandinavia, breastfeeding returned like a boomerang. That it did so, with many other parts of the world following in its wake, was in large measure an achievement of mothers themselves.

When a mother wishes to breastfeed, she is entitled to expect that society will make it possible – both for herself and her baby. The Health Services need to ensure that she can obtain real assistance when she has need of it. Breastfeeding should not require any sacrifice on a mother's part or be feasible only for those who are wealthy, strong, or fortunate, or have a partner enjoying these privileges. Breastfeeding should be accessible for all. We hope this book will contribute to the achievement of that goal.

DEFIANCE, COURAGE, & BREASTFEEDING

The portrait (Figure 15.3) is of Bíbi Vogel, a photo model and organizer of breastfeeding support from Rio de Janeiro (who sadly died in 2004), clad in an expensive fur coat with her one year-old baby. It is perhaps not the idyllic breastfeeding scene that we tend to connect with infant feeding. Instead it expresses both defiance and courage. Bíbi arranged for the portrait to be made by one of Brazil's leading fashion photographers. With her good looks, she earned her living in part by modeling. To her surprise, she later found the portrait on display at one of the photographer's exhibitions. To her even greater surprise, she saw how numerous visitors paused lengthily in front of the picture, often discussing it with other bystanders. Breastfeeding can be provocative – a fact that many have experienced.

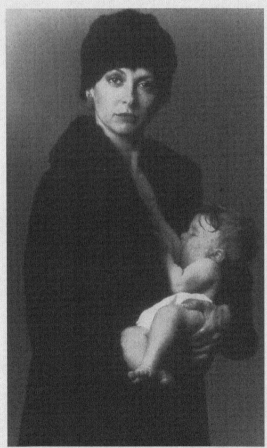

Figure 15.3. *Defiant: Bíbi Vogel with her baby. Photo: Oscar Balducci*

Used with permission.

REFERENCES

Agostoni, C., Braegger, C., Decsi, T., Kolacek, S., Koletzko, B., Michaelsen, K. F., et al. (2009). Breast-feeding: A commentary by the ESPGHAN Committee on Nutrition. *Journal of Pediatric Gastroenterology and Nutrition, 49,* 112-125.

Åkerström, S., Asplund, I., & Norman, M. (2007). Successful breastfeeding after discharge of preterm and sick newborn infants. *Acta Paediatrica, 96,* 1450-1454.

Akre, J. (Ed.). (1989). Infant feeding. The physiological basis. *Bulletin of the World Health Organization, 67,* Suppl. 1-108.

Allain, A. (2002). Fighting an old battle in a new world. How IBFAN monitors the baby food market. *Development Dialogue,* Special Issue, 2, Uppsala: Dag Hammarskjöld Foundation 2005.

American Academy of Pediatrics (AAP), Gartner, L. M., Morton, J., Lawrence, R. A., Naylor, A. J., O'Hare, D., Schanler, R. J., et al. (2005). Breastfeeding and the use of human milk. *Pediatrics, 115,* 496-506.

Amir, L. H. (2001). Maternal smoking and reduced duration of breastfeeding: a review of possible mechanisms. *Early Human Development, 1,* 45-67.

Anderson, S.A., Chinn, H.I. & Fisher, K. D. (1982). History and current status of infant formulas. *American Journal of Clinical Nutrition, 2,* 381–397.

Andersson, P., & Nyholm, K. (1986). *Tjernobyl mätdata (Chernobyl Statistical Data)* . SSI-rapport 86-23. Stockholm: Statens Strålskyddsinstitut.

Apple, R.D. (1987). *Mothers and medicine. A social history of infant feeding 1890–1950.* Madison, Wisconsin: The University of Wisconsin Press Ltd.

Ås, B. (1999). *Master suppression techniques.* A Philippine edition from the Institute of Women's Studies. Manila: St. Scholastica's College.

Attenborough, D. (1992). *The trials of life.* London: Collins, BBC Books.

Auerbach, K. (1990). Sequential and simultaneous breast pumping: a comparison. *International Journal of Nursing Studies, 27,* 257-265.

Baalsrud, E.S. (1992). Det første året:Et foreldreperspektiv (The first year: the perspective of the parents). In S.E. Ulvund, L. Smith, R. Lindemann, A. Ulvund, & E. S. Baalsrud (Eds.), *Lettvektere. Om for tidlig fødte barn (Light weighters. A book about preterm babies)* (pp. 152-169). Oslo: Universitetsforlaget A/S.

Baby Friendly Canada. (2011). World Health Organization continues to recommend exclusive breastfeeding for six months. Retrieved on August 2, 2011, from http://www. babyfriendlynl.ca/2011/01/25/world-health-organization-continues-to-recommend-exclusive-breastfeeding-for-six-months/.

Bærug, A., Solberg, L., & Kjærnes, U. (1991). Amming i Finnmark – levekår og tilrettelegging. (Breastfeeding in Finnmark - standards of living and support). *Fylkeslegens skriftserie, 2.*

Baker, J.L., Gamborg, M., Heitmann, B.L., Lissner, L., Sørensen, T.I., & Rasmussen, K.M. (2008). Breastfeeding reduces postpartum weight retention. *The American Journal of Clinical Nutrition, 6,* 1543-51.

Ball, H.I. (2011). *Breastfeeding, bed-sharing and infant safety.* Durham University, Department of Anthropology, Parent-Infant Sleep Lab. www.dur.ac.uk/sleep.lab.

Beeton, I. (1859). *Beeton's book of household management.* London: S.O. Beeton.

Binkiewicz, A., Robinson, M.J., & Senior, B. (1978). Pseudo-Cushing syndrome caused by alcohol in breast milk. *The Journal of Pediatrics, 6,* 965-967.

Bolling, K., Grant, C., Hamlyn, B., & Thornton, A. (2007). *Infant feeding survey 2005.* Information Centre, Government Statistical Service, UK Health Departments, London.

Bonet, M., Blondel, B., Agostino, R., Combier, E., Maier, R.F., Cuttini, M., et al. (2010). Variations in breastfeeding rates for very preterm infants between regions and neonatal units in Europe: results from the MOSAIC cohort. *Archives of Disease in Childhood. Fetal and Neonatal Edition.* Epub ahead of print.

Brambell, M.R., & Jones, D.M. (1997). The management of young mammals. In M. Peaker (Ed.), *Comparative aspects of lactation. Symposia of the Zoological Society of London No. 41* (pp. 333-339). New York: Academic Press.

Brandtzaeg, P. (2010). Food allergy: separating the science from the mythology. *Nature Reviews. Gastroenterology & Hepatology, 7,* 380-400.

Brinchmann, A. (1929). *Barnets første år* (The Child's First Year). Oslo: Gyldendal Norsk Forlag.

Brinchmann, A. (1943) *Barnets første år* (The child's first year) (5th ed.). Oslo: Gyldendal Norsk Forlag.

Brundtland, G.H. (1997). *Mitt liv 1929-1986* (My life 1929-1986). Oslo: Gyldendal Norsk Forlag.

Bystrova, K., Widström, A.M., Matthiesen, A.S., Ransjö-Arvidson, A.B., Welles-Nyström, B., Wassberg, C., et al. (2003). Skin-to-skin contact may reduce negative consequences of "the stress of being born:" a study on temperature in newborn infants, subjected to different ward routines in St. Petersburg. *Acta Paediatrica, 92,* 320-326.

Camurdan, A.D., Ilhan, M.N., Beyazova, U., Sahin, F., Vatandas, N., & Eminoglu, S. (2008). How to achieve long-term breast-feeding: factors associated with early discontinuation. *Public Health Nutrition, 11,* 1173-1179.

Canivet, C.A., Ostergren, P.O., Jakobsson, I.L., Dejin-Karlsson, E. & Hagander, B.M. (2008). Infantile colic, maternal smoking and infant feeding at 5 weeks of age. *Scandinavian Journal of Public Health, 3,* 284-291.

Cattaneo, A., Davanzo, R., Uxa, F., & Tamburlini, G. (1998). Recommendations for the implementation of Kangaroo Mother Care for low birthweight infants. International Network on Kangaroo Mother Care. *Acta Paediatrica, 87,* 440-445.

Charpak, N., Ruiz, J.G., Zupan, J., Cattaneo, A., Figueroa, Z., Tessier, R., et al. (2005). Kangaroo mother care: 25 years after. *Acta Paediatrica, 94,* 514-522.

Christensson, K., Siles, C., Moreno, L., Belaustequi, A., De la Fuente, P., Lagercrantz, H., et al. (1992). Temperature, metabolic adaptation and crying in healthy full-term newborns cared for skin-to-skin or in a cot. *Acta Paediatrica, 81,* 488-493.

Cignacco, E., Hamers, J.P., Stoffel, L., van Lingen, R.A., Gessler, P., McDougall, J., et al. (2007). The efficacy of non-pharmacological interventions in the management of procedural pain in preterm and term neonates. A systematic literature review. *European Journal of Pain, 11,* 139-152.

Cobo, E. (1973). Effects of different doses of ethanol on the milk-ejecting reflex in lactating women. *American Journal of Obstetrics and Gynaecology, 6,* 817-821.

Collins, C.T., Ryan, P., Crowther, C.A., McPhee, A.J., Paterson, S., & Hiller, J.E. (2004). Effect of bottles, cups, and dummies on breast feeding in preterm infants: a randomised controlled trial. *BMJ, 329,* 193-198.

Colonial Medical Report No. 71. (1917). *Journal of Tropical Medicine and Hygiene, 20.*

Colson, 2011. *Biological nurturing.* Retrieved May 18, 2011, from http://www.biologicalnurturing.com/pages/beliefs.html.

Colson, S. (2010). *An introduction to biological nurturing - new angles on breastfeeding.* Amarillo, TX: Hale Publishing.

Colson, S.D., Meek, J.H., & Hawdon, J.M. (2008). Optimal positions for the release of primitive neonatal reflexes stimulating breastfeeding. *Early Human Development, 84,* 441-449.

Cotterman, K.J. (2004). Reverse pressure softening: a simple tool to prepare areola for easier latching during engorgement. *Journal of Human Lactation, 20,* 227-237.

Cowie, A.T. (1972). Lactation and its hormonal control. In C.R. Austin & R.V. Short (Eds.), *Reproduction in mammals: 3. Hormones in Reproduction.* Cambridge: The University Press.

Czank, C., Mitoulas, L.R., & Hartmann, P.E. (2007). Human milk composition - Fat. In T.W. Hale & P.E. Hartmann (Eds.), *Textbook of human lactation* (pp. 49-67). Amarillo, TX: Hale Publishing, L.P.

Dahl, A. (1964). *Jeg er blitt mor. En håndbok til hjelp ved barnestell.* (I've become a mother. A handbook for assisance in child care.) Oslo: Det lille universitet, Fredhøis forlag A/S.

Dall'Oglio, I., Salvatori, G., Bonci, E., Nantini, B., D'Agostino, G., & Dotta, A. (2007). Breastfeeding promotion in neonatal intensive care unit: impact of a new program toward a BFHI for high-risk infants. *Acta Paediatrica, 96,* 1626-1631.

Davis, T.A., Nguyen, H.V., Garcia-Bravo, R., Fiorotto, M.L., Jackson, E.M., Lewis, D.S., Lee, D.R., & Reeds, P.J. (1994). Amino acid composition of human milk is not unique. *The Journal of Nutrition, 124,* 1126-1132.

de Onis, M., Onyango, A.W., Borghi, E., Garza, C., & Yang, H. (2006). Comparison of the World Health Organization (WHO) Child Growth Standards and the National Center for Health Statistics/WHO international growth reference: implications for child health programmes. *Public Health Nutrition, 9,* 942-947.

Dennis, C.L. (2002). Breastfeeding initiation and duration: a 1990-2000 literature review. *Journal of Obstetetric, Gynecologic, and Neonatal Nursing, 31,* 12-32.

Dewey, K.G., Nommsen-Rivers, L.A., Heinig, M.J., & Cohen, R.J. (2003). Risk factors for suboptimal infant breastfeeding behavior, delayed onset of lactation, and excess neonatal weight loss. *Pediatrics, 112,* 607-619.

Dewey, K.G., Heinig, M.J., Nommsen, L.A., & Lönnerdal, B. (1991). Maternal versus infant factors related to breast milk intake and residual milk volume: the DARLING study. *Pediatrics, 87*(6), 829-837.

Di Lallo, D., Bertollini, R., Berrucci, C.A., Campos Venuti, G., Risica, R., & Simula, S. (1987). Radioactivity in breast milk in Central Italy in the aftermath of Chernobyl. *Acta Paediatrica Scandinavica, 3,* 530-531.

DiGirolamo, A.M., Grummer-Strawn, L.M., & Fein, S.B. (2008). Effect of maternity-care practices on breastfeeding. *Pediatrics, 122 Suppl 2,* S43-S49.

do Nascimento, M.B., & Issler, H. (2005). Breastfeeding the premature infant: experience of a baby-friendly hospital in Brazil. *Journal of Human Lactation, 21,* 47-52.

Drake, T.G.H. (1940). The wet nurse in France in the eighteenth century. *Bulletin of the History of Medicine, 8,* 934-948.

Dukes, M.N.G. (2005). *The law and ethics of the pharmaceutical industry.* Amsterdam: Elsevier.

Eberhard-Gran, M., Nordhagen, R., Heiberg, E., Bergsjø, P., & Eskild, A. (2003). Barselomsorg i et tverrkulturelt og historisk perspektiv (Infant care in a cross-cultural and historical perspective). *Tidsskrift for den Norske Lægeforening, 24,* 3553–3556.

Edmond, K., Zandioh, C., Quigley, M.A., Amenga-Etego, S., Owusu-Agyei, S., & Kirkwood, B. (2006). Delayed breastfeeding initiation increases risk of neonatal mortality. *Pediatrics 117,* 380-386.

Eide, I., Heiberg, E., Helsing, E., & Paalgard Pape, K. (2003) *Ammeundersøkelsen år 2000. Mor, barn og materutiner ved norske fødeenheter* (The breast feeding survey year 2000. Mother, child and feeding routines in Norwegian materinty units). Oslo: Helsetilsynet (Norwegian Board of Health).

Einarson, A. & Riordan, S. (2009). Smoking in pregnancy and lactation: a review of risks and cessation strategies. *European Journal of Clinical Pharmacology, 4*, 325-30.

Ekström, A., Widström, A.M., & Nissen, E. (2003a). Breastfeeding support from partners and grandmothers: perceptions of Swedish women. *Birth, 30*, 261-266.

Ekström, A., Widström, A.M., & Nissen, E. (2003b). Duration of breastfeeding in Swedish primiparous and multiparous women. *Journal of Human Lactation, 19*, 172-178.

Erlandsson, K., Dsilna, A., Fagerberg, I., & Christensson, K. (2007). Skin-to-skin care with the father after cesarean birth and its effect on newborn crying and prefeeding behavior. *Birth, 34*, 105-114.

Fairbairn, J.S. (1914). *A text-book for midwives.* London: Oxford Medical Publications.

Fisher, D. (2010). Social drugs and breastfeeding: Handling an issue that isn't black and white. Retrieved on July 22, 2011, from http://www.health-e-learning.com/resources/articles/40-social-drugs-and-breastfeeding.

Flacking, R., Nyqvist, K.H., Ewald, U., & Wallin, L. (2003). Long-term duration of breastfeeding in Swedish low birth weight infants. *Journal of Human Lactation, 19*, 157-165.

Flint, A., New, K., & Davies, M.W. (2007). Cup feeding versus other forms of supplemental enteral feeding for newborn infants unable to fully breastfeed. *Cochrane Database Systemic Reviews*, CD005092.

Food and Nutrition Board (US). National Academy of Sciences, Institute of Medicine. (2010). *Maternal nutrition during lactation.* Washington: National Academic Press.

Fortune 500. (2011). Annual ranking of America's largest corporations. Retrieved on August 2, 2011, from http://money.cnn.com/magazines/fortune/fortune500/2011/index.html.

Friedman, N.J., & Zeiger, R.S. (2005). The role of breast-feeding in the development of allergies and asthma. *The Journal of Allergy and Clinical Immunology, 115*, 1238-1248.

Funk, C. (1912). The etiology of the deficiency diseases. *Journal of State Medicine, 20*, 341-368.

Funkquist, E.L., Tuvemo, T., Jonsson, B., Serenius, F., & Nyqvist, K.H. (2010). Influence of test weighing before/after nursing on breastfeeding in preterm infants. *Advances in Neonatal Care, 10*, 33-39.

Garrison, M.M., & Christakis, D.A. (2000). A systematic review of treatments for infant colic. *Pediatrics, 106*, 184-190.

Gathwala, G., Singh, B., & Singh, J. (2010). Effect of Kangaroo Mother Care on physical growth, breastfeeding and its acceptability. *Tropical Doctor, 40,* 199-202.

Geddes, D.T. (2007). Inside the lactating breast: the latest anatomy research. *The Journal of Midwifery & Women's Health, 52,* 556-563.

Gerstenberger, H.J., & Ruh, H.O. (1919). Studies in the adaptation of an artificial food to human milk. II. A report of three years' clinical experience with the feeding of S.M.A. (synthetic milk adapted). *American Journal of the Diseases of Children, 1,* 1-37.

Gomes, C.F., Trezza, E.M., Murade, E.C., & Padovani, C.R. (2006). Surface electromyography of facial muscles during natural and artificial feeding of infants. *Jornal de Pediatria (Rio J.), 82,* 103-109.

Gray, R. (2011, April 2). Genetically modified cows produce "human" milk. *Daily Telegraph* (London), p.13.

Griffin, T.L., Meier, P.P., Bradford, L.P., Bigger, H.R., & Engstrom, J.L. (2000). Mothers' performing creamatocrit measures in the NICU: accuracy, reactions, and cost. *Journal of Obstetric, Gynecologic, and Neonatal Nursing, 29,* 249-257.

Gupta, A., Khanna, K., & Chattree, S. (1999). Cup feeding: an alternative to bottle feeding in a neonatal intensive care unit. *Journal of Tropical Pediatrics, 45,* 108-110.

Häggkvist, A.P., Brantsaeter, A.L., Grjibovski, A.M., Helsing, E., Meltzer, H.M., & Haugen, M. (2010). Prevalence of breast-feeding in the Norwegian Mother and Child Cohort Study and health service-related correlates of cessation of full breast-feeding. *Public Health Nutrition, 13,* 2076-2086.

Hake-Brooks, S.J., & Anderson, G.C. (2008). Kangaroo care and breastfeeding of mother-preterm infant dyads 0-18 months: a randomized, controlled trial. *Neonatal Network, 27,* 151-159.

Hale, T.W. (2010). *Medications and mothers' milk* (14th ed.). Amarillo, TX: Hale Publishing.

Hall, B. (1975) Changing composition of milk and early development of an appetite control. *Lancet, 1*(7910), 779-781.

Hall, B.M., & Oxberry, J.M. (1977). Comparative studies on milk lipids and neonatal brain development. In M. Peaker (Ed.), *Comparative aspects of lactation. Symposia of the Zoological Society of London, 41.* New York: Academic Press.

Hanson, L.Å. (2004). *Immunobiology of human milk: How breastfeeding protects babies.* Amarillo, TX: Pharmasoft Publishing.

Hanson, L.A. (2007). The role of breastfeeding in the defense of the child. In T.W. Hale & P.E. Hartmann, *Textbook of human lactation* (pp. 159-192). Amarillo, TX: Hale Publishing.

Haschke, F., Pietschnig, B., Karg, V., Vanura, H., & Schuster, E. (1987). Radioactivity in Austrian milk after the Chernobyl accident. *New England Journal of Medicine, 7,* 409-410.

Hedberg, N.K., & Ewald, U. (1999). Infant and maternal factors in the development of breastfeeding behaviour and breastfeeding outcome in preterm infants. *Acta Paediatrica, 88,* 1194-1203.

Heiberg Endresen, E., & Helsing, E. (1995). Changes in breastfeeding practices in Norwegian maternity wards: national surveys 1973, 1982 and 1991. *Acta Paediatrica, 7,* 719–724.

Helsing, E. (2000). Vitamins. In M.N.G. Dukes & J. Aronson (Eds.), *Meylers's side effects of drugs* (14th ed., pp. 1338-1363). Amsterdam: Elsevier Science B.V.

Hendrickse, R.G. (1976). Socio-economic and psychological factors in breast feeding motivation. *Bulletin of the International Pediatric Association, 6,* 37–42.

Hess, J. (1996). *Menschenaffen mutter und kind* (Apes, mother and child). Basel: Friedrich Reinhardt Verlag.

Hillervik-Lindquist, C., Hofvander, Y., & Sjolin, S. (1991). Studies on perceived breast milk insufficiency. III. Consequences for breast milk consumption and growth. *Acta Paediatrica Scandinavica, 80,* 297-303.

Ho, E., Collantes, A., Bhushan, M.K., Moretta, M., & Koren, G. (2001). Alcohol and breastfeeding: Calculation of time to zero level in milk. *Biology of the Neonate, 3,* 219-222.

Hönerbach, F. (2005). Flammschutzmittel in Muttermilch - in Deutschland kein Risiko für Säuglinge. Stillen bleibt die beste Ernährung für Säuglinge. (Flame retardants in breast milk - no risk to infants in Germany. Breastfeeding remains the best nutrition for infants.) Bundesinstitut für Risikobewertung. *Gemeinsame Presseinformation des Umweltbundesamtes und des Bundesinstituts für Risikobewertung, 24.*

Hormann, E. (2006). *Breastfeeding an adopted baby and relactation.* Schaumburg, IL: La Leche League International.

Hörnell, A., Aarts, C., Kylberg, E., Hofvander, Y., & Gebre-Medhin, M. (1999). Breastfeeding patterns in exclusively breastfed infants: a longitudinal prospective study in Uppsala, Sweden. *Acta Paediatrica, 88,* 203-211.

Høst, A. (1994). Cow's milk protein allergy and intolerance in infancy. Some clinical, epidemiological and immunological aspects. *Pediatric Allergy and Immunology, 5,* 1-36.

Høst, A., Halken, S., Muraro, A., Dreborg, S., Niggemann, B., Aalberse, R., et al. (2008). Dietary prevention of allergic diseases in infants and small children. *Pediatric allergy and immunology, 19,* 1-4.

Howard, C.R., Howard, F.M., Lanphear, B., Eberly, S., deBlieck, E.A., Oakes, D., et al. (2003). Randomized clinical trial of pacifier use and bottle-feeding or cupfeeding and their effect on breastfeeding. *Pediatrics, 111,* 511-518.

Hurst, N.M., & Meier, P. (2010). Breastfeeding the preterm infant. In J. Riordan (Ed.), *Breastfeeding and human lactation* (pp. 425-470). Boston: Jones & Bartlett.

Hurst, N.M., Meier, P.P., Engstrom, J.L., & Myatt, A. (2004). Mothers performing in-home measurement of milk intake during breastfeeding of their preterm infants: maternal reactions and feeding outcomes. *Journal of Human Lactation, 20*(2), 178-187.

Hurst, N.M., Valentine, C.J., Renfro, L., Burns, P., & Ferlic, L. (1997). Skin-to-skin holding in the neonatal intensive care unit influences maternal milk volume. *Journal of Perinatology, 17,* 213-217.

Hytten, F.E. (1954). Clinical and chemical studies in human lactation.

I. Collection of milk samples. *British Medical Journal, 1*(4855),175-176;

II. Variations in the major constituents during a feeding. *British Medical Journal, 1*(4855), 176-179;

III. Diurnal variations in major constituents of milk. *British Medical Journal, 1*(4855), 179-182; VI. The functional capacity of the breast. *British Medical Journal, 1*(4867), 912-915;

VIII. Relationship of the age, physique, and nutritional status of the mother to the yield and composition of milk. *British Medical Journal, 2*(4892), 844-845;

VII. The effect of the differences in yield and composition of milk on the infant's weight gain and the duration of breast-feeding. *British Medical Journal. 1*(4876), 1410-1413;

IX. Breast feeding in hospital. *British Medical Journal, 2*(4902), 1447-1452.

Interagency Group on Breastfeeding Monitoring (IGBM). (1997). *Cracking the Code, monitoring the International Code of Marketing of Breast-Milk Substitutes.* London: IGBM.

International Monetary Fund. (April 2011). *World economic outlook database.* Retrieved on August 2, 2011, from http://www.imf.org/external/pubs/ft/weo/2011/01/weodata/index.aspx.

Ip, S., Chung, M., Raman, G., Trikalinos, T.A., & Lau, J. (2009). A summary of the Agency for Healthcare Research and Quality's evidence report on breastfeeding in developed countries. *Breastfeeding Medicine, 4 Suppl 1,* S17-S30.

IPCS (International Programme on Chemical Studies). (1992). Summary of toxicological evaluations performed by the joint FAO/WHO meeting on pesticide residues (JMPR). *International Programme on Chemical Safety WHO/PCS/93.11.* Geneva: World Health Organization.

Istituto di Ricovero. (2003). *Promotion of breastfeeding in Europe: Protection, promotion and support of breastfeeding in Europe: current situation.* Trieste: Istituto di Ricovero "Buro Garofolo."

Ivarsson, A. (2005). The Swedish epidemic of coeliac disease explored using an epidemiologic approach - some lessons to be learnt. *Best Practice & Research. Clinical Gastroenterology, 3,* 425-440.

Jelliffe, D.B., & Jelliffe, E.F.P. (1978). *Human milk in the modern world.* Oxford: Oxford University Press.

Jenness, R. (1979). The composition of human milk. *Seminars in Perinatology, 3,* 225-239.

Johannessen, A.K. (1902). In A. Arstal (Ed.) *Forældre og Børn: En bog om hjemmets oppgaver af forældre og barnevenner* (Parents and children : a book about the tasks in a home, by parents and friends of the child). Kristiania (Oslo): H. Aschehoug & Co.

Jones, E., Dimmock, P.W., & Spencer, S.A. (2001). A randomised controlled trial to compare methods of milk expression after preterm delivery. *Archives of Disease in Childhood. Fetal & Neonatal Edition, 85,* 91-95.

Jones, E.A. (1977.) Synthesis and secretion of milk sugars. In M. Peaker, *Comparative aspects of lactation.* New York: Academic Press.

Kendall-Tackett, K.A. (2007). Violence against women and the perinatal period: the impact of lifetime violence and abuse on pregnancy, postpartum, and breastfeeding. *Trauma Violence Abuse, 8,* 344-353.

Kendall-Tackett, K.A. (2010). *Depression in new mothers: causes, consequences, and treatment alternatives* (2nd ed.). London: New York.

Kent, J.C., Mitoulas, L.R., Cregan, M.D., Ramsay, D.T., Doherty, D.A., & Hartmann, P.E. (2006). Volume and frequency of breastfeedings and fat content of breast milk throughout the day. *Pediatrics, 117,* e387-e395.

Kesäniemi, Y.A. (1974). Ethanol and acetaldehyde in the milk and peripheral blood of lactating women after ethanol administration. *The Journal of Obstetrics and Gynaecology of the British Commonwealth, 1,* 84-86.

Kesho Bora Study Group. (2011). *Preventing mother-to-child transmission of HIV during breastfeeding.* WHO Policy Brief: WHO.RHR/11.01. Geneva: World Health Organization.

King, J., & Ashworth, A. (1987). Historical review of the changing pattern of infant feeding in developing countries: the case of Malaysia, the Caribbean, Nigeria and Zaire. *Social Science & Medicine, 12,* 1307–1320.

Konner, M., & Worthman, C. (1980). Nursing frequency, gonadal function, and birth spacing among ¡Kung hunter-gatherers. *Science, 207,* 788-791.

Kramer, M.S., Chalmers, B., Hodnett, E.D., Sevkovskaya, Z., Dzikovich, I., Shapiro, S., et al. (2001). Promotion of Breastfeeding Intervention Trial (PROBIT): a randomized trial in the Republic of Belarus. *JAMA, 285,* 413-420.

Kristiansen, A.L., Lande, B., Øverby, N.C., & Andersen, L.F. (2010). Factors associated with exclusive breast-feeding and breast-feeding in Norway. *Public Health Nutrition, 13,* 2087-2096.

Kronborg, H., & Vaeth, M. (2004). The influence of psychosocial factors on the duration of breastfeeding. *Scandinavian Journal of Public Health, 32,* 210-216.

Lago, P., Garetti, E., Merazzi, D., Pieragostini, L., Ancora, G., Pirelli, A., et al. (2009). Guidelines for procedural pain in the newborn. *Acta Paediatrica, 98*, 932-939.

Lai, C.T., Hale, T.W., Simmer, K., & Hartmann, P.E. (2010). Measuring milk synthesis in breastfeeding mothers. *Breastfeeding Medicine, 3*, 103-7.

LaKind, J., Berlin, C., & Mattison, D. (2008). The heart of the matter on breastmilk and environmental chemicals: essential points for health care providers, new parents. *Breastfeeding Medicine, 3*, 251-259.

Lande, B., & Frost Andersen, L. (2005). *Landsomfattende kostholdsundersøkelse – Småbarnskost* (National nutrition survey. Young children's diet). Oslo: Helsedirektoratet, Avdeling for ernæring.

Lande, B., Andersen, L.F., Baerug, A., Trygg, K.U., Lund-Larsen, K., Veierød, M.B., et al. (2003). Infant feeding practices and associated factors in the first six months of life: the Norwegian infant nutrition survey. *Acta Paediatrica, 92*, 152-161.

Lande, B., Andersen, L.F., Veierød, M.B., Baerug, A., Johansson, L., Trygg, K.U., & Bjørneboe, G.E. (2004). Breast-feeding at 12 months of age and dietary habits among breast-fed and non-breast-fed infants. *Public Health Nutrition, 7*, 495-503.

Lawrence, R.A. (2011). Breastfeeding in the face of natural disaster and nuclear reactor core damage. *Breastfeeding Medicine, 6*, 53-54.

Lawrence, R.A., & Lawrence, R.M. (2005). *Breastfeeding: A guide for the medical profession* (6th ed., p. 115). New York: Mosby.

Lawton, M.E. (1985). Alcohol in breast milk. *The Australian and New Zealand Journal of Obstetrics and Gynaecology, 1*, 71-73.

Li, R., Zhao, Z., Mokdad, A., Barker, L., & Grummer-Strawn, L. (2003). Prevalance of breastfeeding in the United States. *Pediatrics, 111*, 1198-1201.

Liddiard, M. (1946). *The mothercraft manual or the expectant and nursing mother and baby's first two years.* London: J. & A. Churchill Ltd.

Liestøl, K., Rosenberg, M., & Walløe, L. (1988). Breast-feeding practice in Norway 1860-1984. *Journal of Biosocial Science, 20*, 45-58.

Lindberg, T. (1999). Infantile colic and small intestinal function: a nutritional problem? *Acta Paediatrica Supplement, 88*, 58-60.

Lindemann, R., & Christensen, G.C. (1987). Radioactivity in breastmilk after the Chernobyl accident. *Acta Paediatrica Scandinavica, 6*, 981-986.

Lithell, U.B. (1999). *Små barn under knappa villkor* (Small children under poor conditions). En studie av bakgrunden till minskningen av dödligheten bland spädbarn under förra hälften av 1800- och 1900-talet i Sverige. Karlstad: Universitetstryckeriet.

Little, R.E., Anderson, K.W., Ervin, C.H., Worthington-Roberts, B., & Clarren, S.K. (1989). Maternal alcohol use during breast-feeding and infant mental and motor development at one year. *New England Journal of Medicine, 7*, 425-430.

Liu, J.M., Ren, A., Yang, L., Gao, J., Pei, L., Ye, R., Qu, Q., & Zheng, X. (2010). Urinary tract abnormalities in Chinese rural children who consumed melamine contaminated dairy products: a population-based screening and follow- up study. *Canadian Medical Association Journal, 5,* 439-443.

Ljungberg, T. (1991). *Människan, kulturen och evolutionen. Et alternativt perspektiv.* (Humans, culture and evolution. An alternative perspective.) Nyköping: Exiris.

Lozoff, B., Brittenham, G.M., Trause, M.A., Kennell, J.H., & Klaus, M.H. (1977). The mother-newborn relationship: limits of adaptability. *The Journal of Pediatrics, 91,* 1-12.

Marinelli, K.A., Burke, G.S., & Dodd, V.L. (2001). A comparison of the safety of cupfeedings and bottlefeedings in premature infants whose mothers intend to breastfeed. *Journal of Perinatology, 21,* 350-355.

Marx, K. (1954). *Capital* (Vol. 1, p 372, Section 3.a). Moscow: Progress Publishers.

Matheson, I., & Rivrud, G.N. (1989). The effect of smoking on lactation and infantile colic. *The Journal of the American Medical Association, 1,* 42-43.

Meier, P.P., Furman, L.M., & Degenhardt, M. (2007). Increased lactation risk for late preterm infants and mothers: evidence and management strategies to protect breastfeeding. *The Journal of Midwifery and Women's Health, 52,* 579-587.

Mennella, J.A. (2007). Chemical senses and the development of flavor preferences in humans. In T.W. Hale & P.E. Hartmann (Eds.), *Textbook of human lactation* (pp. 403-413). Amarillo, TX: Hale Publishing, L.P.

Mennella, J.A. (2009). Flavor programming during breast-feeding. *Advances in Experimental Medicine and Biology, 639,* 113-120.

Mennella, J.A., & Beauchamp, G.K. (1991). The transfer of alcohol to human milk. Effects on flavor and the infant's behavior. *The New England Journal of Medicine, 14,* 981-85.

Mennella, J.A. (1997). Infants' suckling responses to the flavor of alcohol in mothers' milk. *Alcoholism, Clinical and Experimental Research, 4,* 581-585.

Merewood, A., Philipp, B.L., Chawla, N., & Cimo, S. (2003). The baby-friendly hospital initiative increases breastfeeding rates in a US neonatal intensive care unit. *Journal of Human Lactation, 19,* 166-171.

Merlin, H. (1994). *Le don de lait maternel en France* (Milk banks in France). *La Revue Prescrire, 140,* 283-286.

Merten, S., Dratva, J., & Ackermann-Liebrich, U. (2005). Do baby-friendly hospitals influence breastfeeding duration on a national level? *Pediatrics, 116,* e702-e708.

Mes, J., Davies, D.J., Doucet, J., Weber, D., & McMullen, E. (1993). Levels of chlorinated hydrocarbon residues in Canadian human breast milk and their relationship to some characteristics of the donors. *Food Additives and Contaminants, 4,* 429-441.

Meyer, H.F. (1968). Breastfeeding in the United States. Report of a 1966 national survey with comparable 1946 and 1956 data. *Clinical Pediatrics, 12,* 708-715.

Meyer, L. (1899). *Den første barnepleje. Populært fremstillet* (Early Infant Care) (3rd ed.). København: Det Nordiske Forlag. Published both in Norway and Denmark.

Milliard, A.V. (1990). The place of the clock in pediatric advice: rationales, cultural themes and impediments to breastfeeding. *Social Science & Medicine, 2,* 211–221.

Ministry of Health and Care Services. (2009). *Forskrift om barns opphold i helseinstitusjon, FOR 2000-12-01 nr 1217. (Regulation of childrens rights when hospitalized.).* Retrieved on August 2, 2011, from http://www.lovdata.no/cgi-wift/ldles?doc=/sf/sf/sf-20001201-1217.html.

Mitoulas, L.R., Kent, J.C., Cox, D.B., Owens, R.A., Sherriff, J.L., & Hartmann, P.E. (2002). Variation in fat, lactose and protein in human milk over 24 h and throughout the first year of lactation. *British Journal of Nutrition, 88*(1), 29-37.

Monrad, S. (1952). *Moderens bog* (The mother's book) (9th ed.). København: Gyldendalske Boghandel, Nordisk Forlag.

Moore, E.R., Anderson, G.C., & Bergman, N. (2007). Early skin-to-skin contact for mothers and their healthy newborn infants. *Cochrane Database of Systematic Reviews,* CD003519.

Neville, M.C., & Neifert, M.R. (1983). *Lactation: Physiology, nutrition and breast-feeding.* New York: Plenum Press.

Newman, J., & Pitman, T. (2000a). Colic. In *The Ultimate Breastfeeding Book of Answers* (pp. 175-199). Roseville: Prima Publishing.

Newman, J., & Pitman, T. (2000b). *The Ultimate Breastfeeding Book of Answers* (1st ed.) Roseville: Prima Publishing.

Newton, M., & Newton, N.R. (1948). The let-down reflex in human lactation. *The Journal of Pediatrics, 33,* 698-704.

New Zealand Ministry of Health. (2002). New Zealand's breastfeeding rates: Statistics from breastfeeding: A guide to action. Wellington: Ministry of Health.

Nissen, E., Widstrom, A.M., Lilja, G., Matthiesen, A.S., Uvnas-Moberg, K., Jacobsson, G., et al. (1997). Effects of routinely given pethidine during labor on infants' developing breastfeeding behavior. Effects of dose-delivery time interval and various concentrations of pethidin/norpethidine in cord plasma. *Acta Paediatrica, 86,* 201-208.

Njå, A. (1965). Guide to infant nutrition and care. Norway: Board of Health.

NOMESCO (Nordic Medico-Statistical Committee). (2005). *Health Statistics in the Nordic Countries 2003.* Copenhagen.

Norwegian Board of Health. (2002). *Smittevernloven: drift og organisering av morsmelkbanker* (Law on immunization: The management and organization of milk banks). Oslo: Norwegian Board of Health.

Norwegian Directorate of Health, Food Insectorate, & University of Oslo. (2009). *Spedkost 2006-2007. Landsomfattende kostholdsundersøkelse blant 6 måneder gamle barn National.* (The Norwegian Infant Nutrition Survey). Retrieved June 7, 2011, from http://www.helsedirektoratet.no/publikasjoner/rapporter/rapport__spedkost_6_m_neder__2008__185414.

Norwegian Resource Centre for Breastfeeding, Rikshospitalet, Oslo University Hospital. (2008). *Breast is beast.* HEALTH-INFO, Video Vital.

Nyqvist, K.H. (2008). Early attainment of breastfeeding competence in very preterm infants. *Acta Paediatrica, 97,* 776-781.

Nyqvist, K.H., Anderson, G.C., Bergman, N., Cattaneo, A., Charpak, N., Davanzo, R., et al. (2010a). Towards universal kangaroo mother care: recommendations and report from the First European Conference and Seventh International Workshop on Kangaroo Mother Care. *Acta Paediatrica, 99,* 820-826.

Nyqvist, K.H., Anderson, G.C., Bergman, N., Cattaneo, A., Charpak, N., Davanzo, R., et al. (2010b). State of the art and recommendations. Kangaroo mother care: application in a high-tech environment. *Acta Paediatrica, 99,* 812-819.

Odent, M. (2004). Nursing the caesarean born. *Midwifery Today with International Midwife,* Spring (69), 40-41.

Odijk van, J., Kull, I., Borres, M.P., Brandtzaeg, P., Edberg, U., Hanson, L.A., et al. (2003). Breastfeeding and allergic disease: a multidisciplinary review of the literature (1966-2001) on the mode of early feeding in infancy and its impact on later atopic manifestations. *Allergy, 58,* 833-843.

Oftedal, O.T. (1997). Lactation in whales and dolphins: evidence of divergence between baleen- and toothed-species. *Journal of Mammary Gland Biology and Neoplasia, 3,* 205-230.

Ohyama, M., Watabe, H., & Hayasaka, Y. (2010). Manual expression and electric breast pumping in the first 48 h after delivery. *Pediatrics International, 52,* 39-43.

Ólafsson, E. (1772). *Reise gjennom Island* (Travel through Iceland). Sorøe: Videnskabernes Selskab.

Øverby, N.C., Kristiansen, A.L., Frost Andersen, L., & Lande, B. (2008). *Spedkost 12 måneder. Landsomfattende kostholdsundersøkelse blant 12 måneder gamle barn.* (The Norwegian nutrition survey among 12 months old children). Oslo: The Board of Health. Available from http://www.helsedirektoratet.no/vp/multimedia/archive/00110/Spedkost_12_m_neder_110659a.pdf.

Peaker, M. (1977). The aqueous phase of milk: ion and water transport. In M. Peaker (Ed.), *Comparative aspects of lactation. Symposia of The Zoological Society of London No. 41* (pp. 113-134). New York: Academic Press.

Pedersen, C.A., & Prange, A.J. (1985). Oxytocin and mothering behavior in the rat. *Pharmacology & Therapeutics, 28,* 287-302.

Pérez-Escamilla, R. (1993). Breastfeeding patterns in nine Latin American and Caribbean countries. *Bulletin of the Pan American Health Organization, 1,* 23-42.

Persson, L.A., Ivarsson, A., & Hernell, O. (2002). Breast-feeding protects against celiac disease in childhood--epidemiological evidence. *Advances in Experimental Medicine and Biology, 503,* 115-123.

Pickthall, M.M. (1948). *The meaning of the glorious Koran.* Beirut: Dar El Fikr.

Pinelli, J., & Symington, A. (2005). Non-nutritive sucking for promoting physiologic stability and nutrition in preterm infants. *Cochrane Database of Systematic Reviews, 4.*

Powers, N.G. (2010). Low intake in the breastfed infant: Maternal and infant considerations. In J. Riordan & K. Wambach (Eds.), *Breastfeeding and human lactation* (pp. 325-363). Boston: Jones & Bartlett.

Prentice, A.M., Goldberg, G.R., & Prentice, A. (1994). Body mass index and lactation performance. *European Journal of Clinical Nutrition, 48* (Supplement 3), S78-S89.

Ramos, R., Kennedy, K.I., & Visness, C.M. (1996). Effectiveness of lactational amenorrhoea in prevention of pregnancy in Manila, the Philippines: non-comparative prospective trail. *BMJ, 313,* 909-912.

Ramsay, D.T., Kent, J.C., Hartmann, R.A., & Hartmann, P.E. (2005). Anatomy of the lactating human breast redefined with ultrasound imaging. *Journal of Anatomy, 206,* 525-534.

Ramsay, D.T., Kent, J.C., Owens, R.A., & Hartmann, P.E. (2004). Ultrasound imaging of milk ejection in the breast of lactating women. *Pediatrics, 113,* 361-367.

Rebuffe-Scrive, M., Crona, L.E.N., Lønnroth, P., Abrahamsson, L., Smith, U., & Bjørntorp, P. (1985). Fat cell metabolism in different regions in women: effect of menstrual cycle, pregnancy and lactation. *Journal of Clinical Investigations, 75,* 1973-1976.

Riordan, J., & Wambach, K. (2010). Women's health and breastfeeding. In J. Riordan & K. Wambach (Eds.), *Breastfeeding and human lactation* (pp. 519-549). Boston: Jones & Bartlett.

Riordan, J. (2010). The biological specificity of breastmilk. In J. Riordan & K. Wambach (Eds.). *Breastfeeding and human lactation* (pp. 117-162). Boston: Jones & Bartlett.

Rocha, N.M., Martinez, F.E., & Jorge, S.M. (2002). Cup or bottle for preterm infants: effects on oxygen saturation, weight gain, and breastfeeding. *Journal of Human Lactation, 18,* 132-138.

Rønneberg, R., & Skåra, B. (1992). Essential fatty acids in human colostrum. *Acta Paediatrica, 81,* 779-783.

Rønnestad, A., Abrahamsen, T.G., Medbø, S., Reigstad, H., Lossius, K., Kaaresen, P. I., et al. (2005). Late-onset septicemia in a Norwegian national cohort of extremely premature infants receiving very early full human milk feeding. *Pediatrics, 115,* e269-e276.

Rotch, T.M. (1890). The management of human breast-milk in cases of difficult infantile digestion. *Transactions of the American Pediatric Society, 2*, 88-100.

Saarinen, U.M., & Siimes, M.A. (1979). Iron absorption from breast milk, cow's milk and iron-supplemented formula: an opportunistic use of changes in total body iron determined by hemoglobin, ferritin and body weight in 132 infants. *Pediatric Research, 13*, 143-147.

Schluter, P.J., Carter, S., & Percival, T. (2006). Exclusive and any breast-feeding rates of Pacific infants in Auckland: data from the Pacific Islands Families First Two Years of Life Study. *Public Health of Nutrition, 9*, 692-699.

Sedgwick, J.P. (1921). A preliminary report of the study of breast feeding in Minneapolis. *American Journal of Diseases of Children, 5*, 455–464.

Shillito Walser, E. (1977). Maternal behaviour in mammals. In M. Peaker (Ed.), *Comparative Aspects of Lactation. Symposia of the Zoological Society of London No. 41* (pp 313-331). New York: Academic Press.

Siimes, M.A., Salmenperä, L., & Perheentupa, J. (1984). Exclusive breast-feeding for 9 months: risk of iron deficiency. *The Journal of Pediatrics, 2*, 196-199.

Skjerve, K. (1916) *Sundhedslære for unge kvinner* (Health Knowledge for Young Women). Oslo: Aschehoug.

Skullerud, K. (1995). Å være nær. En fars beretning om to fødsler (To be close. The father's story of two different birth experiences) Oslo: Exlex forlag.

Slusher, T., Hampton, R., Bode-Thomas, F., Pam, S., Akor, F., & Meier, P. (2003). Promoting the exclusive feeding of own mother's milk through the use of hindmilk and increased maternal milk volume for hospitalized, low birth weight infants (< 1800 grams) in Nigeria: a feasibility study. *Journal of Human Lactation, 19*, 191-198.

Smith, L., & Riordan, J. (2010). Postpartum care. In J. Riordan & K. Wambach (Eds.), *Breastfeeding and human lactation* (pp. 253-290). Boston: Jones & Bartlett.

Somoyogi, A., & Beck, H. (1993). Nurturing and breast-feeding: exposure to chemicals in breast milk. *Environmental Health Perspectives, Suppl 2*, 45-52.

Søndergaard, C., Henriksen, T.B., Obel, C., & Wisborg, K. (2001). Smoking during pregnancy and infantile colic. *Pediatrics, 108(2)*, 342-346.

Stenhammar, A., Ohrlander, K., Stark, U., & Söderlind, I. (2001) *Mjölkdroppen – Filantropi, förmynderi eller samhällsansvar?* (The milk drop [organization] – Philanthropy, guardianship or community responsibility?) Stockholm: Carlsson bokförlag.

Sundal, A. (1944). *Mor og barn* (Mother and baby) (8th ed.). Oslo: Fabritius & Sønner.

Sundal, A. (1939). *Mor og barn* (Mother and child) (2nd ed., p.73). Oslo: Fabritius & Sønner.

Taveras, E.M., Capra, A.M., Braveman, P.A., Jensvold, N.G., Escobar, G.J., & Lieu, T.A. (2003). Clinician support and psychosocial risk factors associated with breastfeeding discontinuation. *Pediatrics, 112*, 108-115.

Taylor, A. (1998). Violations of the international code of marketing of breast milk substitutes: prevalence in four countries. *British Medical Journal (Clinical research edition), 7138*, 1117-1122.

Thygarajan, A., & Burks, A.W. (2008). American Academy of Pediatrics recommendations on the effects of early nutritional interventions on the development of atopic disease. *Current Opinion in Pediatrics, 20,* 698-702.

Truby King, F. (1908). *Feeding and care of baby.* Wellington, New Zealand: Whitcombe and Tombs.

Tufte, E. (2005). *Norske kvinners ammeproblemer* (Breastfeeding problems among Norwegian women). Master of Public Health thesis, MPH 2005:32. Gøteborg: Nordiska högskolan för folkhälsovetenskap.

United Nations. (1990). *Convention on the rights of the child.* Retrieved May 14, 2011, from http://www2.ohchr.org/english/law/crc.htm#art5.

Uvnäs-Moberg, K., & Eriksson, M. (1996). Breastfeeding: physiological, endocrine and behavioral adaptations caused by oxytocin and local neurogenic activity in the nipple and mammary gland. *Acta Paediatrica, 85,* 525-530.

Uvnäs-Moberg, K. (2003). *The oxytocin factor: tapping the hormone of calm, love, and healing.* Cambridge, MA: Da Capo Press.

Van Acker, J., de Smet, F., Muyldermans, G., Bougatef, A., Naessens, A., & Lauwers, S. (2001). Outbreak of necrotizing enterocolitis associated with Enterobacter sakazakii in powdered infant formulas. *Journal of Clinical Microbiology, 1,* 293-297.

Van Look, P.F. (1996). Lactational amenorrhoea method for family planning. *BMJ, 313,* 893-894.

Vaz, R., Slorach, S.A., & Hofvander, Y. (1993). Organochlorine contaminants in Swedish human milk: studies conducted at the National Food Administration 1981-1990. *Food Additives and Contaminants, 4,* 407-418.

Vekemans, M. (1997). Postpartum contraception: the lactational amenorrhea method. *European Journal of Contraception and Reproductive Health Care, 2,* 105-111.

Vorherr, H. (1974.) *The breast-morphology, physiology, and lactation.* New York: Academic Press.

Wagner, G., & Fuchs, A.R. (1968). Effect of ethanol on uterine activity during suckling in post-partum women. *Acta Endocrinologica (Copenhagen), 1,* 133-141.

Wallace, J.P., Inbar, G., & Ernsthausen, K. (1992). Infant acceptance of post-exercise breast milk. *Pediatrics, 89,* 1245-1247.

Webb, B.H., Johnson, A.H., & Alford, J.A. (1974). Fundamentals of dairy chemistry (2nd ed.). Westport, CT: AVI Publishing Company.

Weir, E. (2002). Powdered infant formula and fatal infection with Enterobacter sakazakii. *Canadian Medical Association Journal, 12,* 1570.

Weiser-Aall, L. (1973). *Omkring de nyfødtes stell i nyere norsk overlevering* (Around the care of newborns in recent Norwegian history). Småskrifter fra Norsk Etnologisk Gransking, Nr. 8. Oslo: Norsk Folkemuseum.

West, D., & Marasco, L. (2009). *The breastfeeding mother's guide to making more milk.* New York: McGraw-Hill.

Westcott, T.S. (1900). The scientific modification of milk. *International Clinics, 3,* 235.

Whitelaw, A., & Sleath, K. (1985). Myth of the marsupial mother: home care of very low birth weight babies in Bogota, Colombia. *Lancet, 1,* 1206-1208.

WHO. (2003). *Kangaroo mother care. A practical guide.* Geneva: Department of Reproductive Health and Research, World Health Organization.

WHO. (2009a). *Baby-friendly hospital initiative. Revised, updated and expanded for integrated care.* Geneva: UNICEF and World Health Organization.

WHO. (1981). *Contemporary patterns of breast-feeding. Report on the WHO Collaborative Study on Breast-feeding* (p. 149). Geneva: World Health Organization.

WHO, Edmond, K., & Bahl, R. (2006). *Optimal feeding of low-birth-weight infants: Technical review.* Geneva: WHO Department of Child and Adolescent Health and Development.

WHO. (2001). *The optimal duration of exclusive breastfeeding. Report of an Expert Group.* Geneva: WHO.

WHO. (2009b). *WHO child growth standards.* Retrieved on July 26, 2011, from http://www.who.int/childgrowth/en/.

WHO. (1987). *Weaning food in the 1980ies. Pilot analysis of information material for parents in three European countries.* Copenhagen: Nutrition Unit, WHO Regional Office for Europe1987. ICP/NUT 102/s06.

WHO/CAH. (1998). *Relactation: Review of experience and recommendations for practice.* Document WHO/CAH/98.14. Geneva: World Health Organization, Department of Child and Adolescent Health.

WHO, UNAIDS, UNFPA, & UNICEF. (2010). *Guidelines on HIV and infant feeding. Principles and recommandations for infant feeding in the context of HIV and a summary of evidence.* Geneva: WHO.

Wickes, I.G. (1953). A history of infant feeding: Part IV – Nineteenth century continued. *Archives of Disease in Childhood, 141,* 416–422.

Widström, A.M., Ransjö-Arvidson, A.B., Christensson, K., Matthiesen, A.S., Winberg, J., & Uvnäs-Moberg, K. (1987). Gastric suction in healthy newborn infants. Effects on circulation and developing feeding behavior. *Acta Paediatrica Scandinavia, 76,* 566-572.

Wikipedia. (2011). *List of countries by GDP*. Retrieved on August 2, 2011, from http:// en.wikipedia.org/wiki/List_of_countries_by_GDP_(PPP).

Woodbury, R.M. (1925). Causal factors in infant mortality. *Children's Bureau Publication No 142.* Washington D.C.: US Government Printing Office.

Wyckerheld Bisdom, C.J. (1937). Alcohol and nicotine poisoning in nurslings (abstract). *The Journal of the American Medical Association, 2,* 178.

Zachariassen, G., Faerk, J., Grytter, C., Esberg, B.H., Juvonen, P., & Halken, S. (2010). Factors associated with successful establishment of breastfeeding in very preterm infants. *Acta Paediatrica, 99,* 1000-1004.

APPENDICES

Appendix 1: Sources of Help, Knowledge, and Support

Appendix 2: Recommended Books and Videos

Appendix 3: The International Code of Marketing of Breastmilk Substitutes and Subsequent Relevant World Health Assembly Resolutions: A 10-Point Summary

Appendix 4: The Baby-Friendly Initiative in the Hospital and the Community

Appendix 5: Milk Banks: Contact Addresses

Appendix 6: Human Rights Relevant to Breastfeeding

Appendix 7: The ILO Convention on Maternity Protection

INTRODUCTION

In many countries, there are national or regional bodies providing advice, help, and support to breastfeeding mothers. Many women are likely to find that their own clinic, maternity home, midwifery service, or a lactation consultant can give all the guidance they need. Mothers who would like to look a little further to understand breastfeeding can contact a mother-to-mother support organization that may supply both individual advice and helpful materials, such as informative websites, material on Facebook, breastfeeding blogs, brochures, or videos. The organizations listed below are primarily those working in English-speaking countries; most can readily be contacted by phone or e-mail and have numerous local representatives. At the beginning of this Appendix, we list organizations in many countries providing direct support to mothers, often at the local level.

In addition to mother-to-mother support groups, you will find information about organizations supporting breastfeeding in different ways. *The World Alliance for Breastfeeding Action (WABA)* has links with national associations throughout the world and is developing an electronic "gateway" through which one can identify local support groups. *The International Baby Food Action Network (IBFAN)* is a coalition of voluntary organizations in this field; many of these have their own websites through which they can be contacted. *The International Lactation Consultants Association (ILCA)* is a body bringing together professional lactation consultants to advance the profession of lactation counseling worldwide through leadership, advocacy, professional development, and research.

Appendix 1
SOURCES OF HELP, KNOWLEDGE AND SUPPORT

NATIONAL ORGANIZATIONS

Australia

Australian Breastfeeding Assoc.
Breastfeeding helpline: 1-800-686-2686
1818-1822 Malvern Rd
East Malvern, Victoria 3145
E-mail: info@breastfeeding.asn.au
Website: www.breastfeeding.asn.au

Canada

Canadian Breastfeeding Foundation
Telephone: 514-946-2967
5764 Monkland Ave, Suite 424
Montreal, Quebec, H4A 1E9
E-mail: info@canadianbreastfeedingfoundation.org
Website: www.canadianbreastfeedingfoundation.org

South Africa

La Leche League S.A.
E-mail: nel.esme@gmail.com
Website: www.llli.org*

United Kingdom

National Breastfeeding Helpline
Helpline: 0300-100-0212
Website: www.nationalbreastfeedinghelpline.org.uk/

Association of Breastfeeding Mothers
Enquiries: 020-7813-1481
PO Box 207
Bridgewater, Somerset TA6 7YT
Helpline: 0844-122-949
Website: www.abm.me.uk

Breastfeeding Network
Network: 300-100-310
PO Box 11126
Paisley, Yorkshire, PA2 8YB
Supporterline: 0300-33- 00-771
Website: www.breastfeedingnetwork.org.uk

La Leche League GB
Helpline: 0845-120-2918
PO Box 29
West Bridgeford Nottingham NG2 7NP
Website: www.llli.org*

National Childbirth Trust
Breastfeeding helpline: 0300-330-0771
Alexandra House
Oldham Terrace
Acton, London, W3 6NH
Enquiries: 0300-330-0770
Website: www.nct.org.uk

New Zealand

La Leche League NZ
Enquiries: 04-471-0690
PO Box 50780
Porirua 5240
E-mail: help@lalecheleague.org.nz
Website: www.llli.org*
and local groups

United States

La Leche League
Helpline: 845-120-2918
PO Box 4079
Schaumburg, IL 60168-4079
USA
Website: www.llli.org*
and local groups

* To find your closest La Leche League support, use the map or the list of countries at the website, for the U.S.A., use the list of states.

Other countries: Use the "emap" to find your mother-to-mother support groups at the homepage for www.waba.org, www.breastfeedinggateway.org, or www.llli.org. Use the map or the list of countries at the website, for the U.S.A. the list of states, to find your closest help.

INTERNATIONAL ORGANIZATIONS

La Leche League International (LLLI)
Telephone: 1-800-LALECHE (525-3243)
PO Box 4079
Schaumburg, IL 60168-4079
USA
Fax: 1-847-969-0460
Website: www.llli.org

International Baby Food Action Network (IBFAN)
Telephone: (60-4) 890 5799
Penang, Malaysia
Website: www.ibfan.org

World Alliance for Breastfeeding Action (WABA)
Telephone: (60-4) 658 4816
PO Box 1200
10850 Penang, Malaysia
Website: www.waba.org.my

Note: WABA is currently developing a worldwide directory of breastfeeding support sites for both parents and professionals. This "Breastfeeding Gateway," currently in experimental operation, provides access to many organizations in this field and is accessible on the Internet at www.breastfeedinggateway.org.

International Lactation Consultants Association (ILCA)
Website: www.ilca.org

Baby Milk Action Coalition (BMAC)
Website: www.babymilkaction.org

USEFUL WEBSITES ON BREASTFEEDING AND RELATED ISSUES

Bright Future Lactation Resource Centre Ltd
Website: www.bflrc.com

Biological Nurturing
Website: www.biologicalnurturing.com

Kellymom – breastfeeding and parenting
Website: www.kellymom.com

Ted Greiner's Breastfeeding Website
Website: www.tedgreiner.info

A site for breastfeeding advice
Website: www.breastfeeding.com

All you need about breastfeeding
Website: www.breastfeedingonline.com

Dr. Jack Newmans website
Website: http://www.breastfeedinginc.ca

The kangaroo method
Website: www.kangaroomothercare.com

Healthy Children
Website: www.healthychildren.org
(choose Ages&stages>breastfeeding)

Centers for Disease Control, US government
Website: www.cdc.gov
(choose breastfeeding)

Baby carrying – non profit organization
Website: www.babywearinginternational.org

Baby-Friendly Hospital Initiative
Websites: www.unicef.org & www.who.org
(search for BFHI on both sites)

Baby-Friendly Hospital Initiative in the U.S.A.
Website: www.wellstart.org

Baby-Friendly Hospital Initiative in United Kingdom
Website: www.babyfriendly.org.uk

Infant feeding action coalition in Canada:
Website: www.infactcanada.ca

Breastfeeding Gateway
Website: www.breastfeedinggateway.org
(support, knowledge & organizations)

Appendix 2:
RECOMMENDED BOOKS AND VIDEOS

BOOKS FOR MOTHERS

Bergman, J., & Bergman, N. (2010). *Hold your premie!* Kangaroo Mother Care Promotions (148 pages). Available from: www.kangaroomothercare.com.

Hormann, E. (2007). *Breastfeeding an adopted baby and relactation.* Schaumburg, IL: La Leche League International, (66 pages).

Wiessinger, D., West, D., Pitman, T & La Leche League International. (2010). *The womanly art of breastfeeding* (8th ed.). Ballantine Books (576 pages).

McKenna, J. (2007). *Sleeping with your baby: A parent's guide to cosleeping.* Washington, DC: Platypus Media (128 pages).

Mohrbacher, N. & Kendall-Tackett, K. A. (2010). *Breastfeeding made simple. Seven natural laws for nursing mothers* (2nd ed.). Oakland: New Harbinger Publications, Inc. (337 pages).

Mohrbacher, N. (2005). *The breastfeeding answer book: Pocket guide edition.* Schaumburg, IL: La Leche League International (262 pages).

Newman, J., & Pitman, T. (2006). *The ultimate breastfeeding book of answers* (Rev. ed.). Three Rivers Press (352 pages).

Nylander, G. (2002). *Becoming a mother. From birth to six months.* Berkeley, CA: Ten Speed Press (260 pages).

Pryor, G., & Huggins, K. (2007). *Nursing mother, working mother* (Rev. ed.). Boston, MA: Harvard Common Press (237 pages).

Peterson, A., & Harmer, M. (2009). *Balancing breast and bottle: Reaching your breastfeeding goals.* Amarillo, TX: Hale Publishing (169 pages).

Sears, M., & Sears, W. (2000). *The breastfeeding book: Everything you need to know about nursing your child from birth through weaning.* New York and London: Little, Brown & Co (272 pages).

Uvnäs-Moberg, K. (2003). *The oxytocin factor: Tapping the hormone of calm, love, and healing.* Cambridge, MA: Da Capo Press (240 pages).

West, D., & Marasco, L. (2009). *The breastfeeding mother's guide to making more milk.* New York: McGraw-Hill (304 pages).

West, D. (2001). *Defining your own success. Breastfeeding after breast reduction surgery.* Illinois: La Leche League International.

BOOKS FOR HEALTH PROFESSIONALS

Cadwell, K., & Turner-Maffei, C. (2011). *Case studies in breastfeeding. Problem-solving skills & strategies.* Boston: Jones & Bartlett (195 pages).

Cadwell, K., & Turner-Maffei, C. (2004*). Continuity of care in breastfeeding.* Sudbury MA: Jones & Bartlett Publishers (168 pages).

Colson, S. (2010). *Biological nurturing - New angles on breastfeeding.* Amarillo, TX: Hale Publishing (136 pages).

Genna, C.W. (2007). *Supporting sucking skills.* Boston: Jones & Bartlett (355 pages).

Hale, T.W., & Hartmann, P.E. (2007). *Textbook of human lactation.* Amarillo, Texas: Hale Publishing (662pages).

Hale, T.W. (2010). *Medications and mothers' milk* (14th ed.). Amarillo, TX: Hale Publishing (1262 pages).

Hanson, L.Å. (2004). *Immunobiology of human milk: How breastfeeding protects babies.* Amarillo, TX: Pharmasoft Publishing (241 pages).

Jelliffe, D.B., & Jelliffe, E.F.P. (1979). *Human milk in the modern world.* Oxford: Oxford University Press (510 pages).

Lang, S. (2002). *Breastfeeding special care babies.* Edinburgh: Baillèire Tindall (200 pages).

Lauwers, J., & Swisher, A. (2010). *Counseling the nursing mother* (5th ed.). Sudbury, MA: Jones & Bartlett Publishers (799 pages).

Lauwers, J. (2008). *Quick reference for the lactation professional.* Sudbury, MA: Jones & Bartlett Publishers (176 pages).

Lawrence, R.A., & Lawrence R.M. (2010). *Breastfeeding: A guide for the medical profession* (7th ed.). Maryland Heights, MO: Elsevier Mosby (1128 pages).

Merewood, A., & Philipp, B.L. (2001). *Breastfeeding - conditions and diseases. A reference guide* (1st ed.). Amarillo, TX: Pharmasoft Publishing (267 pages).

Mohrbacher, N., & Stock, J. (2003) *The breastfeeding answer book.* Schaumburg, IL: La Leche League International (720 pages).

Neville, M.C., & Neifert, M.R. (1983). *Lactation: Physiology, nutrition and breast-feeding.* New York NY: Plenum Press (466 pages).

Riordan, J., & Wambach, K. (2010). *Breastfeeding and human lactation* (4th ed.). Boston: Jones & Bartlett (912 pages).

Walker, M. (2009): Breastfeeding management for the clinician: Using the evidence (2nd ed.). Sudbury MA: Jones & Bartlett Publishers (550 pages).

West, D., & Hirsh, E.B. (2008). *Breastfeeding after breast and nipple procedures.* Amarillo, TX: Hale Publishing (60 pages).

Wilson-Clay, B., & Hoover, K. (2008). *The breastfeeding atlas* (4th ed.). Austin, TX: Lactnews Press (206 pages).

RECOMMENDED VIDEOS AND DVDS

Many videos about breastfeeding can be found on the Internet; some can be viewed directly, while others have to be purchased. Do realize that not all videos are equally trustworthy; some are intended to promote particular ideas, and some seem to be designed to advertise products, such as breastmilk substitutes. Some of the best videos are those produced by recognized breastfeeding organizations –search on their websites.

DVD	Year/language in addition to English	Available from
Biological Nurturing	2010	biologicalnurturing.com
Breast is Best (45 min)	2008/ many others	HELSE-INFO@videovital.no
Breastfeeding (30 min)	Norwegian	HELSE-INFO@videovital.no www.ammehjelpen.no/video
Is it possible?...a film about breastfeeding babies with cleft lip and palate (23 min)	Norwegian	HELSE-INFO@videovital.no
Breastfeeding: Mom and I can do that (20 min)	2006	www.iBreastfeeding.com
Baby-Led Breastfeeding. The Mother-Baby Dance (16 min)	2007	www.geddesproduction.com
Breast feeding Techniques That Work! First Attachment (34 min)	1986/2005/Spanish	www.geddesproduction.com
Hold Your Prem!	2010	www.kangaroomothercare.com

Appendix 3:

THE INTERNATIONAL CODE OF MARKETING OF BREASTMILK SUBSTITUTES AND SUBSEQUENT RELEVANT WORLD HEALTH ASSEMBLY RESOLUTIONS: A 10-POINT SUMMARY*

1. Aim: The Code aims to protect and promote breastfeeding by ensuring appropriate marketing and distribution of breastmilk substitutes.

2. Scope: The Code applies to breastmilk substitutes when marketed or otherwise represented as a partial or total replacement for breastmilk. Breastmilk substitutes include foods and beverages such as:

   • Infant formula

   • Follow-up milks

   • Other milk products

   • Baby juices and teas

   • Cereals and vegetable mixes

The Code also applies to feeding bottles and teats.

Since exclusive breastfeeding is recommended for six months, all complementary foods marketed or otherwise represented for use before six months are breastmilk substitutes.

3. Advertising: No advertising of above products to the public.

4. Samples: No free samples to mothers, their families, or healthcare workers.

5. Healthcare facilities: No promotion of products, i.e., no product displays, posters, calendars, or distribution of promotional materials. No use of mothercraft nurses or similar company-paid personnel.

6. Healthcare workers: No gifts or samples to healthcare workers. Product information must be factual and scientific.

7. Supplies & Donations: No free or low-cost supplies of breastmilk substitutes to any part of the healthcare system.

8. Information: Information and educational materials must explain the benefits of breastfeeding, the health hazards associated with bottle-feeding, and the costs of using infant formula.

9. Labels: Product labels must clearly state the superiority of breastfeeding, the need for the advice of a healthcare worker, and a warning about health hazards. No pictures of infants, other pictures, or text idealizing the use of infant formula.

10. Quality: Unsuitable products, such as sweetened condensed milk, should not be promoted for babies. All products should be of a high quality (Codex Alimentarius standards) and take account of the climatic and storage conditions of the country where they are used.

* Code Essentials 1: Annotated International Code of Marketing of Breastmilk Substitutes and subsequent WHA resolutions. ICDC (International Code Documentation Center), Penang, Malaysia, 2008.

Appendix 4:
THE BABY-FRIENDLY INITIATIVE IN THE HOSPITAL AND THE COMMUNITY

INTRODUCTION

The Baby-Friendly Hospital Initiative (BFHI) was developed by the World Health Organization and the United Nations Children's Fund (UNICEF) as a worldwide venture designed to promote breastfeeding and close and early contact between mother and child. In the light of research findings and practical experience, the two organizations drew up a set of ten criteria that would need to be met if a birthing unit was to be recognized as baby friendly.

Following the launch of the Initiative in 1991, however, it soon became clear that if breastfeeding was to enjoy sufficient support and the venture was to have real impact, it should not be limited to hospitals. Supportive care is of great importance in pediatric practice, neonatal intensive care units, and physicians' offices, and more widely in the community. This broader approach is particularly necessary since in some countries mothers and their babies are discharged from the hospital much earlier than was formerly the case. It is reflected in a revised document issued by WHO in 2009 entitled "Baby-Friendly Hospital Initiative: Revised, Updated and Expanded for Integrated Care." [8*]

Because the structure of birthing care has traditionally differed from country to country, the introduction of BFHI principles has not followed precisely the same pattern everywhere. The description that follows reflects in part experience in Norway where the "National Resource Centre for Breastfeeding," under the able leadership of Gro Nylander and Anne Bærug, has been charged with the introduction of the Initiative and

---

8   [*] WHO, UNICEF (2009): Baby-friendly Hospital Initiative: Revised, updated and expanded for integrated Care. ISBN 978 92 4 159495 0.

ensuring adherence to its standards; similar arrangements have been made in many other countries.

You can expect the following standard of care from a Baby Friendly Hospital:

Arrangements for breastfeeding will be clear, and will be set out for parents in a readily understood form. The Unit will provide its staff with breastfeeding training, so you can expect complete and up-to-date guidance from all the staff working with you.

During your pregnancy, the benefits of breastmilk will be explained to you, and you will be shown how to start breastfeeding and how to continue it.

- Immediately after delivery, you can expect your baby to be laid close to you (skin-to-skin) for an hour or so, or until you have given the first breastfeed.

- If you have had a cesarean or you experience any complications during delivery, your baby will be given to you as soon as you are able and ready to be close to it, and not more than half an hour after you have said that you are ready.

- The staff will see to it that you succeed in starting to breastfeed. You can rely on getting all the guidance you need as often as you want. If you have any difficulties, you will get help to solve them and to become self-reliant.

- If, for any reason, you and your baby are separated for a while, you will be shown how to express your milk by hand or how to use a pump, and you will learn how you can make sure that your milk production is kept up.

- Your newborn baby will, at this time, be given no food or drink other than breastmilk, unless there is some medical reason to do so.

- In the birthing unit, it is possible and desirable for your baby to stay with you day and night. If you need to be relieved of the responsibility now and again, just ask for help. The staff will look after you so that you gain the strength you need to look after your baby.

- You will be encouraged to breastfeed whenever the baby indicates that it is ready for it. You can continue as long as the baby shows interest, naturally within reasonable limits and without doing more than you feel you can.

- If your baby is sleepy and seems too tired to feed, you will be told to take it up in your arms, stimulating it and offering the breast as you do so. You can wake a sleepy baby and put it to the breast if you need to breastfeed, for example, if you feel that your breasts are becoming overfilled with milk.

- The birthing unit will not provide pacifiers or feeding bottles. You will be advised to avoid using them at least until breastfeeding is well established and your milk production is sufficient.

- Mothers who cannot breastfeed or don't succeed in getting breastfeeding established will be given all the support they need.

- You will be told which Maternal and Child Health center will provide you with support after you leave the birthing unit; where you can rely on getting expert help with any problems you may experience. You will also get information on the nearest breastfeeding support organization and, if necessary, be shown how to contact them.

You can expect the following standard of care from a Baby-Friendly Neonatal Unit (example from Norway):

The same principles as a baby-friendly hospital apply here, but with a few additions and adjustments:

- Pregnant women admitted to a hospital with an expected transfer of the infant to a neonatal intensive care unit (NICU) will be given information about the parents' access to the NICU. They will also be told how to start milk production early and effectively using a pump or with the help of the baby, depending on its health. Just how these things are handled will depend on the mother's wishes and on the baby's condition and prospects.

- Printed information on pumping and hand milking should be provided.

- The NICU will encourage and facilitate early skin-to-skin contact between parents and baby, beginning as soon as possible, once the baby is stable enough. The kangaroo method should preferably be used throughout the whole period of the hospital stay.

- The parents must have the opportunity to be together with their baby throughout the day and night. The NICU must ensure that this is feasible for at least one of the parents. They must have the opportunity to take their meals, rest, and spend the night in the hospital.

- The baby should, irrespective of its maturity and weight, be encouraged to have early contact with the mother's breast. The unit will encourage a free choice of feeding times (semi-demand feeding) as soon as the baby's health renders this possible.

- Where supplementary feeding is indicated, this can be provided using a gastric tube, cup, spoon, or a nursing supplementer.

- You can expect to be offered the chance to return home with the possibility to come back to the NICU if necessary, or to be discharged early with the help of a home support team if this exists. After you have been discharged, you can still ring the NICU to get whatever guidance you may need on breastfeeding.

- In the neonatal unit, you may find that a pacifier is used to relieve discomfort or pain, as a means of helping the baby to settle down or sleep, or to stimulate digestion when a gastric tube is used and the mother's breast is not available. Using a pacifier may lead to reduced stimulation of milk production, especially when it has not yet been well established. If the baby is separated from its mother, the milk production is stimulated using a pump. The use of a pacifier under these conditions are not shown to upset milk flow. However, when one gets to the point of semi-demand or demand feeding, the problems may recur: excessive use of a pacifier at this time may mask the baby's hunger signals and therefore mean that the mother's breast is insufficiently stimulated.

You can expect the following standard of care from the Baby-Friendly Community Health Service (example from Norway):

- A written breastfeeding policy known by all the staff in the Maternal and Child Health center.

- The staff has been trained in skills necessary to implement this policy.

- During pregnancy, the staff gives information about the benefits of breastfeeding and how to succeed.

- Links between centers providing pregnancy care, maternity units, and Maternal and Child Health centers, so they all work together to provide consistent help and advice.

- Information on available mother-to-mother support groups (Ammehjelpen).

- Good advice on how to start breastfeeding and how to maintain your milk production.

- The help and support you need to be able to breastfeed exclusively for six months if it is what you and your baby want to do.

You can read more about the Norwegian BFHI on: www.oslo-universitetssykehus.no/ammesenteret, choose "In English."

Other links to Baby-Friendly Hospital Initiative:

www.unicef.org and www.who.org – search for BFHI

Baby-Friendly Hospital Initiative in U.S.A.: www.wellstart.org

Baby-Friendly Hospital Initiative in United Kingdom: www.babyfriendly.org.uk

Appendix 5:
MILK BANKS-CONTACT ADDRESSES

There are about 160 milk banks worldwide, active in a range of countries. They took over when the wet-nurse disappeared around 1900. Today human milk available though milk banks is usually given to high risk cases, such as premature babies, who are considered to do much better on human milk than on any substitute.

Since human milk is similar all over the world, there is considerable contact between the milk banks worldwide, even though there is considerable variation in the routines followed.

MILK BANKING WEB SITES:

Human Milk Banking Association of North America (HMBANA, includes Canada & Mexico): www.hmbana.org

European Milk Banking Association (EMBA): www.europeanmilkbanking.com

International Milk Banking Initiative (IMBI): www.internationalmilkbanking.org

United Kingdom: www.ukamb.org

Australia: www.mercybreastmilkbank.com.au

New Zealand: www.mothersmilk.org.nz

Appendix 6:
HUMAN RIGHTS RELEVANT TO BREASTFEEDING

THE RIGHTS OF THE CHILD:

Children have the right to:

- Enjoyment of the highest attainable standard of health (Art. 24(I) CRC)

- Enjoyment of the highest attainable standard of physical and mental health (Art. 12 ICESCR)

- Primary health care (Art. 24(2)(b) CRC)

- Adequate food (Art. 1 (1) ICESCR)

- Adequate nutritious food (Art. 24(2)(c) CRC)

- A standard of living adequate for the child's physical, mental, spiritual, moral, and social development (Art. 27(1) CRC)

THE RIGHTS OF THE MOTHER:

Mothers have the right to:

- Appropriate post-natal care (Art. 24(2)(d) CRC)

- Education and support in use of basic knowledge of child health and nutrition, the advantages of breastfeeding (Art. 24(2)(e) CRC)

- Access to information, education regarding child-spacing (Art. 16(e) CEDAW)

- Appropriate assistance in their child-rearing responsibilities (Art. 18 CRC)

- Access to health care services, including ... provision of appropriate services in connection with pregnancy, confinement, and the post-natal period (Art. 12(2) CEDAW)

- The highest attainable standard of health (Art. 12 ICESCR)

- Adequate nutrition during pregnancy and lactation (Art. 12(2) CEDAW)

- Special protection during a reasonable period of time before and after childbirth..., working mothers should be accorded paid leave or leave with adequate social security benefits (Art. 10 ICESCR)

- Maternity leave with pay or comparable social benefit (Art. 11(2)(b) CEDAW)

Sources:

ICESCR: International Covenant on Economic, Social and Cultural Rights
CEDAW: Convention on the Elimination of all forms of discrimination Against Women
CRC: Convention on the Rights of the Child

Appendix 7:
THE ILO CONVENTION ON MATERNITY PROTECTION

The International Labour Organization (ILO, www.ilo.org) is a UN body dealing with the relationships between workers and employers, both in the public and the private sector. Of particular interest to breastfeeding mothers are questions such as the duration of maternity leave and the right to paid breaks for breastfeeding during working hours. Two legal instruments deal with such questions:

- ILO Convention No. C183 (Maternity Protection Convention, 2000)

- Recommendation No. R191 (Maternity Protection Recommendation, 2000).

In 2000, when earlier standards were revised, the minimum duration of maternity leave was set as not less than 14 weeks (up from 12 weeks), but with the recommendation that the parties should endeavor to extend this to at least 18 weeks (up from 16 weeks). This seems reasonable given that the WHO recommends exclusive breastfeeding for six months.

Further, it was recommended that breastfeeding breaks during working hours be paid, and that the breastfeeding facilities in the workplace be of a satisfactory hygienic standard.

It is actually remarkable that the standards formulated in 2000 were adopted at all, since an earlier convention and recommendation had not been ratified by more than a handful of countries. None the less, the present Convention has been influential, and even countries that have not to date ratified it are studying its provisions.

It is worth noting that human rights are now explicitly brought into the convention, and breastfeeding breaks are recognized as a woman's *right.*

INDEX

AUTHOR BIOS

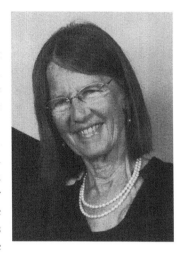

Elisabet Helsing's children were born in 1965 and 1967, and throughout her career, she has worked on various matters relevant in one way or another to breastfeeding. In 2003 in Norway, she was awarded "The King's Gold Medal for Public Service," as an acknowledgement of her achievements. Holder of a doctorate in nutrition policy, she was active for many years as Regional Officer for Nutrition in the World Health Organization's European Office for Europe. She was also a staff member of the Norwegian Board of Health and continues to advise the Norwegian Resource Centre for Breastfeeding on issues that include the Baby-Friendly Hospital Initiative. She was among the founders of the International Baby Food Action Network (IBFAN) and was for many years a member of the Board of the World Alliance for Breastfeeding Action (WABA). She also served a term as President of the Federation of European Nutrition Societies.

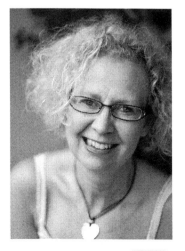

Anna-Pia Häggkvist has been concerned with breastfeeding matters since the first of her two children was born in 1986. She started her breastfeeding career as a peer counselor in the Norwegian mother-to-mother support group "Ammehjelpen" in 1986, where she still is an active member. She is a popular lecturer and has written both articles and guidelines, as well as contributing to books and brochures. Trained as an intensive care nurse, she has a master's degree in health sciences and is an Internationally Board-

Certified Lactation Consultant (IBCLC), with specialized experience over many years in supporting the breastfeeding of premature and ill newborn infants. She has been deeply involved in the Norwegian Baby-Friendly Hospital Initiative since 1993 and is employed at the Norwegian Resource Centre for Breastfeeding.

Graham Dukes, husband of Elisabet, is a lawyer, physician, and author who prepared the English translation of Elisabet and Anna-Pia's Norwegian book "*Amming*," that forms the basis of the present volume.

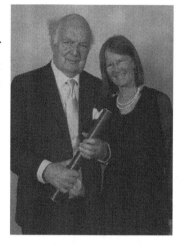

ORDERING INFORMATION

Hale Publishing, L.P.

1712 N. Forest Street

Amarillo, Texas, USA 79106

8:00 am to 5:00 pm CST

Call » 806.376.9900

Toll free » 800.378.1317

Fax » 806.376.9901

Online Orders

www.ibreastfeeding.com